Measuring Up

IMPROVING HEALTH SYSTEM PERFORMANCE IN OECD COUNTRIES

OECD

ORGANISATION FOR ECONOMIC CO-OPERATION AND DEVELOPMENT

THE ORGANISATION FOR ECONOMIC CO-OPERATION AND DEVELOPMENT (OECD)

Pursuant to Article 1 of the Convention signed in Paris on 14th December 1960, and which came into force on 30th September 1961, the Organisation for Economic Co-operation and Development (OECD) shall promote policies designed:

- to achieve the highest sustainable economic growth and employment and a rising standard of living in Member countries, while maintaining financial stability, and thus to contribute to the development of the world economy;

- to contribute to sound economic expansion in Member as well as non-member countries in the process of economic development; and

- to contribute to the expansion of world trade on a multilateral, non-discriminatory basis in accordance with international obligations.

The original Member countries of the OECD are Austria, Belgium, Canada, Denmark, France, Germany, Greece, Iceland, Ireland, Italy, Luxembourg, the Netherlands, Norway, Portugal, Spain, Sweden, Switzerland, Turkey, the United Kingdom and the United States. The following countries became Members subsequently through accession at the dates indicated hereafter: Japan (28th April 1964), Finland (28th January 1969), Australia (7th June 1971), New Zealand (29th May 1973), Mexico (18th May 1994), the Czech Republic (21st December 1995), Hungary (7th May 1996), Poland (22nd November 1996), Korea (12th December 1996) and Slovak Republic (14th December 2000). The Commission of the European Communities takes part in the work of the OECD (Article 13 of the OECD Convention).

Publié en français sous le titre :

Être à la hauteur
MESURER ET AMÉLIORER LA PERFORMANCE DES SYSTÈMES DE SANTÉ DANS LES PAYS DE L'OCDE

FOREWORD

This report examines progress and challenges in the effective measurement and application of performance indicators to improve health systems. Measuring and improving health system performance is a key priority for OECD countries. In May 2001, OECD Ministers noted that "health systems are an important element in social cohesion and represent the largest service sector in many OECD countries. Their efficiency, effectiveness and equity consequences, their impact on public finances, and their ability to meet the challenges of medical advances, ageing populations and rising expectations require creative policy approaches".

Annual healthcare costs in OECD countries have topped US$2.3 trillion – almost 10 per cent of GDP. Health systems play a crucial role in promoting people's well-being. They are also major employers of skilled workers and an important source of demand for high-tech industries such as pharmaceuticals, diagnostic and imaging products and biotechnology. However, OECD health systems are coming under increasing pressure, and additional funding alone will not be enough to respond to steadily rising demands. There is an on-going need to improve the cost-effectiveness of health care spending.

In response to requests from Member governments, the OECD launched in 2001 a new *Health Project*. The main theme of this project is performance measurement and improvement in OECD health systems. Through comparing experiences across OECD countries, the project will seek to address the challenge of deciding the appropriate amount of resources to be devoted to health care as well as ways in which these resources should be financed and allocated.

As part of this new *Health Project*, the OECD and Health Canada held a conference entitled "Measuring Up: Improving health system performance in OECD countries", on 5-7 November 2001 in Ottawa. The conference brought together more than 400 participants from OECD countries and other international organisations, to discuss good practices in measuring key components of health system performance and to share experiences on how best to report and use performance measures to build more effective health systems. The conference assembled not only experts and policy-makers, but also representatives from civil society and key actors directly involved in the functioning of health care systems, be they patients, health care professionals or managers of health care institutions. The views of these different actors in health care systems were factored into the conference deliberations through the active participation of a "Commentary Panel" which provided useful inputs at different points during the meeting. The conference ended with a Ministerial Roundtable discussion, which provided an opportunity for Ministers from several OECD countries to share views about the political challenges their countries face in developing and applying performance measures. This report contains the main papers presented at the conference together with the highlights of the Ministerial Roundtable.

The Ottawa Conference was an important milestone in OECD's work on health system performance. It provided a marvellous opportunity to discuss practical ideas on ways to measure and improve the efficiency and equity of health care systems. It also demonstrated strong political commitments to international co-operation in developing performance measurement frameworks that support on-going health systems improvement.

Donald J. Johnston
Secretary-General of the OECD

Allan Rock
Former Minister of Health, Canada

Acknowledgements

The OECD would like to thank all those who contributed to the Ottawa conference and to this volume. It would like to express particular gratitude to the Government of Canada and the former Canadian Minister of Health, Allan Rock, for hosting this conference. Thanks go to Denis Gauthier, David Kelly, David Hoye, and François Sauvé in Health Canada and to Peter Scherer, Jeremy Hurst, Stéphane Jacobzone and Gaétan Lafortune in the OECD Secretariat for their contributions in planning and organising this conference. Special thanks go also to Peter Smith from the Centre for Health Economics at the University of York in the United Kingdom, for assuming the responsibility of Editor of these conference proceedings. The contributions of Geoff Anderson from the Department of Health Policy, Management and Evaluation at the University of Toronto in Canada and Tom Reilly from the Agency for Healthcare Research and Quality in the United States as members of the Conference Advisory Group, are also gratefully acknowledged.

TABLE OF CONTENTS

EDITOR'S PREFACE

by

Peter Smith[*]

The concern with measuring the performance of health systems and health care is not recent. In the 1860s Florence Nightingale pioneered the systematic collection, analysis and dissemination of comparative hospital outcomes data in order to understand and improve performance. Fifty years later, Ernest Codman promoted the need for scrupulous collection and public release of surgical outcome data (Spiegelhalter, 1999). However, there were many practical, professional and political impediments to making such principles operational. It is only in the last ten years that the vision of using large-scale data sources to help improve health system performance has become a reality.

A number of developments have led to this recent transformation. Most importantly, the accelerating advances in medical technology have led to enormous potential for new interventions and methods of delivering and organising health care, with a concomitant pressure on expenditure levels. There is therefore an urgent need to check that innovations – of whatever sort – promote system objectives and avoid adverse side-effects. At the same time, popular expectations have become ever more demanding, not least in the accountability and transparency they demand of their health systems. In this respect, performance information serves as a fundamental tool of communication. Finally, developments in information technology have revolutionised the capacity to capture almost instantaneously many measures of process and outcome in a way that was until recently unimaginable.

The interest in system performance was given added impetus by the *World Health Report* 2000 produced by the World Health Organisation, entitled "Health systems: improving performance" (World Health Organisation, 2000). The debate initiated by WHR2000 has been dominated by responses to the league tables of national health system performance presented in its statistical annexes. However the main body of the report raises fundamental issues associated with defining, measuring and promoting health system performance.

In this context, performance data have two broad functions: to identify in general "what works" in promoting the objectives of the health system; and to identify the functional competence of specific practitioners or organisations. These correspond, respectively, to the research and managerial roles of performance data. In whichever role, such data can then be used to promote continuous improvement, by enabling policy makers to adopt the most cost-effective technologies, and helping practitioners to identify opportunities for personal or organisational improvement.

This volume seeks to reflect the current "state of the art" in performance measurement across OECD health systems. It is organised into seven sections, reflecting different perspectives on the performance measurement process. Part I sets the scene. Naylor, Iron and Handa (Chapter 1) summarise progress to date, emphasizing the simple but powerful truth that we cannot manage what we do not measure. Hurst (Chapter 2) surveys the issues and challenges faced by OECD countries as they seek to measure and improve their health system's performance. He pays particular attention to the role of international comparisons, in which the pioneering work of the OECD has played a central role (OECD, 2001).

---

[*]   Centre for Health Economics, University of York.

Part II of the book summarises developments in five contrasting OECD countries. Smee (Chapter 3) describes the move towards a philosophy of "performance management" in the English National Health Service, the archetypal centralised health system, an approach that relies heavily on the massive compulsory provision of reliable, comprehensive and timely performance data. In contrast, Rehnqvist (Chapter 4) presents the Swedish case, in which responsibility for the health system is devolved to local government, and the provision of performance data relies on clinically led collaboratives known as quality registers, to which subscription is voluntary. The US health system has a uniquely strong focus on consumers and the market, and Reilly, Meyer and colleagues (Chapter 5) summarise experience with public release of performance data to inform consumer choice. They report that – although consumers appear to take little notice of such data – the public release nevertheless stimulates important improvement efforts by providers. A more formal approach to performance management amongst providers is the Dutch experience with "guided" self-regulation, presented by Klazinga, Delnoij and Kulu-Glasgow (Chapter 6). They note that the key challenge is to translate the undoubted progress made in clinically based performance measurement to the more ambitious agenda of managing whole system performance. Finally, Wolfson and Alvarez (Chapter 7) summarise the enormous progress made towards integrating information systems in Canada, and the promise it holds for performance monitoring.

Part III examines the methodological issues raised when seeking to make international performance comparisons. Jacobzone, Moise and Moon (Chapter 8) describe one of the OECD approaches towards international comparison, which concentrates on micro data for specific conditions. The intention is to use the natural experiment of international variations to secure an improved understanding of the links between technology adoption and clinical outcome. Evans (Chapter 9) describes some of the methodological issues pursued by the World Health Organisation since publication of *World Health Report* 2000, in particular the problem of securing comparability when interpreting survey results from different countries. Coulter and Cleary (Chapter 10) examine the complex issue of measuring the patient's experience. They emphasize the importance of this dimension of health care, but note the methodological difficulties involved in developing reliable and comparable indicators of system responsiveness. Van Doorslaer, Koolman and Puffer (Chapter 11) summarise their work on the important issue of measuring horizontal equity, in the sense of equal treatment for equal need. They confirm that – even in health systems that explicitly seek to promote equity and solidarity – there exist important unexplained variations in treatment associated with income levels.

In Part IV the book turns to a series of key measurement issues. De Pouvourville and Minvielle (Chapter 12) describe the rich experience of seeking to develop indicators of hospital performance, based mainly on US research. The principal methodological challenges are to develop adequate patient outcome measures and to adjust satisfactorily for variations in the complexity of the hospital's case-mix. Long term care for people with physical or mental disability is a key policy issue for many OECD countries, and the provision of good quality performance data is a prerequisite for the development of effective policy. The advantage in this sector is that – compared with hospitals – the client groups are relatively homogeneous, and Ikegami, Hirdes and Carpenter (Chapter 13) report a great deal of progress on a range of quality indicators. To conclude part four, Smith (Chapter 14) examines the issues that arise when seeking to combine individual indicators into a single composite measure of system performance. There may often be a need to construct such composites, but to date the methodology underlying such efforts has been weak.

Although most of the papers in the first four parts of the book concentrate on methodological topics, many make reference to the key issue of how performance data can be used to secure health system improvement. It is not enough merely to produce the performance data. They must be embedded in a system that uses them to best effect (and avoids unintended dysfunctional consequences). In Part V, Leatherman (Chapter 15) outlines the range of levers that exist to secure performance improvements, grouped into five categories: external oversight, professional development and education, empowering consumers, incentives, and regulation. She concludes that the gaps in our evidence base make it imperative to employ a blend of approaches that give rise to complementary effects.

The conference from which these proceedings are taken provided a wealth of material. In *Part* VI, Girard and Minvielle (Chapter 16) seek to synthesize the experience, and situate the performance measurement movement within a democratic context. The messages they distil from the proceedings are that performance measurement is first a legitimate undertaking, underpinned by public expectations of a better health system and enhanced accountability of that system; second, a difficult undertaking, reflecting the complexity of the health system; and third a political undertaking, requiring conscious involvement of political institutions.

Indeed, as the *World Health Report* 2000 noted, almost all performance improvement activity eventually relies on the preoccupations and actions of politicians charged with stewardship of the health system. The conference concluded with a round table (Part VII, Chapter 17) at which ministers from Canada, France, Mexico, the United Kingdom and the United States presented their views on health system performance measurement. They highlight many consistent themes emerging from diverse health systems, including the key role of information technology, the need to engage health professionals, the heightened concern with measuring difficult areas (such as clinical quality, population health and disparities of outcome and access), the rising expectations of citizens, the need to find effective ways of disseminating information to citizens, and the central importance of international comparisons and shared experience.

The progress reported in this book suggests that the vision set out by pioneers such as Nightingale and Codman is (not before time) starting to become a reality. Most health systems are still at an early stage in implementing effective methods of performance measurement and improvement. However, a remarkable consensus regarding the need for such methods is emerging, and there is strong evidence of a heightened recognition of this need amongst policy makers. There is much to be learnt from the great variety of early experience, and the work of organisations such as OECD will be crucial in seeking out, analysing and disseminating "what works". I suspect that I am not alone in looking forward to seeing whether the high hopes expressed in many of the chapters are realised.

Editing this book has been a great pleasure and honour. I should like to thank the OECD for giving me the opportunity to contribute, and to acknowledge the unstinting help given by Jeremy Hurst, Gaétan Lafortune and Peter Scherer. I am also indebted to Geoff Anderson and Tom Reilly, who shared the editorial responsibilities with great generosity and wisdom. Finally, I should like to thank the authors for their alacrity, forbearance and flexibility.

REFERENCES

OECD (2001),
> OECD *Health Data* 2001: *comparative analysis of 30 countries*, OECD and CREDES, Paris.

SPIEGELHALTER, D. (1999),
> "Surgical audit: statistical lessons from Nightingale and Codman", *Journal of the Royal Statistical Society*, Series A, Vol. 162, pp. 45-58.

WORLD HEALTH ORGANISATION (2000),
> *The World Health Report* 2000. *Health systems: improving performance*, World Health Organisation, Geneva.

Part I
OVERVIEW OF ISSUES AND CHALLENGES

Chapter 1

MEASURING HEALTH SYSTEM PERFORMANCE: PROBLEMS AND OPPORTUNITIES IN THE ERA OF ASSESSMENT AND ACCOUNTABILITY

by

C. David Naylor[*], Karey Iron[**] and Kiren Handa[**]

Abstract

A common goal among the health systems of OECD nations is to optimise the health of individual patients and populations in an equitable, efficient and effective manner that is acceptable to patients, providers and administrators. No "magic bullets" have been found that will achieve this goal through reforms of service delivery or finance. Instead, improvement appears to require incremental change at all levels of health systems. This evolutionary process, in turn, depends on systematic measurement of health system performance, coupled to decision-making processes grounded in evidence.

Broad measures of population health are confounded by factors that cannot be managed through the health care system, and composite indices of system-specific performance can be imprecise and misleading. To drive change within the system, it will be more useful to develop accurate and reliable data systems, at a micro- and meso-level, with performance indicators that are aligned to expensive, complex, or high-priority services, particularly those that are unevenly delivered. Ascertaining the needs and views of all health system users – patients, providers, administrators and policy-makers – is essential to the development of data collection systems. The creation of continuous, audience-specific reporting systems is also important to facilitate change. In the latter respect, harnessing information to consumer choice does not appear effective in driving change at the procedure- or provider-specific level, but may be a powerful tool at a macro-level in an environment of competing health plans.

Supply-side drivers of change include regulatory frameworks and the alignment of funding with performance. Implementation of reforms, however, is ultimately dependent on collaborative action by professionals and administrators aimed at identifying and implementing best practices. With enhanced information structures, measures and mechanisms, the use of health system performance information will ensure that health services reflect the best policies and practices, in addition to community contexts and values.

Introduction

We sometimes forget that interest in measuring elements of health system performance can be traced back many decades. For example, early luminaries in the field include England's Florence Nightingale (1820-1910), still renowned as a pioneering nurse-administrator, and Boston surgeon Ernest Codman (1869-1940) who laid the groundwork for modern outcomes research. Governmental fascination with health care performance was already the butt of satiric humour on BBC television twenty years ago.

---

[*] Dean, Faculty of Medicine, University of Toronto and Adjunct Senior Scientist, the Institute for Clinical Evaluative Sciences.
[**] Research co-ordinators, the Institute for Clinical Evaluative Sciences.

In a 1981 episode of "Yes, Minister", the Honourable James Hacker is concerned that St. Edward's hospital has been launched with 500 administrators and secretaries, but no providers or patients (Jay and Lynn, 1981). The following dialogue about the new hospital ensues:

Jim Hacker: "You think it is functioning now?"

Mrs. Rogers: "Minister, it is one of the best-run hospitals in the country. It is up for the Florence Nightingale Award."

Jim Hacker: "And what is to praise that?"

Mrs. Rogers: "It is won by the most hygienic hospital in the area."

Misplaced zeal in assessing and rewarding health system performance, however, has until relatively recently been less common than relative neglect. This conference accordingly signals a welcome culture shift that has swept across the nations of the OECD during the last decade.

1. Why measure health system performance?

Although health systems across the OECD are varied in their history and configurations, every system arguably shares one goal. That goal is the equitable, efficient, and effective delivery of services that patients want and need, in a manner acceptable to patients and providers alike. Each system seeks to maximise its positive impact on the health of both individual patients and communities, at a cost that is acceptable to those who must directly or indirectly finance health services.

Over the last three decades we have seen waves of health care reform wash across every OECD nation. The recurring variables are the extent of private or public financing and delivery, as well as overall levels of expenditure; but mechanisms of reform have varied. Some countries have tried internal markets and decentralization, while others imposed tighter central controls. Some have contracted out more services, while others moved to contain the role of private enterprise in publicly-financed systems. Some have embraced user fees while others focused on enhancing access to a wider range of citizens. As different countries have gone different routes, a hard reality has emerged: there are no "magic bullets" to be had in health care reform.

One conclusion, which may be taken as depressing, liberating, or a bit of both, appears to be that improvements in health care are not contingent on the drafting of grand blueprints or the ability of politicians and public servants to pull big policy levers. Health care improvement starts from the ground up. It requires tenacious work to understand what does and does not work in real life, and the engagement of countless providers and patients, institutions and communities. Similarly, most policy movement seems likely to be incremental, driven by experience and evidence, rather than theory or ideology.

There, in a nutshell, lies the importance of health system performance measurement and reporting. We cannot manage what we do not measure. We cannot understand and address the ubiquitous variations in practice and performance within and across OECD countries without better assessment methods and sharing of information. Assessment of performance is the only means by which we can understand what we are doing well, where we are falling short, and what kinds of solutions have been found effective in other jurisdictions.

Health services will always reflect not just evidence about best policies and practices, but also local and national contexts or circumstances, and the values or preferences of different communities and polities. Indeed, the degree of variation in health service delivery within and across jurisdictions constitutes a set of both purposive and inadvertent experiments from which a great deal can be learned. However, variations in healthcare culture across the OECD have been eroded by the standardisation of scientific and analytical methods, the obvious commonality of human biology, the convergence of medical sociology, advances in transportation, and, perhaps most importantly, the enormous impact of electronic communication and the World Wide Web. In sum, we have much to learn from each other, now and on a continuing basis.

This movement is clearly not a passing administrative or political fad. Citizens are demanding evidence of value-for-money in their role as taxpayers, surfing the web for information on all aspects of health care, and more generally insisting on a higher level of transparency and accountability regarding the services they consume. They have also become highly aware of medical errors, and more inclined to litigate and advocate when they and their loved ones are the victims of negligence, incompetence, miscommunication, or even minor departures from the outcomes apparently achievable by leading practitioners in leading centres.

Coupled to mounting public expectations is the growing cost and complexity of medical technologies. We may hope that, as Lewis Thomas put it, medicine and health care are simply mired in a transient phase of expensive and risky "half-way technologies" which palliate or mitigate a disease process, but do not offer either a definitive cure, or a transformation and permanent improvement in health status (Thomas, 1977). It is conceivable that post-genomic (New York Times, 2000) or molecular medicine will have a transformative impact on the efficiency and effectiveness of current care models, permitting individualised drug therapy, targeted prevention, and definitive interventions for many conditions that are now palliated rather expensively. But an alternative scenario for this new era of genetic medicine is far more plausible. In that scenario, breakthroughs will enable safe, cheap, and curative interventions against some diseases, while the costs and risks of treating other diseases mount dramatically. The result for at least two or three decades is likely to be a more dichotomous set of medical tools – some blunt, others razor-sharp, with all the same challenges that we now face. Moreover, to paraphrase Bertrand Russell, habits of thought change more slowly than techniques, with the result that, as skill mounts, wisdom recedes. Measurement of performance will therefore be an essential part of creating and maintaining wise oversight of our health care systems for some time to come.

Let us not paint too gloomy a picture. As Jeremy Hurst noted in the WHO Bulletin in 2000, OECD nations remain incredibly privileged as regards their health systems (Hurst, 2000). Our populations enjoy a relatively high health status that has increased over time (Figure 1). We have embraced more or less equitable financing systems in which the healthy support the sick, the young support the old and the rich support the poor. Providers do tend to view funding as inadequate everywhere. But the fact remains that OECD economies have generally succeeded in supporting levels of social and health expenditures

Figure 1. **Average life expectancy at birth in 13 OECD countries, 1960-96**

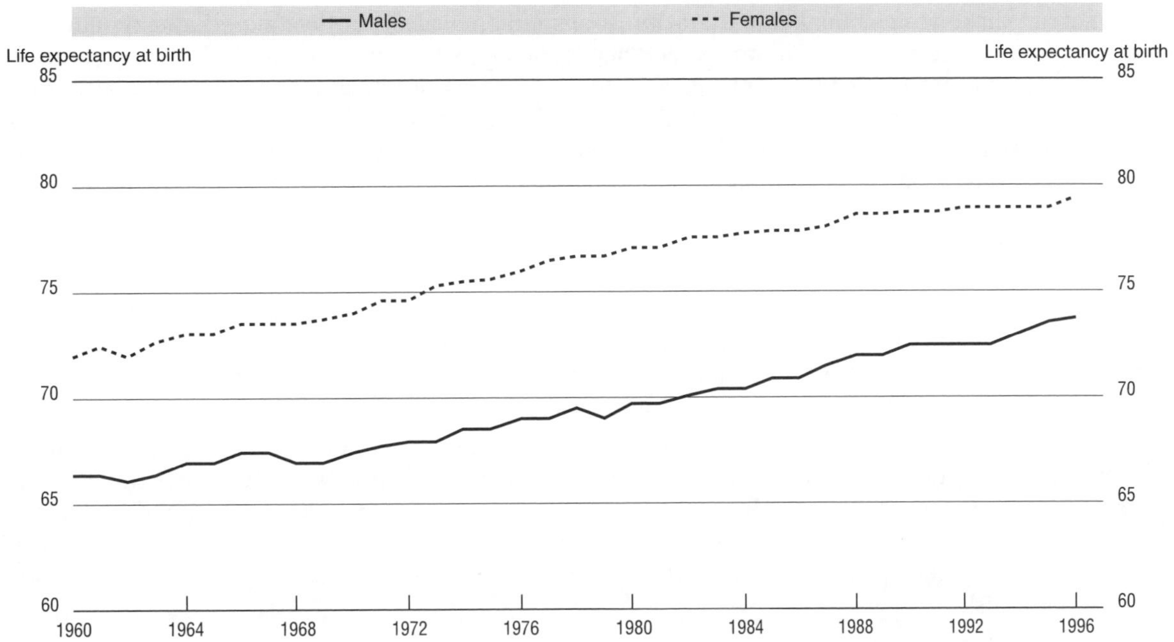

Source: Hurst (2000).

adequate to improve a variety of population health indicators, reduce disease-specific morbidity and mortality, and achieve moderately high levels of satisfaction among those who use the system.

Together we can take great pride in what our varied health systems have achieved. But for all the reasons outlined above, every nation must now redouble its efforts to assess system performance at multiple levels. Assessment must go from appropriate use of medications in a single clinic, to costs per patient day across a set of acute care hospitals in a region, and on to broad markers of population health and system efficiency and equity. Without such information and indicators, health systems across the OECD will continue to vary more by institutional culture, political geography and historical happenstance, than by explicit evidence-based design.

2.   Measuring health care versus measuring health status

In a wonderful essay called "Doing better, feeling worse: The Political Pathology of Health Policy" published 25 years ago, Aaron Wildavsky wrote: "According to the great equation, medical care equals health. But the great equation is wrong" (Wildavsky, 1977). This is a lesson that we seem to re-learn every few decades.[1] The corollary of Wildavsky's proposition is that we must be cautious about drawing inferences from measures of health system performance that are admixed with broad population health indices. In the reductio ad absurdum, one cannot measure the success of cancer care by tallying the incidence of cancer or even the potential years of life lost due to cancer in a population.

Put another way, population health indices are clearly affected by determinants such as social and educational policies, socio-economic conditions, disparities in income and education, the health of local and national economies, environmental standards, and public health or health promotion activities. These influences are neither deeply embedded in the health system nor readily manageable through system-focused performance measurement. This suggests a rather daunting examination question: "Health care has only modest effects on population health status. Should measures of health system performance include population health indicators as outcomes or as confounders? Please answer in 200 words or less". Howsoever one answers that question, there is unquestionably a "signal and noise" problem in measurement. Take large populations and general health status measures, and one concludes that the marginal returns of more health expenditure are likely to be limited. Assess sub-populations at specific risk, using more specific outcome measures, and the marginal yields of medical care become more apparent.

What are those yields? Bunker and Frazier published an analysis in 1994 aimed at estimating the effects of medical care on overall life expectancy (Bunker, 1995; Bunker et al., 1994). They selected preventive and therapeutic interventions for which strong evidence of efficacy was available from randomised controlled trials (RCTs) and conditions with a high enough prevalence that some meaningful impact on community health status might result from more or less intensive application of the relevant intervention.[2] Their best guess was that medical care might account for 17-18 per cent of the increases in life expectancy in America and Britain over the last century. Intriguingly, Hurst has since noted that there is some correlation between life expectancy and increases in numbers of physicians per capita, admissions to hospital and real expenditure on pharmaceuticals, over and above the correlation of these markers with per capita GDP. There is also strong evidence for sustained improvements in quality of life resulting from the treatment of non-self-limited conditions such as depression, heart disease, arthritis and joint diseases, migraines, osteoporosis, inflammatory bowel disease, asthma, cataracts, hearing impairments, and scores of other conditions (Bunker, 1995; Bunker et al., 1994).

We can reasonably conclude that the majority of clinical interventions can be correlated more closely with quality of life and functional status, than with indices of broader population health such as life expectancy or age-specific mortality rates. These life-enhancing interventions are greatly valued by patients, families, and communities. For that reason, more attention must be given to health indices that capture functional status and quality of life, both in the general population and for specific sub-populations at risk.[3]

These lines of argument bear on measuring health system performance in another direction. Since performance measurement is itself resource intensive, our first priority in measurement should perhaps be to assess whether those health services with a demonstrably big impact on community health status are being provided equitably, effectively, and efficiently. Even small shortfalls in highly cost-effective services should surely be a cause for local or national concern. Next in priority might be those services that have a marked effect on general or disease-specific quality of life, or that have modest effects but are extremely expensive or risky. Services with a high degree of variation, because of provider discretion, planned pluralism, or usual-and-customary chaos, must also be examined.

There is a flip-side to this issue of the disjunction between health status and health care. Work by Alter *et al.* published in 1999 sheds some light on this issue. The authors used linked administrative data to follow about 50 000 Canadians for one year from their respective dates of hospitalisation for acute myocardial infarction (AMI). Patients were divided into five neighbourhood income groups. As shown in Figure 2, there was a dramatic impact of socio-economic status on the baseline incidence of heart disease: a massive inequality in health status. This is consistent with other published work. That said, the Canadian system is widely praised for equitable access, and the patients all suffered a sentinel event that could be presumed to level the playing field in terms of anticipated outcomes. One might expect outcomes after treatment to be similar. In fact, the survival results varied as shown in Figure 3. Each line represents an income quintile with thousands of patients. The highest median household income was approximately C$29 000; the lowest, C$16 000. For each increase in neighbourhood income of C$10 000, the relative risk of death fell by 10 per cent. Notwithstanding a universal first-dollar health insurance system without any parallel private plans, there were also income-related variations in access to and use of invasive cardiac procedures. Additional research is underway to understand why these disparities occur.

Four inferences can be drawn from this train of thought. First, the same markers outside the health system that are associated with broad inequities in health status may have a surprising impact when micro-level or disease-specific assessments of system performance are undertaken. Second, and as a corollary, providers who serve relatively higher numbers of disadvantaged patients must not be penalised if performance measures show that their patients have poorer outcomes. Third, and most importantly, we must begin to integrate the broad population health perspective with a health services

Figure 2. **Number of acute myocardial infarction cases by income quintile in Ontario, 1994 to 1997**

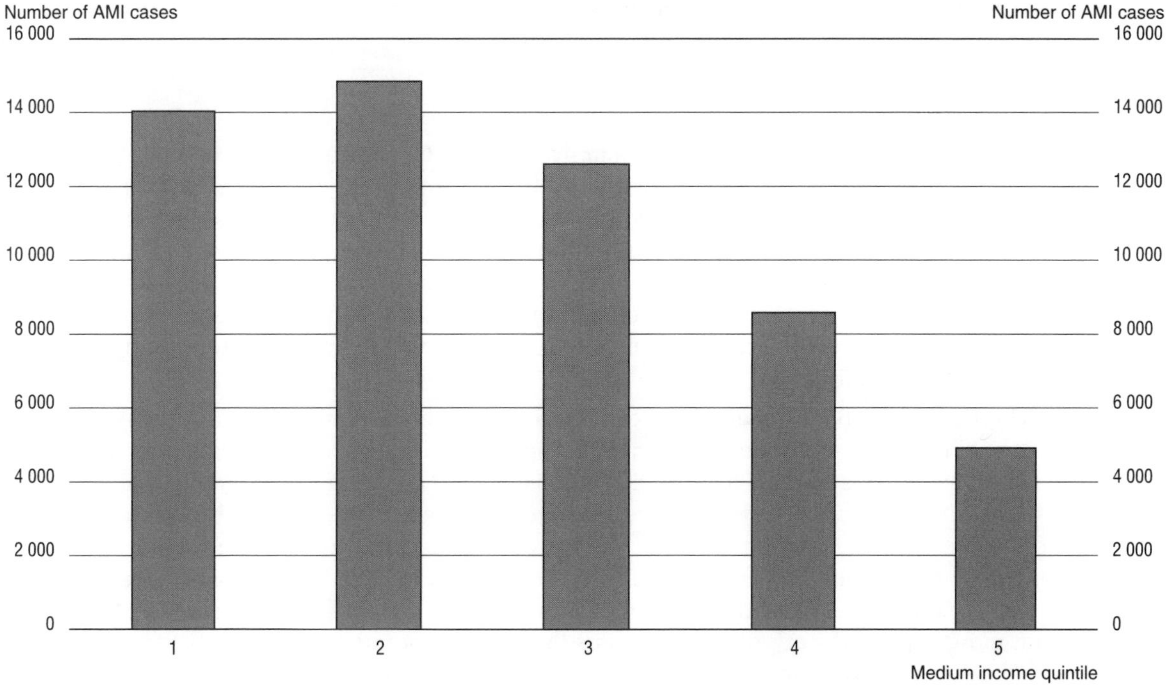

Number of AMI cases
16 000

Number of AMI cases
16 000

Medium income quintile

Source: Alter *et al.* (1999).

Figure 3. **Survival post-AMI by socio-economic status**

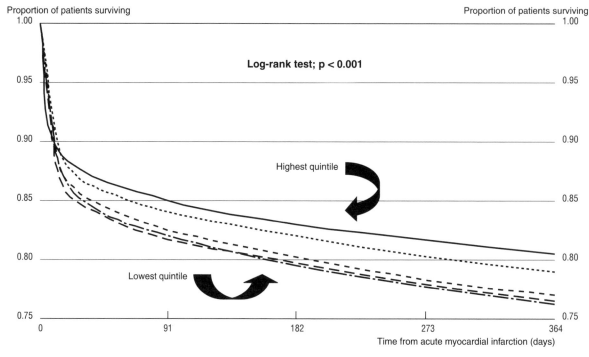

Source: Alter *et al.* (1999).

perspective. Researchers must elucidate the causal pathways that determine why some people are healthier than others and determine the relative impacts on health status to be expected from interventions inside and outside the health system. Above all, we must begin benchmarking and sharing information about our relative success in reducing health status inequities through a variety of social policy, health promotion, and health service reforms.

3. Seductive reductionism

Health systems, as we all know, are extraordinarily complex. In consequence, one must beware the seductive reductionism of devising a single measure to capture all dimensions of health status, let alone health system performance. A balanced approach with an array of indicators is desirable, as each set of stakeholders will need a different type of information to make better decisions (Smith, Part IV, Chapter 14 of this volume; Hurst, Part I, Chapter 2 of this volume). For example, if I am a hospital administrator or a trauma surgeon or a nurse-manager in France or Norway or Australia, does it really matter whether the World Health Organisation (WHO) has ranked my health system number one or number eleven or number thirty-two?

The WHO report exemplifies a regrettable tendency for health system performance measures to be reduced to ordinal rankings or ordered categories (World Health Organisation, 2000; Murray and Frenk, 2001; Evans *et al.*, 2001). This approach simplifies messages and concentrates minds usefully, but the criticism of the WHO rankings goes beyond concern about the "league table" approach. Among the points of debate have been the weights in the index, the uncertain relationship of conventional population health measures to health service performance, and the question of how best to assess health system equity. Navarro, for one, has agreed that countries should be ranked, but on disaggregated indicators such as infant mortality, deaths at work, waiting lists for serious operations or other indicators that are more likely to be comparable across countries and linked to policies or practices (Navarro, 2000; Navarro, 2001).

We are among those who strongly disagree with the analytical framework for country rankings adopted by the WHO. However, Murray and his colleagues from the WHO team deserve credit for moving the goalposts with their provocative analysis. The recent round of consultation in Europe exemplifies the positive impact of the WHO exercise. To colleagues who have dismissed this work as "social marketing", we would say only that better social marketing of health system performance measures is overdue, and the debate engendered by the WHO rankings will ultimately be the most valuable result of that exercise.

More generally, the advantage of composite indices and rankings is that they give policy-makers and high-level managers some efficient decision-tools. A hospital CEO, regional manager, or senior public servant can use composite indices as a snapshot of system performance before drilling down to determine where change is desirable or feasible. For example, as Clive Smee will later report, during the 1980s the British NHS developed a massive array of health and health system indicators that overwhelmed decision-makers (Smee, Part II, Chapter 3 of this volume). Eventually indicators were set aside and/or grouped into six categories which bear mention here: health improvement; fair access; effective delivery of appropriate healthcare; efficiency; patient/care-giver experience; health outcomes related to care within the health service.

In a paper prepared for this conference, Peter Smith provides a careful analysis of the strengths and weaknesses of composite indicators that we do not wish to pre-empt. Two challenges, however, merit brief elaboration here (Smith, Part IV, Chapter 14).

The first is dubious precision. Every composite measure compounds the imprecision of its component measures. A useful analogy can be drawn between composite measures of health system performance and cost-utility ratios. Cost-utility analysis involves only three measures: the costs, utilities, and life-expectancies associated with one intervention strategy compared to another. As O'Brien et al. have demonstrated (see Figure 4), the zone of uncertainty around any cost-utility ratio is disturbingly large if one views the components as stochastic rather than absolute point estimates (O'Brien et al., 1994). Composite measures of health system performance combine uncertain weighting systems, imprecision arising from the potential non-comparability of component measures, and misleading reliability in the form of whole-population averages that mask distributional issues.

The last-mentioned concern leads directly to a second general challenge. The distillation of even disaggregated data to means and medians can be misleading. This is a general statistical problem that emerges when the goal of measurement is not to explain a phenomenon but to change behaviours or performance. There is substantial evidence of fluctuation in performance measures at the level of the individual practitioner, clinic, institution, or region. We cannot always use a "Shewhart-style" control chart approach to reduce variation, nor can we accept the conventional definitions of "statistical significance" (Mohammed et al., 2001). Instead, we must define the degree of variation in process or outcome measures that is unacceptable to different groups of stakeholders.

For example, let us imagine addressing the widespread problem of long waiting lists in public systems for hip and knee replacements. One can simply publish crude waiting list data by surgeon, hospital or region. Better still, one can publish these data adjusted for, or categorised by, the severity of symptoms or impairment of function among those waiting. That at least begins to take us towards clinical significance. One can even go further and ask: How important are the differences in waiting times to patients themselves? In this respect, one could ask patients to scale the acceptability of different maximal waiting times in relation to symptoms. Or, one could find a way to force patients to make trade-offs that are pertinent to the waiting list experience.

Our group has tried to determine patients' maximal acceptable waiting times using trade-off methodologies. In one study, we asked patients in the queue for hip or knee replacement to consider waiting one month for a surgeon with 2 per cent post-operative mortality as opposed to a 6-month wait for a surgeon with 1 per cent post-operative mortality (Llewellyn-Thomas et al., 1998). The results varied widely: some patients were highly mortality-averse, while others were strongly symptom driven. We have performed similar exercises to assess breast cancer patients' willingness to travel for shorter waiting times for radiotherapy (Palda et al., 1997). Although the evidence linking radiotherapy to

Figure 4. **Cost-effectiveness quasi-confidence interval**

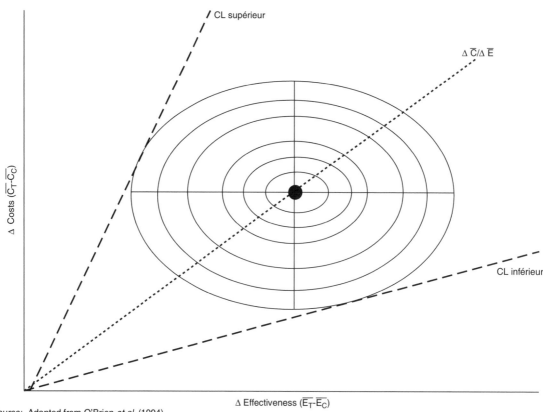

Source: Adapted from O'Brien *et al.* (1994).

improved survival after breast cancer was weak at the time, patients showed a surprising willingness to travel far from their families for faster access to radiotherapy. On the other hand, there are published data showing that other types of patients would accept increased post-operative mortality rather than travel elsewhere for major cancer surgery.

For policy-makers, the test may not be clinical significance but policy relevance, measured by budgetary impact, population health yields, number of "identifiable victims", or perhaps the font size of the adverse headlines in major newspapers! The lesson is that one cannot always predict the impact of health information on different audiences, particularly patients. Creative methods are needed to help distil out what is and is not meaningful to each audience.

A corollary is that every measure and situation must be assessed in terms of the impact of outlier versus "herd" effects. The canon of CQI and TQM tells us that we should focus less on "bad apples" and mostly on moving the entire group to a higher level of efficiency, safety, or effectiveness (Malenka *et al.*, 1995). On the other hand, a focus on outliers may be appropriate at times, because a few outlying institutions or providers can cause considerable harm or exert a major adverse influence by undermining professional standards and eroding public confidence in the system.

In sum, reporting on health system performance should be undertaken with a variety of aggregated and disaggregated indicators that are targeted to the needs of different audiences. Composite indices or aggregated indicators have the merit of allowing us to relate inputs and outputs in a fashion that can inform decision-making by system managers and governors. However, it is prudent to disaggregate any composite indicator and show the separate components so as to avoid black-box inferences. The uncertainty associated with any composite or aggregate indicator should always be acknowledged. Last, the distribution of performance measures may be more important than any measure of central tendency. As the old adage goes, statistics are like bathing suits: what they reveal is intriguing; but what they conceal is vital.

4. Getting it right: data, measures, comparisons, messages

4.1. *Data considerations*

Other authors will be addressing system-wide indicators, economic measures, and the sometimes-tenuous links between health services and population health status. For reasons already given, we believe that a great deal of the improvement to be achieved in health systems involves decidedly unglamorous micro-level and meso-level benchmarking and comparisons. This is difficult terrain. In industrial design, the old slogan used to be: "Good, Fast, Cheap" – pick any two and optimise; try for all three and fail. In assessing health system performance, we face similar trade-offs. The tensions that exist are myriad: comprehensiveness versus parsimony; population health measures versus a patient-focused paradigm rooted in health services; assessment of processes versus outcomes; and confidential provider-focused reporting systems versus public report cards that are more market-oriented or consumer-oriented. Keeping these trade-offs in mind, what general axioms might govern our collection of data for health system performance? We suggest six that are closely linked.

i) *Focus on assembling accurate, reliable, and relevant data*

Huge amounts of money can be wasted in collecting health data. In many countries, we go on requiring the assembly of massive computerised datasets for one-up administrative reporting without a great deal of thought as to whether and how our data collection should be limited or expanded to meet specific analytical goals. We have all seen reports arising from administrative data analysis within and between the OECD nations, and worried about the comparability of data across institutions, regions, or nations. We need to increase the profile and importance of health records professionals and emphasise the importance of accurate charts and records to all those working in our health services.

ii) *Talk with different audiences about their data needs and concerns before designing an information system*

Some health data systems seem to be designed for administrative "bean-counting", not for modern and dynamic management of health care. Patients, providers, lay governors, local managers, and system managers all have different information needs, and our data systems should be designed accordingly. A word about providers and local or institutional managers: unless the data systems are designed with their input and buy-in, the credibility of every performance report will be attacked. Physicians, in particular, are masters at the "Yes but" response: "Yes but you didn't account for the occurrence of acute-on-chronic undifferentiated Buzzard's disease in my patients". Or, in the same vein, "Yes but you forgot that those surgeons send the easiest cases to the private system so they can make more money". And on it goes.

iii) *Standardise and fill the "black holes" in health info-structure*

Many health systems have "black holes" where information systems tend to be limited and greater investments are needed along with renewed efforts at standardisation. An adequate level of detail to characterise patients and services, along with consistency of definitions, is crucial for credibility of information to providers as well as patients and general public (including governors). Frequent data lacunae include waiting list information systems, primary and ambulatory care services where discrete and concrete diagnoses are often difficult to apply, and long-term care and rehabilitation services that are rapidly gaining importance in every health system.

We do want to put forward one caveat to the foregoing three points. There are no perfect data and no perfect data systems, but some providers and managers will demand both before accepting performance measurement. The fastest way to improve the quality of data collection is to make it clear that the information derived from available data will be reported to decision-makers or the general public. The implication, with apologies to Shakespeare, follows: It is sometimes better to have measured with imperfect data, than never to have measured at all.

iv)   Launch more projects to supplement existing data systems on a time-limited basis with specific analytical goals

The principle here is obvious. Pick the services where there is an opportunity or a tangible gain from enhancing quality, access or efficiency. Focus resources on them, and supplement existing systems so that the data are more useful. In this respect, retrospective data collection through chart audits is difficult and expensive. However, time-limited development of prospective registries targeting specific aspects of the health system may be a very cost-effective way of enhancing existing data, so that we can learn more from each other.

v)   Drill down into system performance with data that follow patients throughout episodes of illness and across the care continuum

Many health systems in the OECD are incompletely integrated in management and finance. Similarly, they lack integrated data collection mechanisms that can shed light on inputs and outputs, or on structures, processes, and outcomes of care. Data linkage exercises that draw together administrative databases in universal healthcare systems are one partial solution to this problem, but as mentioned, these data are sometimes unreliable or insufficiently detailed. Integration and upgrading of health info-structure could be a driver of functional integration, which in turn will have positive consequences in terms of quality and health services efficiency. We cannot move beyond delivery silos if our information systems reinforce administrative insularity and professional territoriality.

vi)   Take advantage of technology and upgrade info-structure as necessary

In our view the state of health information across many OECD nations has lagged hugely behind the available technology. The "Holy Grail" of health info-structure enhancement is the Electronic Client Record. We can all imagine essential information embedded in personal digital devices, or "smart card systems" that allow health information to accrue as a client moves through the private and public health and social services systems of our countries. The confidentiality and privacy concerns with such integrated and digitised health info-structures cannot be ignored. However, we suggest that if patients are themselves given greater control over those records, and if appropriate electronic security systems are put in place, confidentiality and privacy could well be enhanced, not compromised.

4.2. Picking the measures

Measures of health system performance can be readily categorised by: who, what, when, where, and how.

"*Who*" refers first to the providers whose behaviour, perceptions, or beliefs are under study but also extends to the target audience for the performance measures. Most health systems indulge in some mindless measurement and ritual publication of data. It is essential to think about target audiences and points of potential pay-off in performance measurement (Coulter and Cleary, Part III, Chapter 10 in this volume; Leatherman, Part V, Chapter 15 in this volume). What measures will inform members of a board of directors of a health region or a hospital that the operation is meeting its objectives? Those indicators will be different than the measures that galvanise a nurse administrator to change his/her hiring practices.

"*What*" refers to the data themselves. What data are we collecting, and what are the limitations of those data for the purposes we have in mind? Causal pathways in health system performance require careful consideration when deciding what to measure. It may be helpful to consider data collection as a 3 x 3 matrix. We may collect economic, clinical, or population-based health indicators. And, after Donabedian, we can decompose the other axis into elements of structure, process and outcomes (Naylor, 1997). Structure refers to static or technical elements. These can range from disconnect alarms on anaesthesia apparatus in operating rooms, to a requirement that a neurosurgeon have a certain number of years of training and pass a specified examination before receiving hospital privileges. Process refers to whether we are doing the right thing for the right patient at the right time for the right reason (some analysts would add an economic rider – at the right cost, which is subsumed under the proposed matrix). Outcome refers to the impact of a service on the health status of a patient or a population (Naylor, 1996).

"Where" is self-evident. We may take a macro-geographic perspective, examining performance at the level of a country, or a region, or county. Alternatively, we may profile the performance or behaviour of institutions, physicians, administrators, patients, and policy-makers. Hospital or regional analyses, in particular, allow professionals and administrators to compare themselves to similar settings and share best practices (Naylor, 1994; Naylor, 1996).

For the concept of "When", it is vital to consider whether we are assessing performance using a cross-sectional or longitudinal framework. In many cases, there are time lags between interventions and outcomes, and more importantly, limitations in the info-structures of many OECD nations impose time lags due to data availability. Information must be available on a rapid-cycle basis to support change on the front lines of service, and the temporal factor in causality must always be considered.

Last, on the matter of "How", we must consider the ways that the data can be used to catalyse change. This goes well beyond putting a coloured cover on a mind-numbing statistical compendium, or reducing complex data to a league table or star-ranking system that will be more accessible a wide readership. What we must begin to do is to align information systems, selection of performance measures, reporting systems, organisational or professional culture, and implementation mechanisms.

Returning to the category of "What" measures: One hears a great deal of emphasis on "outcomes measurement". In fact, the most efficient indicators of health system performance at the micro-level are usually process-based.[4] This is partly because existing data systems tend not to capture key outcomes such as the quality-of-life benefits of modern health and social services. More generally, there are strong epidemiological grounds for this approach.[5] In a nutshell, identification of flawed processes pinpoints where change should occur, rather than generating an acrimonious debate about causes and confounders. We would suggest that for sub-system performance measurement, outcomes data collection be focused on three domains:

1. High-volume relatively homogeneous procedures that are technically demanding. The rationale is obvious. We are seeking to ensure that inadequately skilled or equipped providers are either brought up to standard or put out of business. Epidemiological or statistical input is necessary to adjust for imbalances in patient or population characteristics across the providers under study, thereby helping to ensure that comparisons occur on a level playing field.

2. High-volume relatively homogeneous diagnoses where the causal connection between interventions and outcomes is sharply delineated and reasonably short-term. The same rationale and caveats apply here as for the first category.

3. Otherwise-heterogeneous populations whose outcomes may be tracked back to a common causal pathway or environmental factor. Obvious measures here would be the rates of post-operative infection or various measures of patient satisfaction.

Last, on the interface of "Who" and "What", we would like to underscore a message that others will bring in this volume. One of the great under-developed areas for performance assessment is the elicitation of the perspective of patients or more generally the public. As Angela Coulter will emphasise, we are in this business to be responsive to patients' needs as well as to optimise population health (see, Part III, Chapter 10 in this volume). We should all urge providers to meet regularly with patient representatives about measurement issues, so there can be agreement on the outcomes that matter; the two perspectives are surprisingly disparate. Moreover, public polls and patient surveys are not only important at a micro-level or meso-level; they are also invaluable as screening tests for systems issues. In this respect, consider the results from a recent five-nation survey of randomly chosen households by a Harvard team led by Donelan and Blendon (Donelan *et al.*, 1999). Respondents were asked to estimate the duration of their last visit to a primary care physician. As

Figure 5. **Length of most recent doctor visit**

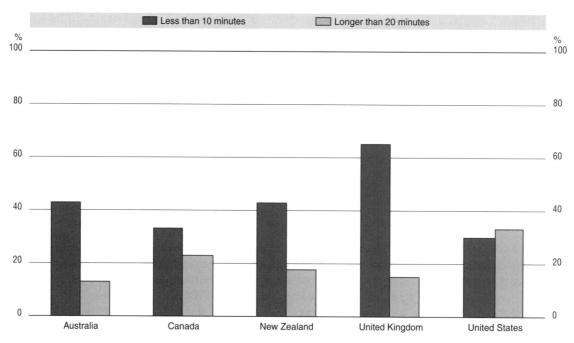

Source: 1998 Commonwealth Fund International Policy Health Survey.

shown in Figure 5, Americans clearly led the way with long visits. But when the researchers asked the citizens if they were getting enough time with their doctor, Americans were again leading the way in an unanticipated direction (see Figure 6). A reasonable conclusion is that managing public expectations may be as important as managing resources in our health care system!

4.3. International comparisons: a procedure-specific case study

Later chapters will illuminate the value of international comparisons at a general and disease-specific level. To help set the stage, the following examples encapsulate some of our own experiences with cross-border comparisons in North America, focused on coronary heart disease and related procedures.

New York State does about twice as much coronary bypass surgery per capita as Ontario, Canada, even though the incidence of coronary disease is similar in the two jurisdictions (Tu, Naylor *et al.*, 1997). Figure 7 shows the rates of bypass surgery for Ontario and New York, broken down by the severity of the underlying arterial blockages, and their impact on life expectancy, and by the age of the patients. For left mainstem and multi-vessel disease, where surgery is expected to prolong life, we see rather disturbingly that Ontario has much lower rates of surgery on a per capita basis. However, the big differences are for single vessel disease where no life expectancy gains have been demonstrated with randomised trials. This is quality-of-life-enhancing surgery. New York State does 17 times as many bypasses as Ontario on patients in this subgroup aged 75 and over. Ontario has the highest provincial rate of bypass surgery in Canada; New York State, almost the lowest of the 50 states in America. It is clear that this comparison, if anything, underestimates the dramatic differences in practice patterns between the two countries. Data like these help illustrate why America spends so much more than Canada on health care.

What are the implications of these differences in access or utilisation for outcomes? We analysed linked administrative data for all senior citizens in Ontario and the United States who had recently been hospitalised with an acute myocardial infarction (Tu, Pashos *et al.*, 1997). We measured how often they

Figure 6.   **Respondents reporting time their doctor spent with them was too short**

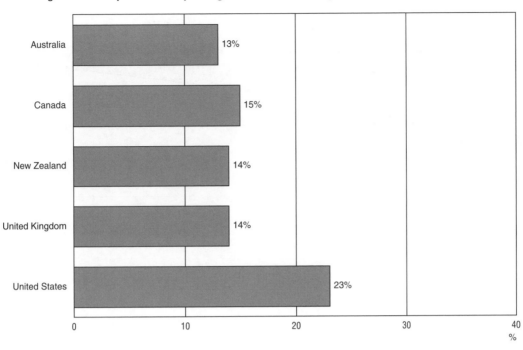

Source: 1998 Commonwealth Fund International Policy Health Survey.

Figure 7.   **Coronary surgery: Ontario *vs* New York**

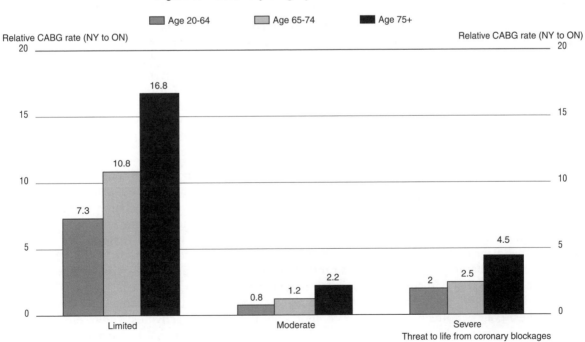

Source: Tu, Naylor *et al.* (1997).

Figure 8. **Mortality after myocardial infarction for elderly patients in the US and Ontario, 1991**

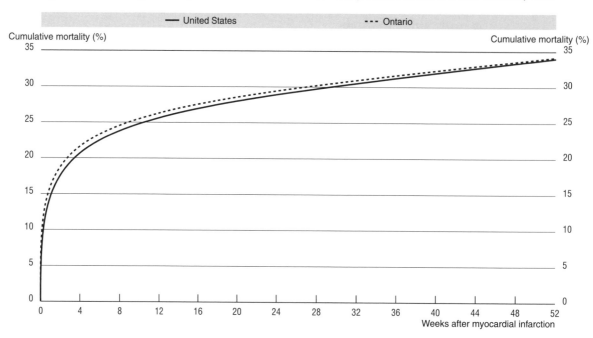

Source: Tu, Pashos *et al.* (1997).

received expensive tertiary services, including bypass surgery, coronary angiograms, and balloon angioplasties. American seniors were up to eight times more likely to get these procedures within 30 days after a heart attack. And even after six months, Americans were still four times more likely to have undergone a major procedure, a huge difference in resource consumption. What was the impact on mortality, when all of these patients were followed for a year? As shown in Figure 8, absolutely none.

As noted earlier, death is certainly not the only outcome that matters. A major study was recently reported in *The Lancet* on this exact topic (TIME Investigators, 2001). This was a careful randomised trial including European patients aged 75 and over with symptoms of coronary disease. It compared a very aggressive surgical strategy to normal conservative care. The authors reported this study as dramatically positive, given the prevention of downstream hospitalisations for acute coronary syndrome and nonfatal infarctions 6 months following surgery. Moreover, elderly patients undergoing routine surgery had fewer symptoms and better functional status. On the other hand, the death rates actually favoured the conservative arm rather dramatically as the number of deaths were almost half of those reported in the group receiving invasive surgery.

Non-randomised studies have anticipated these findings by showing that American heart attack patients have better quality of life outcomes than Canadians without mortality advantages. However, it is not that simple. The most extensive study undertaken was led by investigators from Duke University, and involved researchers across the United States, along with many of us in Canada (Mark *et al.*, 1994). It examined the array of quality of life and economic outcomes shown in Table 1, and followed a large group of Canadians and Americans who had been part of a major worldwide study of clot-lysing drugs for acute myocardial infarction. Americans predictably underwent many more expensive procedures than the Canadian trial participants. They were also far more likely to see specialists than Canadians, who relied instead on family physicians for ongoing care. We did find that Canadians were more likely to have chest pain symptoms. They had more limitations in their daily activities. They were even more likely to be somewhat depressed. But, when asked to rate their overall health, Canadians responded virtually identically to Americans. And when we assessed work status, Canadians were just as likely as Americans to be back working full time.

Table I. **Domains and economic/resource consumption indicators assessed in the EQUOL GUSTO study**

Domains
Quality of life
Functional status
Employment status/role functioning
Symptoms (chest pain, dyspnea)
Psychological well-being
Time trade – off (QALY)
General health status

Economic/resource consumption indicators
Hospitalisations
Cardiac catheterisation
Revascularisation

Source: Mark *et al.* (1994).

One interpretation is that Canadians are simply more stoic than our flamboyant and good friends to the south. Then, again, to paraphrase H.L. Mencken, for every complex problem, there is a simple solution and it is almost always dead wrong. So let us consider another interpretation that is more complex and probably more accurate. Consistent with the view of health care as a field where half-way technologies predominate, neither surgery nor angioplasty offers much benefit on average to patients at medium risk of major cardiac events. Instead, the vast majority would still be alive ten years later if they had simply been given drugs. The first consequence of marshalling half-way technologies, in a climate of uncertainty within highly variable local and national health systems, is a great deal of variation in practice patterns and resource consumption. The second consequence is the phenomenon of diminishing marginal impacts on health status (Naylor, 1997).

We may start with a near linear relationship between service investments and improvements in population health status. But as service intensity rises, more and more resources are poured into achieving smaller and smaller gains. Our great challenge, from the health policy standpoint, is to decide where along the flattening part of the curve we stop expending public resources on health services per se. At what point would we be better off making investments in public infrastructure or in post-secondary education, or in social policy initiatives to improve the life chances of our children? Each nation will make its own choices, but we submit to you that one of the great values of international comparisons is to spark rigorous research that will help delineate the balance of benefits and harms for various programs and services, and to throw these crucial trade-offs into high relief.

4.4. *Reporting on performance measures*

As managers, we have all been taught how to do performance appraisal with individual staff in a way that catalyses change rather than provoking defensive responses. Unfortunately, the same principles are sometimes forgotten when performance assessments are put before providers, managers, public servants, or the general public. The goal of measurement, after all, is to "move and improve" the system, not to "name, shame, and blame" individuals or institutions. Moreover, if the target audiences are involved in selecting the measures, it will be much easier for them to accept the messages.

One key strategy in presenting performance information is to freely acknowledge any limitations of the data and any associated analyses, including lack of timeliness. Otherwise, as we all know, those who dislike the findings will make the same arguments very quickly indeed. A second strategy is to avoid excess interpretation, and let the debate flow. This can be a little harrowing, particularly if the media get active. The headline shown in Figure 9 appeared in Canada's largest daily newspaper after our group identified major geographic variations in the use of pharmacological versus surgical castration for metastatic prostate cancer (*Toronto Star*, 1994). The point was to raise the possibility that the variations

27

Figure 9. *The Toronto Star*, March 4, 1994

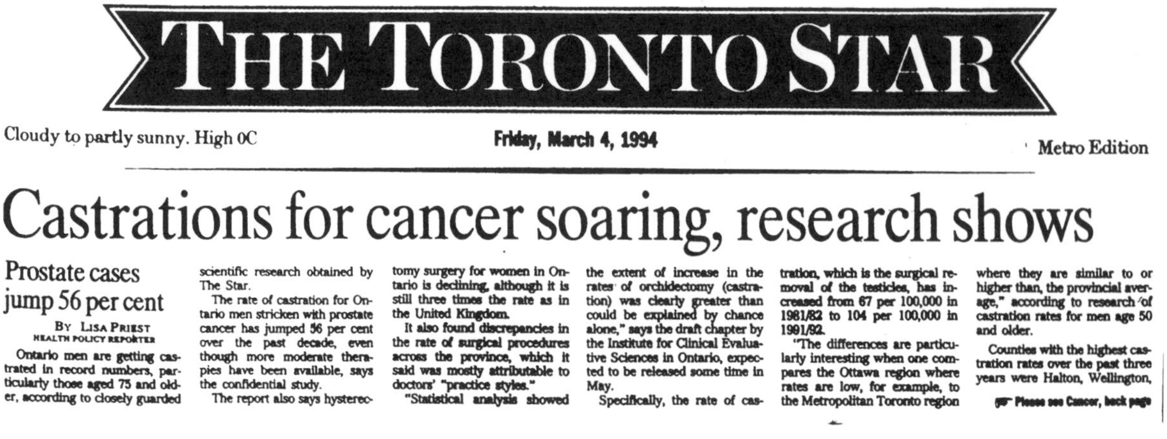

THE TORONTO STAR

Cloudy to partly sunny. High 0C   **Friday, March 4, 1994**   Metro Edition

Castrations for cancer soaring, research shows

Prostate cases jump 56 per cent

BY LISA PRIEST
HEALTH POLICY REPORTER

Ontario men are getting castrated in record numbers, particularly those aged 75 and older, according to closely guarded scientific research obtained by The Star.

The rate of castration for Ontario men stricken with prostate cancer has jumped 56 per cent over the past decade, even though more moderate therapies have been available, says the confidential study.

The report also says hysterec-tomy surgery for women in Ontario is declining, although it is still three times the rate as in the United Kingdom.

It also found discrepancies in the rate of surgical procedures across the province, which it said was mostly attributable to doctors' "practice styles."

"Statistical analysis showed the extent of increase in the rates of orchidectomy (castration) was clearly greater than could be explained by chance alone," says the draft chapter by the Institute for Clinical Evaluative Sciences in Ontario, expected to be released some time in May.

Specifically, the rate of cas-tration, which is the surgical removal of the testicles, has increased from 67 per 100,000 in 1981/82 to 104 per 100,000 in 1991/92.

"The differences are particularly interesting when one compares the Ottawa region where rates are low, for example, to the Metropolitan Toronto region where they are similar to or higher than, the provincial average," according to research of castration rates for men age 50 and older.

Counties with the highest castration rates over the past three years were Halton, Wellington,

☞ Please see Cancer, back page

reflected practice styles rather than respect for patients' preferences (Klotz *et al.*, 1994). The story was reasonable, but the headline was more exciting than we had expected!

The challenge of media reportage highlights the tension between ensuring broad accessibility of information to the public, the political uses of that information, and profiling performance in a way that is credible and fair to providers and managers. We have seen a tremendous proliferation of disease- or procedure-specific league tables of performance, as well as simple "star" rankings of hospitals or regions across the OECD nations. When a dozen British hospitals received a rating of zero stars out of three, Canada's Medical Post reported on what were near-classic responses from the government and providers (M*edical Post*, 2001). Alan Milburn, the Health Secretary, was quoted as stating that "there has always been a convenient excuse when there is a problem, but these tables explode the myth once and for all". In contrast, Peter Hawker, Chairman of the BMA Consultants' Committee was quoted as follows: "I worry that strident reporting of a hospital's weaknesses can dent the confidence of the community in its local hospital, adversely affect recruitment and further damage the morale of clinical staff".

Controversy continues about the impact of public dissemination of such information, but we view it as essential to make performance findings understandable to a wide audience (Schneider and Epstein, 1998; Marshall *et al.*, 2000; Leatherman, Part V, Chapter 15 in this volume). If the citizen in the street can understand a report, then volunteer governors, lay managers, and politicians can understand it as well. The result is that information asymmetry is reduced and professional accountability enhanced.

One little-addressed issue is the commercialisation of performance measurement and the potential impact on messages received by either patients or providers. Investor-owned interests have entered this field with a variety of proprietary algorithms that are not accessible to those whose performance is under scrutiny – not an ideal situation. One company, which shall remain nameless, uses American administrative data to do internet-accessible performance profiling for a wide variety of procedures and diseases. It has plans to publish on-line ratings for nursing homes, hospices, home health agencies, fertility clinics and linkages to data for health plans and providers. The "value proposition" here seems to be that the free profiles concentrate providers' minds on redemption that may be best achieved by purchasing the management consulting services of the same firm. Officials in OECD nations may wish to put their minds to these issues at some point in future.

Perhaps the most important reflection on performance reporting is that, to bastardise McLuhan, the medium, context, and implications are more important than the message itself . For example, Schneider and Epstein (1998) surveyed patients undergoing cardiac surgery in Pennsylvania to determine the impact of the highly-publicised state-wide consumer guide to the performance of both hospitals and individual surgeons. Only 12 per cent of the patients were aware of the guide before undergoing a coronary artery bypass graft (CABG) procedure. And less than 1 per cent knew the correct rating of their hospital or surgeon, or reported that such information had any meaningful influence on the selection of a provider for open-heart surgery. In contrast, both public and confidential reports on cardiac surgery performance have been shown to be similarly effective at galvanising improvements in processes and outcomes of care, as long as provider organisations sanction the need for change (Malenka *et al.*, 1995; Bentley and Nash, 1998).

It is perhaps not surprising, then, that a systematic review by Marshall *et al.* published in JAMA (2000) suggested that public report cards about specific diseases or procedures have had little measurable impact. On the other hand, as Gregg Meyer (Part II, Chapter 5 in this volume) will explicate, balanced score-cards on health systems or subsystems can indeed have an impact on consumer choice among health plans in nations like America where multiple private providers compete. The distinction is important. We surmise that patients are indeed willing to make broad choices on the basis of performance data, but do not have the time or inclination to benchmark every practitioner and encounter within a given system. That leads logically to our "final frontier".

5. Change: the final frontier

Knowledge may be power, and information may be catalytic, but change will be stalled by professional and organisational inertia in the absence of specific steps to make change both necessary and possible. Changes in aspects of system performance can be surprisingly difficult to effect in the desired directions. Professional self-regulation sometimes serves provider interests, not the public interest. Citizens vary across the OECD nations in their consumerism as regards health issues, and professionals may either dismiss performance data or respond in unanticipated ways, such as avoiding high-risk patients who actually have the most to gain from their services. Indeed, the unintended costs of mismeasurement include misdirected effort, defensive medicine, and demoralisation. Blunt financial and regulatory instruments may have perverse effects, as already noted. To repeat an earlier point which we cannot over-emphasise: we must understand how measurement relates to behaviour change and *vice versa*. This requires alignment of the factors and forces shown in Table 2.

The ways that performance measurement can drive change will be reviewed in much greater detail by other authors, particularly by Sheila Leatherman. As summarized in Table 3, drivers of change may be economic or non-economic factors. The mechanisms whereby information is brought to bear on the system may be regulatory, administrative/professional, or market-based. And the actors whose behaviour is changed by information may be consumers, purchasers or funders, professionals/ administrators, or central managers. Often two or more of these elements are operational in any dimension. For example, Britain's NHS has taken extraordinary and commendable steps to marry performance measurement to budgetary rewards as well as administrative autonomy. In effect, the incentives for good performance are both economic and non-economic. Performance information for American employees and employers allows them to choose among competing health plans, leading to a market-driven approach based on the alignment of consumers and purchasers, with impact on professionals and administrators in the diverse plans. Even for the simple procedure-specific report cards mentioned earlier, the drivers of change range from regulatory responses designed to close low-volume programs to collaborative action by professionals and administrators aimed at identifying and implementing best practices across a network of institutions.

Table 2.   **Alignment for improvement of health care**

1. **Align information systems**
2. **Align performance measures**
3. **Align reporting systems**
4. **Align organisational/professional culture**
5. **Align implementation mechanisms**

Table 3. **Drivers of change**

1. **Incentives**
    a) Economic
    b) Non-economic

2. **Actors**
    a) Consumers
    b) Purchasers/funders
    c) Professionals/managers

3. **Mechanisms**
    a) Regulatory
    b) Administrative/professional
    c) Market-based

Money is a powerful incentive, but it is also worth reminding ourselves what the available evidence tells us about non-economic methods for altering the behaviour of health professionals (Table 4). Results of a definitive overview by Davis *et al.* from 1995 show that one-off interventions have little impact, be it in the form of feedback about past performance or information about new research evidence that might bear on future behaviour. Even consistent performance feedback has only a modest impact. Instead, what seems to work best is a combination of factors. Professionals change more readily when the available research evidence is strong and when the clinical issues are sharply drawn. In many cases, our health systems actively reward providers for doing the wrong things, or impede change by failing to provide the requisite technology or staff support. Addressing barriers to change is therefore important. Finally, multi-modal interventions can be used to drive positive change, including: the training or recruiting of opinion leaders and local champions to convince peers of the merits of responding to evidence such as performance profiles; the development of information systems that give real-time feedback on the relevant practice patterns; and, engagement of other members of the healthcare team, including administrators, to reinforce the desired behaviour. In our view, these non-economic factors must be aligned whenever possible with financial levers, either through market mechanisms or public administration. This is still the exception rather than the norm. For example, in Canada's health system, most of the funding mechanisms for professionals, institutions, and regions are at best indifferent to indicators of quality, equity, and efficiency in service delivery.

Table 4. **Non-economic methods for changing professional behaviour**

1. **Minimal impact**
    a) One-off information sessions
    b) Intermittent performance feedback

2. **Bigger impact**
    a) Consistent performance feedback
    b) Point-of-decision information tools for patients or providers
    c) Training and supporting opinion leaders
    d) Repeated education interventions

3. **Biggest impact**
    a) Strong evidence or burning issues (overwhelming evidence of large net benefit or avoidable harms)
    b) Identify and address barriers to change (perverse incentives, technology, staffings, etc.)
    c) Multimodal approaches (information systems, culture shift, local champions, administrative commitment)

Source: Davis *et al.* (1995)

6. Conclusion

The current commitment to performance measurement is overdue and merits the support of all those who work in health care, or who fund or administer it. There is already ample evidence of inexplicable variations in structures, processes, and outcomes within and between our national health systems. There is also evidence of unacceptable clinical and economic impacts from unwanted variation in our systems at all levels. But by conjoining the systematic assessment of research evidence to the rigorous measurement of health care performance, these variations can be transformed from problems to benchmarking opportunities. With enhanced info-structure, the right measures, the right mechanisms, and variously the requisite political will or the right market forces, healthcare performance information can and will make a vast difference to the quality, accessibility, and efficiency of our diverse health care systems. As part of making a difference, we know all the participants will take from this Conference a sense of spectacular opportunities for us to learn from each other, not just at the systems-level but at the coal-face of clinical service delivery and management. Onwards and upwards – may we all be ready to measure and manage better than ever.

NOTES

1. Public health activists and social democrats in the 19th century argued for reducing class-related variation in health status through better public and occupational health measures, relative income equality, and a strong social safety net. These insights gained prominence again in the Great Depression as links between health and unemployment became clear. McKeown's seminal work in the 1960s provided a quantitative foundation for this line of argument, illustrating the lack of correlation between indices of population health and medical care advances. In Canada, the Lalonde report of 1974 signalled that mainstream political thinking had embraced this "New Perspective" with its emphasis on the multiple determinants of health status outside the health system per se. Meanwhile, important work by Marmot *et al.* in the United Kingdom (Marmot, 2000; 2001) and Symes *et al.* in the United States provided deeper and stronger evidence for the impact of social factors on health status. Today, a small industry has grown up to investigate, elaborate on, and popularize this latest incarnation of a wider-angle view of health determinants. One can only hope that we do not lose sight of this valuable and oft-forgotten framework in the rush to embrace molecular medicine or the "next new thing" in some future decade.

2. The tally included preventive interventions such as screening for hypertension and cervical cancer, smoking cessation, and immunizations for diphtheria, polio, tetanus, smallpox, flu, pneumococcus, and hepatitis B. Also considered were treatment of conditions such as cervical cancer, colorectal cancer, peptic ulcer, ischemic heart disease, renal failure, infant respiratory diseases, appendicitis, diabetes, complications of pregnancy, pneumonia and flu, tuberculosis, and trauma (Bunker *et al.*, 1994).

3. Note that even community surveys aimed at measuring self-rated general health status may be divorced from the actual impacts of medical care. There is now a moderate-sized literature showing that generic measures of self-rated health, functional status, and quality of life, are insensitive to variations in processes and outcomes of clinical care. Those same variations, however, are associated with measurable impacts on disease-specific quality of life measures.

4. As per G.M. Brown Lecture (Naylor, 1997), a concrete example: "From overviews of randomized placebo-controlled trials we know that beta-blockers confer about a 25 per cent relative reduction in mortality in the first year after a myocardial infarction. For a cohort of medium-risk patients, this equates to an absolute reduction in cumulative post-discharge mortality from 4 to 3 per cent. To show such a mortality difference on a comparative audit of two practices (80 per cent power, 2-sided alpha of 0.05), we require over 5 000 patients per practice; but a 1 per cent mortality difference presumes absolutely no use of beta-blockers in the practice with poorer outcomes. A more realistic assumption would be that about 70 per cent of eligible patients receive beta-blockers in the practice with worse outcomes; based on the randomized trials, this equates to a 0.2 per cent increase in mortality. To detect such a small difference in mortality would require over 100 000 patients per practice! In contrast, we could simply examine charts to see whether patients were getting beta-blockers or not – a process-of-care audit. If a better practice had over 90 per cent beta-blocker prescriptions, versus 70 per cent in the other practice, we would only need to examine 75 charts in each practice for a reliable assessment. This latter audit is simple in another respect. We can basically use randomized trial inclusion and exclusion criteria to decide who should be getting the drug, make sure there are no obvious contraindications or medication intolerances documented on the medical record, and tally whether patients are getting the treatment that they ought to be getting."

5. Again, as per the G.M. Brown Lecture (Naylor, 1997): "The key place to measure outcomes assiduously is not in effectiveness research, but in efficacy research where randomized trials with clinically meaningful outcomes can help us understand what we ought to be doing for our patients. In ordinary practice, as opposed to randomized studies, patients receive different treatment according to their characteristics rather than according to the play of chance. Such case selection for treatment or referral is an integral part of good clinical judgement in routine care. Thus, in the absence of randomization or a prospective study designed to isolate a potentially causative variable of interest, it will be hard to know if the outcomes observed are due to a process-of-care variable, including provider skill, or to imbalances in the prognostic characteristics of patients themselves."

REFERENCES

ALTER, D., NAYLOR, D., AUSTIN, P. and TU, J. (1999),
"Effects of socio-economic status on access to invasive cardiac procedures and on mortality after Acute Myocardial Infarction", *New England Journal of Medicine*, Vol. 341, No.18, pp.1359-1367.

BENTLEY, J. and NASH, D. (1998),
"How Pennsylvania hospitals have responded to publicly released reports on Coronary Artery Bypass Graft Surgery", *Journal on Quality Improvement*, Vol. 24, No. 1, pp. 40-49.

BUNKER, J. (1995),
"Medicine matters after all", *Journal of the Royal College of Physicans of London*, Vol. 29, No. 2, pp. 105-112.

BUNKER, J., FRAZIER H. and MOSTELLER, F. (1994),
"Improving health: Measuring effects of medical care", *Millbank Quarterly*, Vol. 72, No. 2, pp.225-258.

DAVIS, D., THOMSON, M., OXMAN, A. and HAYNES, B. (1995),
"Changing physician performance: A systematic review of the effect of continuing medical education strategies", JAMA (*Journal of the American Medical Association*), Vol. 274, No. 9, pp. 700-705.

DONELAN, K., BLENDON, R., SCHOEN, C., DAVIS, K. and BINNS, K.(1999),
"The cost of health system change: public discontent in five nations", *Health Affairs (Millwood)*, Vol. 18, No. 3, pp. 206-216.

EVANS, D., TANDON, A., MURRAY, C. and LAUER, J. (2001),
"Comparative efficiency of National Health Systems: Cross-national econometric analysis", *British Medical Journal*, Vol. 323, No. 11, pp. 307-310.

HURST, J. (2000),
"Challenges for health systems in member countries of the Organisation for Economic co-operation and Development", *Bulletin of the World Health Organization*,Vol. 78, No. 6, pp. 751-760.

JAY, A. and LYNN, J. (2001),
"Yes, Minister", *British Broadcasting Corporation*, 1981. In *www.yes-minister.com*, September 16, 2001.

KLOTZ L., TO, T., ISCOE N. and NAYLOR D. (1994),
"Orchidectomy as a treatment for prostate cancer", in Naylor, C.D., Anderson, G.M. and Goel, V. (eds.), *Patterns of Health Care in Ontario*, The ICES Practice Atlas, 1st edition, Canadian Medical Association, Ottawa, pp. 111-115.

LALONDE, M. (1974),
"A new perspective on the health of Canadians: A working document", Government of Canada, Department of Health and Welfare.

LLEWELLYN-THOMAS, H., ARSHINOFF, R., BELL, M., WILLIAMS, J., NAYLOR, D. and The Ontario Hip and Knee Replacement Project Team (1998),
"In the queue for total joint replacement: Patients' perspectives on waiting times", *Journal of Evaluation in Clinical Practice*, Vol. 4, No. 1, pp.63-74.

MALENKA D., O'CONNOR, G. and The Northern New England Cardiovascular Study Group (1995),
"A regional collaborative effort for CQI in cardiovascular disease", *Journal of Quality Improvement*, Vol. 21, No. 11, pp. 627-633.

MARK, D., NAYLOR, D., HLATKY, M., CALIFF, R., TOPOL, E., GRANGER, C., KNIGHT, J., NELSON, C., LEE, K., CLAPP0173CHANNING, N. *et al.* (1994),
"Use of medical resources and quality of life after Acute Myocardial Infarction in Canada and the United States", *New England Journal of Medicine*, Vol. 331, No. 17, pp. 1130-1135.

MARMOT, M. (2001),
"Inequalities in health", *New England Journal of Medicine*, Vol. 345, No. 2, pp. 134-136.

MARMOT, M. (2000),
"Social determinants of health: from observation to policy", *Medical Journal of Australia*, Vol. 172, No. 8, pp. 379-382.

MARSHALL, M., SHEKELLE, P., LEATHERMAN, S. and BROOK, R. (2000),
"The public release of performance data: What do we expect to gain? A review of the evidence", JAMA (*Journal of the American Medical Association*), Vol. 283, No. 14, pp. 1866-1874.

McKEOWN, T. (1979),
"The role of medicine: Dream, mirage or nemesis?", Princeton University Press, Princeton, New Jersey.

MEDICAL POST (2001),
"Rating of Zero Stars for a Dozen British Hospitals", October 16.

MOHAMMED, M., CHENG, K., ROUSE, A. and MARSHALL, T. (2001),
"Bristol, Shipman, and clinical governance: Shewhart's forgotten lessons", *Lancet*, Vol. 357, pp. 463-467.

MURRAY, C. and FRENK, J. (2001),
"World Health Report 2000: A step towards evidence-based health policy", *Lancet*, Vol. 357, pp.1698-1700.

NAVARRO, V. (2000),
"Assessment of the World Health Report 2000", *Lancet*, Vol. 356, pp. 1598-1601.

NAVARRO, V. (2001),
"World Health Report 2000: Responses to Murray and Frenk", *Lancet*, Vol. 357, pp. 1701-1702.

NAYLOR, D. (1998),
"Benchmarking the provision of coronary artery surgery", *Canadian Medical Association Journal*, Vol. 158, No. 9, pp.1151-1153.

NAYLOR, D. (1997),
"G. Malcolm Brown Lecture: Assessing processes and outcomes of medical care", *Annals of the Royal College of Physicians and Surgeons of Canada*, Vol. 30, No. 3, pp.157-161.

NAYLOR, D. (1996),
"Variations in selected surgical procedures and medical diagnoses", in Goel, V., Williams, J.I., Anderson, G.M., Blackstein-Hirsch, P., Fooks, C. and Naylor, C.D. (eds), *Patterns of Health Care in Ontario*, The ICES Practice Atlas, 2nd edition, Canadian Medical Association, Ottawa, pp. 51-54.

NAYLOR, D. and GUYATT, G. for the Evidence-based Medicine Working Group. (1996),
"Users' guide to medical literature X. How to use an article reporting variations in the outcomes of health services", JAMA (*Journal of the American Medical Association*), Vol. 275, No. 7, pp. 554-558.

NAYLOR, D. (1994),
"Introduction", in Naylor C.D., Anderson, G.M. and Goel, V. (eds.), *Patterns of Health Care in Ontario*, The ICES Practice Atlas, 1st edition, Canadian Medical Association, Ottawa, pp. 1-5.

NEW YORK TIMES (2000),
"Genetic Code of Human Life is Cracked by Scientists", June 27.

O'BRIEN, B., DRUMMOND, M., LABELLE, R. and WILLAN, A. (1994),
"In search of power and significance: Issues in the design and analysis of stochastic cost-effectiveness studies in health care", *Medical Care*, Vol. 32, No. 2, pp. 150-163.

PALDA, V., LLEWELLYN-THOMAS, H., MACKENZIE R., PRITCHARD K. and NAYLOR, D. (1997),
"Breast cancer patients' attitudes about rationing postlumpectomy radiation therapy: applicability of trade-off methods to policy-making", *Journal of Clinical Oncology*, Vol. 15, No. 10, pp. 3192-3200.

SCHNEIDER, E. and EPSTEIN, A. (1998),
"Use of public performance reports: A survey of patients undergoing cardiac surgery", JAMA (*Journal of the American Medical Association*), Vol. 279, No. 20, pp. 1638-1642.

THOMAS, L. (1977),
"On the science and technology of medicine", in Knowles, J.H. (ed.), *Doing Better and Feeling Worse*, W.W. Norton, New York, pp. 35-46.

TIME INVESTIGATORS (2001),
"Trial of Invasive vs Medical Therapy in elderly patients with chronic symptomatic coronary artery disease (TIME): A randomized trial", *Lancet*, Vol. 358, pp. 951-957.

TORONTO STAR (1994),
"Castration Rates for Cancer Soaring, Research Shows", March 4.

TU, J., NAYLOR, D., KUMAR, D., DEBUONO, B., McNEIL, B. and HANNAN, E. (1997),
"Coronary artery bypass graft surgery in Ontario and New York State: Which rate is right?", *Annals of Internal Medicine*, Vol. 126, No. 1, pp. 13-19.

TU, J., PASHOS, C., NAYLOR, D., CHEN, E., NORMAND, S-L, NEWHOUSE, J. and McNEIL, B. (1997),
"Use of cardiac procedures and outcomes in elderly patients with myocardial infarction in the United States and Canada", *New England Journal of Medicine*, Vol. 336, No. 21, pp. 1500-1505.

WILDAVSKY, A. (1977),
"The political pathology of health policy", in Knowles, J.H. (ed.), *Doing Better and Feeling Worse*, W.W. Norton, New York, pp. 105-123.

WORLD HEALTH ORGANISATION (2000),
The World Health Report 2000 – Health Systems: Improving Performance, World Health Organisation, Geneva.

Chapter 2

PERFORMANCE MEASUREMENT AND IMPROVEMENT IN OECD HEALTH SYSTEMS: OVERVIEW OF ISSUES AND CHALLENGES

by

Jeremy Hurst[*]

Abstract

OECD health systems are under stress. That stress arises from the combination of the buoyant demand for health services and the continuing private and public desire for limitation of the rate of growth of health expenditure. It also arises from concern about continuing inequities in health and in access to health care.

As a consequence, there is much interest among policy makers in improving the performance of health systems where "performance" includes both efficiency and equity goals. More particularly, there is interest in pursuing what is, in effect, a performance measurement and improvement "cycle" where measurement of performance would be followed by appropriate actions, such as raising the performance of poorly performing providers or selecting better policies to promote efficiency and equity.

Considerable progress is being made in developing better measures of performance but challenges remain – particularly in measuring the quality of care and the determinants of good quality.

When it comes to actions, it is necessary to recognise that OECD health systems and subsystems vary in their institutional and incentive characteristics. As a result, they differ both in their strengths and weaknesses and in their ability to take advantage of better information.

A number of examples are provided of completion of the performance measurement and improvement "cycle" in relation to particular health policy problems in particular OECD countries.

Tentative conclusions include the following:

- there is great potential to improve performance by better alignment of information, incentives and action with appropriate policy objectives;

- the measurement of health outcomes (safety and efficacy) remains a major challenge both for evidence-based medicine and for evidence-based policy;

- to further the measurement of outcomes, there may be a general case for more government support of clinical self-regulation and scrutiny combined with greater openness about the results;

- there is a role for international work to develop better measures of performance and to improve understanding of which incentive and institutional arrangements best promote good performance in health systems.

---

[*] Head, Health Policy Unit, OECD Secretariat.

Introduction

OECD health systems are under stress. The tensions arise from well-known sources. There is buoyant demand for services from patients driven by: the ageing of populations, coverage by almost universal public and private health insurance and rising public expectations. There is controlled supply because public health expenditure is limited by the unpopularity of tax increases while private health expenditure is limited by resistance to premium and price increases. Waves of improvements in medical technology add to the pressure. Although they bring welcome advances in treatments, the new procedures are often more expensive than the old procedures that they replace. In addition, although there have been widespread improvements in average health status in all OECD countries, there is everywhere evidence of persistent health inequalities.

The specific form in which these tensions reach the agendas of Member governments differs between countries, partly because health care is organised and governed in varied ways in different countries. In some, it may be public criticism of the quality or timeliness of services which is the leading problem. For example, long waiting lists for elective surgery are a pressing problem in at least a third of OECD countries. In others, it may be rising real health expenditure, sometimes accompanied by growing deficits in public insurance schemes, that is the leading issue. In others, it may be difficulties with staff morale and recruitment that are the greatest challenge. In yet others, inequities in health or in access to health services may be the chief matter for concern.

Such strains have led to increasing interest among health policy makers in ways of encouraging health systems to improve their performance, where performance is to be measured against quality, efficiency and equity goals. Improving performance has the potential to reduce the tensions between rising demand and limited resources and to make systems fairer. Rising productivity is now expected annually in OECD economies. Can similar expectations be applied to health systems?

As a consequence, many OECD countries have been reviewing and reforming their arrangements for measuring and improving health system performance. Several have developed "performance measurement frameworks" in recent years and have encouraged or required public reporting of performance data.

Such attempts to increase transparency and accountability have sometimes become linked to reassessments of the universal and long-standing division of labour between professional self-regulation (of clinical performance) and government regulation (of health systems in relation to broad matters of efficiency and equity). This division of labour arose because of the asymmetry of knowledge between professionals and patients (and other lay people) about the indications for, and effectiveness of, medical interventions. In effect, because of the difficulty consumers have in judging quality of care, they have to trust health care professionals to act for them as "agents". And because of the difficulty governments have in regulating quality of care, they have given each health profession a monopoly of care in its respective field in exchange for "professional" behaviour, including the profession's commitment to act in the interests of patients and to maintain high standards of care by suitable training, certification and peer review of practice. Peer review has typically taken place behind closed doors. The open reporting of performance data can call into question some aspects of this "incomplete" contract between governments and professions, depending on the extent of clinical detail and identification of individual providers by performance indicators.

This paper is devoted to an overview of the issues and to the challenges facing new attempts to measure and improve health system performance in OECD countries. It is organised around the concept of a performance measurement and improvement "cycle" – a continuous feedback loop involving setting objectives for health systems, measuring performance against these objectives, and acting to improve performance where it is found lacking. The paper is written from an international perspective. It explores similarities and differences in the performance measurement and improvement agenda across OECD countries. Some case studies of apparently successful and unsuccessful use of performance measurement and improvement activities in different countries are identified. References are made to a few specifically international studies and some provisional conclusions are drawn.

1. The performance measurement and improvement cycle

In many cases, improvements to health systems are based on ideology and "experience" rather than on measurement and analysis. However, this paper is devoted mainly to the role of measurement and analysis in performance improvement – that is to evidence-based medicine, evidence-based management and evidence-based policy. Of course, measurement and analysis will often be combined with ideology and experience when changes are contemplated.

The steps that should be taken, ideally, in any health system to improve performance with the help of performance measurement, can be described in terms of a performance measurement and improvement "cycle". Such a cycle is depicted in Figure 1 (following Nutley and Smith, 1998). On the left of the diagram is the health system for which improvements in performance are sought. Weaknesses in performance identified by policy makers and managers will vary from system to system. At the top of the diagram is "conceptualisation and measurement". It is necessary to be clear about the objectives of the health care system and to measure relevant aspects of achievement against these objectives if unambiguous actions to improve performance are to be taken. It is also desirable to measure the structures and processes which give rise to differences in attainment if an understanding of the potential levers of change is to be obtained. At the right of the diagram is "analysis and evaluation". Evaluation is desirable, *ex ante*, to identify, for example, the causes of weaknesses in performance and the cost-effectiveness of steps which could be taken to tackle them. Evaluation is desirable, *ex post*, to monitor and to evaluate the results of taking action and to add to the "evidence-base" for future decisions. At the bottom of the diagram is "action". There are typically at least four key sets of actors in health systems: consumers, providers, managers and governors; and, depending on the problem to be tackled, it will require actions or changes in behaviour among some or all of these sets of actors for improvements in performance to be realised.

This "cycle" can be used to describe the appropriate steps to be taken in clinical initiatives aimed at improving performance. Here, the relevant entities will be, typically, patients, diseases and interventions. The relevant measurement will be of impacts of alternative interventions on the incidence and prevalence of diseases and of any side effects both at the patient and at the population level. The relevant analysis will include, *ex ante*, health technology assessment, which can often be based on randomised controlled trials, and the alternative interventions will often include choices between prevention, cure and care. The relevant actions, which will be taken mainly by health care professionals, will include promulgation of new clinical guidelines and adoption of approved new

Figure 1.   **The performance measurement and management cycle**

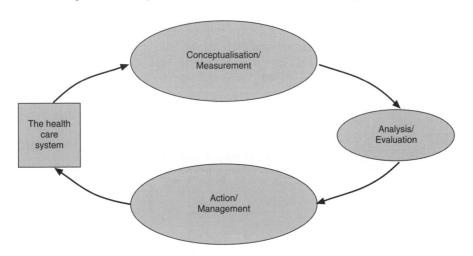

Source: Adapted from Nutley and Smith (1998).

technologies. Ex *post*, it is desirable that surveillance and monitoring is undertaken of the impact of interventions and of adverse events associated with them at patient and at population level.

The same "cycle" can also be used to summarise the appropriate steps to be taken in health policy and management initiatives aimed at improving performance. Here the relevant entities will be, typically, the general level or distribution of health status ("need") and the satisfaction of the population or subgroups of it with health services and policies to promote these. Relevant measurement will be of the impact of alternative health policies and of any perverse effects. Relevant analysis will include, *ex ante*, health policy assessment, usually based on observational studies and uncontrolled "experiments", cost effectiveness analysis and comparisons of the productivity and equity of different financing and service delivery arrangements. Relevant actions, which will be taken mainly by governors and managers, may include improvements in information, incentives or financing, and reform of health care institutions. Ex post, evaluation of the impact of policy initiatives and of any perverse effects is desirable.

Health systems have multiple objectives and adopting particular interventions will often involve tradeoffs between these ends. Needless to say, a health system will only perform well if both clinical decision-makers and mangers and governors are working effectively together towards the same ends.

The various stages in this cycle are explored in more detail below from an international perspective.

2. Conceptualisation of objectives

It is necessary to be clear about the objectives of health systems if performance is to be measured appropriately. Table 1, which has been adapted from a proposal put forward by WHO (Murray and Frenk, 2000), suggests a set of strategic objectives for any health care system. Three goals are proposed: health outcomes (and status); responsiveness to consumers; and health expenditure (for which, less is better, subject to satisfactory attainment of the first two goals). Both the average levels of attainment of each of these three goals (column 1) and their distribution across the population (column 2) are important. Note that in the first row, "health outcomes" is intended to relate only to the level of attainment of the goal (in column 1) and "health status" is intended to relate only to its distribution (in column 2).

"Efficiency" is written at the bottom of the first column. It includes technical, cost and allocative efficiency. It requires, in principle, that a weighted sum of the first two goals should be maximised subject to a given level of health expenditure. It also requires that total health expenditure be set at a level where the value of the marginal gains from extra health services equals the value of the marginal sacrifices from the alternative goods and services foregone. In practice it is hard to operationalise these concepts in the case of health systems, partly because of difficulties in measuring outcomes (see below). In general, efficiency is determined both by micro- and macro- (or government) behaviour in the health system. The role of government is peculiarly important in most OECD health systems. Governments invariably play an important regulatory role in relation to health care. In addition, they are usually the dominant funder of health care and increasingly play an active rather than a passive role in the determination of the level of public spending on health care. On average 75 per cent of health expenditure in the OECD area is public. "Equity" is written at the bottom of the second column – it includes equity of health status, equity of responsiveness and equity of the financial contributions by the population to health expenditure.

Table 1. **OECD proposed health system performance framework**

	Average level	Distribution
Health improvement/outcomes (+)	✔	✔
Responsiveness and access (+)	✔	✔
Financial contribution/health expenditure (–)	✔	✔
	Efficiency	Equity

Source: Adapted from Murray and Frenk (2000).

Assessment of the overall performance of health systems is inescapably value-laden and may also require judgements about facts. The value judgements must come either from consumers or from governments on behalf of consumers. Estimation of efficiency requires explicit or implicit pricing (or weighting) of health services and of the value of outputs foregone. The setting of equity goals is highly political and the political judgements are likely to vary between countries. The role of the health statistician, analyst or adviser is to inform all such judgements.

There is particular interest in measuring the quality of health care. In this framework, quality is captured in the first two rows of Table 1, in the form of health outcomes and responsiveness. These objectives have been unpacked in a recent report of the US Committee on the National Quality Report on Health Care Delivery (Hurtado *et al.*, 2000). In relation to health outcomes, the Committee distinguishes two "components of health care quality": safety and effectiveness. In relation to responsiveness, it distinguishes between patient centeredness and timeliness. In addition, the Committee distinguishes four "consumer perspectives on health care needs over the lifecycle": staying healthy, getting better, living with illness or disability and coping with the end of life. The matrix obtained from combining the Committee's four "components of quality" and four "consumer perspectives on health care needs" could be used to expand the first two rows of Table 1.

3. Measurement issues

Measuring the performance of health care against dimensions such as those set out above is an activity which is still in its infancy. Various OECD countries are developing national performance measurement frameworks and are beginning to populate them with suitable performance indicators. Four such examples have been reviewed in Hurst and Jee-Hughes (2001). Smee (Part II, Chapter 3 in this volume) and Reilly and Meyer (Part II, Chapter 5 in this volume) provide further details of two of these examples. In all these cases, there is an emphasis on achieving a "balanced scorecard" – that is on covering most or all of the areas set out above with a selection of indicators. However, progress along some dimensions has been faster than along others.

3.1. Health outcomes

For performance purposes, health outcomes can be defined narrowly as those changes in health status strictly attributable to the activities of health systems. In other words, we are interested not in so much in health status itself, which depends on many determinants, but in changes in health status, both positive and negative, attributable to health care.

Several OECD countries have now developed long lists of indicators of the effectiveness and safety of health care and have begun to publish relevant data. These have been reviewed in the OECD paper referred to above (Hurst and Jee-Hughes, 2001). The indicators include measures such as: avoidable mortality; avoidable hospitalisations; survival rates following acute, life-threatening events, such as heart attacks; and vaccination and screening rates.

However, close examination of these indicators by a group of experts convened by the Commonwealth Fund of New York, suggests that many so far proposed are ambiguous as measures of health outcome. Most are measures either of health status, where it is believed that the condition would have been avoidable, given appropriate medical care, or of interventions where it is believed that the process concerned is either appropriate or inappropriate. Unfortunately, "avoidable" mortality and morbidity regularly proves to depend on determinants of health apart from current medical care, such as the social and economic status of the patients concerned. The same limitation applies to some process measures of performance (Giuffrida, 1999). Furthermore, although a growing list of health care interventions is backed by evidence of effectiveness (and, indeed, cost effectiveness) as a result of health technology assessments, the way in which drugs and procedures are utilised in routine clinical practice, is often very different from the way in which they are tested on carefully selected, well-diagnosed patients under controlled conditions. Many new technologies diffuse far beyond the classes of patients and range of disease indications on which they were originally tested. In that case, little can be said any longer about their marginal effectiveness or cost-effectiveness on the basis of the original, controlled trials.

The fact that there are high levels of variation in many medical procedures across small geographical areas, variations which cannot be explained on the basis of differences either in morbidity or in resource levels, suggests that among clinicians there remains much underlying uncertainty about health outcomes for many treatments used in routine care. For some procedures, it could be said that we observe symmetry of ignorance across the medical and lay communities, rather than an asymmetry of knowledge.

3.2. Effectiveness

Despite the somewhat gloomy remarks, above, there are encouraging signs of forward progress in measuring health outcomes, viewed from an international perspective. Part of the progress stems from the fact that some OECD countries do link some of their administrative data – for example, within cancer registries – which allows for the estimation of rates of survival following the diagnosis of certain life-threatening conditions. Further study is required to ascertain to what extent survival rates represent health outcomes, reasonably free from confounding factors. The "Tech" project has reported on variations in treatment rates following heart attack across a number of OECD countries (Tech Research Network, 2001) and will go on to investigate links with survival rates. The OECD's Ageing Related Diseases Project (Jacobzone et al., Part III, Chapter 8 in this volume) is undertaking cross national studies of the causes and consequences of variations in treatment levels for three conditions: heart attack, stroke and breast cancer. Again, survival data will be examined for those countries which are able to supply it.

Further progress is in prospect if more countries choose to link their diagnostic, intervention and death records for individuals to allow longitudinal analysis of interventions in relation to the course of diseases – and hence the estimation of comparative health outcomes. There are sometimes confidentiality barriers to that and there are always cost barriers – although the latter may come down as electronic patient records are used more widely. There is also the prospect of progress in gathering process measures of effectiveness. For example, WHO is planning to collect "effective coverage" data for perhaps 100 interventions in many countries, probably via health interview surveys. The aim would be to identify interventions which are known to be effective and then to estimate the ratio of those receiving each intervention to those in need of each intervention, respectively. Childhood immunisation rates – which are widely available across countries – already provide examples of such measures.

When it comes to "living with illness and disability", considerable progress has been made with developing and using measures of the quality of long term care in institutional and community settings (Ikegami, Part IV, Chapter 13 in this volume). These cover both health outcome characteristics and responsiveness characteristics.

3.3. Safety

The first injunction that can be placed on health care providers is, "Do no harm". Unfortunately, in recent years evidence has emerged from small scale, local research studies in several OECD countries that medical care is far from safe. Two studies in the US have found rates of medical errors or "adverse events" for hospitalisation ranging from 2.9 to 3.7 per cent. Between 7 and 14 per cent of these adverse events lead to death. Extrapolated nationally, such rates imply that medical errors are a more important cause of death in the US than motor vehicle accidents or breast cancer or AIDS (Kohn et al., 2000). In Australia, a study found adverse events in 16.6 per cent of hospital admissions (Wilson et al., 1995). In New Zealand a study in three hospitals found adverse events in 10.7 per cent of hospital admissions (Davis et al., 2001). In many cases, the cause was medical care prior to hospitalisation. In the United Kingdom, a study in two hospitals found adverse events in 10.8 per cent of admissions (Vincent et al., 2001). These studies should not be compared directly because of differences in the methodologies adopted. Clearly, given standardisation of measurement, there is a place for routine reporting of such adverse events in performance measurement systems.

3.4. Responsiveness

Responsiveness can be measured by patient satisfaction, part of the outcome of care, or as patient experience, part of the process of care. "Patient satisfaction" measures attempt to capture patients' subjective happiness or unhappiness with the responsiveness of care. "Patient experience" measures attempt to capture factual aspects of responsiveness, such as how long patients waited for attention and the extent to which staff provided helpful information. The former will be affected by expectations and are often subject to a "gratitude" effect – typically 90 per cent or more of patients express satisfaction with health care, *ex post*. An illustration of the difference between these two types of measure can be derived from the Commonwealth Fund's survey of public discontent with health care in five countries (Donelan *et al.*, 1999). A sample of citizens in each of the five countries reported both factually on their length of their waiting times for non-emergency surgery and, subjectively, on whether they were "very worried", "somewhat worried" or "not too worried" about waiting too long to get non-emergency medical care. There was no correlation across countries between the average reported waiting times and the expressions of worry about waiting. Indeed, the country with the longest average reported waiting time, the UK, was the country with the lowest proportion of respondents saying they were "very worried" about waiting. Both measures of responsiveness are likely to be of interest to consumers and policy makers.

There has been considerable progress in measuring the responsiveness characteristics of several OECD health systems in recent years. Increasing numbers of countries which experience significant waiting times for non-emergency surgery are now collecting relevant data at hospital and sometimes physician level and are reporting it to consumers. Other types of experience data have been collected for samples of hospitals in the US and various European countries (Coulter and Cleary, Part III, Chapter 10 in this volume). The WHO is collecting data on six dimensions of responsiveness (dignity, autonomy, communication, confidentiality, prompt attention, access to social support, quality of basic amenities and choice) for a selection of their Member countries. Indeed, it is easier to see progress being made in collecting responsiveness data than it is in seeing progress being made in collecting health outcome data.

3.5. Health expenditure

In principle, the collection of health expenditure data for performance purposes is relatively straightforward. However, there are a number of practical problems to be overcome. First, there are different approaches to setting the boundaries of health systems (Evans, Part III, Chapter 9). Many OECD countries are now collecting health expenditure data according to the boundaries proposed in A *System of Health Accounts* (OECD, 2000). In terms of Evans' definitions, these boundaries encompass "personal medical" and "non-personal" health services. Secondly, there is the problem of disaggregating expenditure into volume and price. One difficulty is that of estimating incremental costs in relation to anticipated or realised changes in activities. The increasing availability of DRG cost estimates for inpatient hospital care is helpful, here. Another difficulty is that of identifying relative price changes specific to health care to allow for reliable estimation of changes in real health expenditure through time.

3.6. Efficiency

A necessary condition for efficiency is that a weighted sum of health improvements and responsiveness is maximised in relation to any given level of health expenditure. Unfortunately, because of the incompleteness, so far, of health improvement and responsiveness data, it is difficult to operationalise this outcome-related concept of efficiency.

The WHO (in its *World Health Report*, 2000) has developed a measure of the micro-determined efficiency of health systems which comes close to the concept set out above. In the absence of health outcome data, the WHO used health status data. Using econometric analysis, WHO estimated an upper and a lower frontier for health status across countries, after allowing for the level of health expenditure and the level of education (the latter, a proxy for all the other factors that affect health) in each country. WHO estimated how far each country's health status lay above the minimum frontier as a fraction of the difference between the upper and lower frontiers. The resulting efficiency measure lies between 0 and 1.

In the 1980s, the UK developed a less ambitious, process-related measure of micro-determined efficiency for hospital and community health services in England – the ratio of: annual changes in activity (inpatient admissions, outpatient attendances, etc.) weighted by unit costs; to annual changes in real health expenditure. This productivity change measure was used to set targets for annual gains in efficiency from the early 1990s with interesting results (see Section 7 on examples, below).

Although the main engine of efficiency in health systems is to be found, arguably, in micro behaviour, to a greater or lesser extent it is determined "top-down" by governments seeking to set the "right" level of total expenditure on health services. On average, 75 per cent of health expenditure is publicly funded in the OECD area. Most governments now take an active role in controlling the level of such expenditure. However, it is possible for governments both to overspend or to underspend on health services, especially if they seek at the same time to influence the level of private health expenditure. In principle, the "right" level of total health expenditure is the level at which the value of the marginal gains from extra health services equals the value of the marginal sacrifices from the alternative goods and services foregone. That cannot be operationalised fully, but the necessary judgements, by governments and the electorate, can be informed to a greater or lesser extent by international comparisons of comparative costs and comparative benefits.

It is part of the performance measurement agenda to inform such judgements. One activity which may be of some help is to monitor the ratio of the actual to the expected share of GDP devoted to health expenditure in a particular country on the basis of a regression line linking such shares to GDP per capita across OECD countries. However, this will be of limited use unless it is combined with international comparisons of health outcome and responsiveness data. An example of how the acquisition of such data may have affected a public expenditure decision in the UK is given in the "action" section, below.

3.7. Equity

In relation to the performance of health systems, equity can be investigated along several dimensions including equity of health status, equity of responsiveness (and access) and equity of the financial contributions by the population to health expenditure. Full equity of health status is unlikely to be achievable in any OECD country (if only because of genetic variations among individuals in each population) but it is a goal that can be pursued through improving equity of access to health care, among other social programmes.

There are a number of population characteristics which give rise to interest in equity. They include income, social status, age, disability status and geographical location.

The measurement of equity is problematic both in terms of deciding what is "equitable" and in terms of data because of its multidimensional character. There is not space to discuss the topic in any depth here. Suffice it to say that the measurement of equity is advancing steadily across OECD countries. There has been considerable conceptual clarification (see, for example, Culyer and Wagstaff, 1993). Also, much empirical progress has been made in measuring equity of finance (van Doorslaer et al., 1999) and equity of delivery (van Doorslaer et al., 2000) across European countries and the US. The WHO has published its own estimates of the equity of health, responsiveness and finance across countries in the World Health Report (2000).

4. Analysis

There has already been some coverage of the analysis of performance data, above, since it is not possible to estimate measures of attainment of complex objectives such as microeconomic efficiency and equity without embarking on considerable analysis of data. This section addresses three further analytical issues: developing composite indicators of performance; finding the causes of variations in performance; and assessing the cost effectiveness of interventions.

4.1. Composite indicators

Not only do health systems have multiple objectives – as indicated above – but also they have multiple providers and multiple outputs. A common problem encountered by those devising and using performance indicators for health systems is that of "drowning in numbers".

A number of ways have been suggested for controlling the number of indicators for those expected to act upon them. One is to try to identify "key" indicators, in the hope that they will be representative of performance across the board. Another is to develop composite indicators which, by way of weighting, reduce longer lists of indicators to summary measures. The measure of microeconomic efficiency proposed above is one such composite. These and others have been reviewed by Smith (Part IV, Chapter 14 in this volume).

5. Causes of variations and policy levers

If differences in performance have been identified, and it is not possible simply to walk away from poor performers, it will be necessary to obtain an understanding of the causes, with an emphasis on identifying the levers which might be pulled to improve performance. The subject of the determinants of health service performance is a large one, which will be dealt with only in a summary way here. Various authors have put forward suggestions about the key determinants of variations in the performance of health systems. For example, in a Working Paper for the IMF, Hsiao (2000) has suggested that a government has five main instruments or "control knobs" for improving the performance of a health system: financing and its institutional organisation; the macro organisation of health service provision; incentives for consumers and providers; regulations; and information and advertising. The WHO has suggested in its *World Health Report* 2000 that there are four key functions which help to determine health system performance: service provision and organisation; methods of paying for health systems; investment in creating resources; and government stewardship. Leatherman (Part IV, Chapter 15) has suggested five main levers: external oversight; knowledge/skill enhancement of providers; empowering consumers; incentives; and regulation. Detailed examination of the texts concerned suggests that none of these lists include setting the level of (public) resources for health services. The approach at the Health Policy Unit at the OECD has been to work with four groups of policy levers for health services: the level of resources; the mixes of services and real resources; institutional characteristics and incentives; and regulation and self-regulation. Performance measurement itself may be included in the last group.

There has been only limited work on the determinants of variations in performance across countries. Econometric analysis by Or (2000) suggests that the level of physician numbers is a highly significant determinant of various types of mortality across OECD countries, after allowing for other determinants of mortality including GDP per capita, occupation, and alcohol and tobacco consumption. When a variety of institutional and incentive characteristics were introduced into the analysis, such as methods of paying ambulatory care doctors and methods of paying hospitals, there was little sign that they had a significant effect on mortality. On the basis of single variate analysis, there have been reports of a significant positive association between total health spending per capita and five-year relative survival rates following a diagnosis of breast cancer; and of a significant negative association between total health spending per capita and waiting times for coronary artery bypass grafting (Anderson *et al.*, 2000). The influence of the incentive and institutional characteristics of health systems on treatments and outcomes for three major diseases across OECD countries has been explored more thoroughly in the Ageing Related Diseases Project (Jacobzone, Part IV, Chapter 8 in this volume).

5.1. *Assessing the cost effectiveness of interventions*

Few interventions to improve performance are likely to come without costs and unwanted side effects. It is desirable, *ex ante*, to attempt to make estimates both of the likely gains from interventions and of the likely costs and side effects. Such an approach has become well established for the introduction of new medical technologies, in the form of health technology assessment, but it is less well established in the policy field, partly because of the difficulty of conducting controlled experiments. Ex *post*, it is desirable, in the interests of establishing an evidence base for future policy development, to evaluate the implementation of policies to see whether the intended effects were realised or not.

6. Action

Often, the most difficult part of improving health system performance is to put into action policies for improving performance. In general, successful action will involve changes in the behaviour of the actors in the health system. The aims of the actors may not be the same as the aims of those trying to influence them. Leatherman (Part V, Chapter 15 in this volume) has discussed action to improve performance using each of the five "levers" mentioned above. This paper reviews similar territory from a different angle.

It is possible to distinguish four key sets of actors in any health care system: consumers; professional providers; managers; and governors. In some systems it is important to make an additional distinction between provider managers and purchasing or insurance managers – those involved in third party financing.

Improvements in information about performance may be a necessary condition for behaviour change but they are by no means sufficient. Appropriate incentives and ability to act are required if suitable action is to take place. In general, performance improvement requires actors to be empowered, for their incentives to be aligned with policy goals and for them to be well informed about the consequences of their actions. Some of these conditions are often missing in health systems.

OECD health systems and subsystems vary considerably in their institutional and incentive characteristics. As a consequence, they differ in their characteristic problems and in their ability to respond to given policy interventions, including the provision of better information. Attempts to improve performance with the development of better performance data should recognise these differences. Three main types of subsystem and their characteristic strengths and weaknesses are discussed in the following section.

6.1. *Three types of subsystem*

All OECD health systems are made up of different mixes of a handful of subsystems of financing and delivery of health care (OECD, 1992). Most systems are dominated by one or two of these subsystems. For the purposes of this paper it is sufficient to consider three of these dominant subsystems: 1) private health insurance with private providers; 2) social health insurance with mixed private and public providers; and 3) general tax funding with public providers. The US has a mixed system but is dominated by 1). Several European countries, Japan and Korea are dominated by 2). The Nordic countries and the UK, among others, are dominated by 3).

The three tables which follow are intended to depict, for different health care subsystems, characteristic interactions between: (on the left) the key actors in the systems, consumers, professional providers, managers and government; and (on the top) the main objectives for which improvements in attainment are sought, responsiveness, health outcomes, prices, health expenditure (which together determine efficiency) and equity. The placing of an "L" (for "largely") in a cell indicates that the actors concerned are well informed, appropriately incentivised and fully empowered to act in relation to the objective concerned. The placing of an "M" (for "moderately") in a cell indicates that these conditions are met partially or most of the time. The placing of an "S" (for "slightly") in a cell indicates that these conditions are met only very partially or some of the time. An empty cell indicates the absence of one or more of these conditions.

Table 2 illustrates how key actors tend to relate to objectives in subsystems based mainly on private, voluntary, indemnity-type, health insurance and private providers paid by fee for service. In these subsystems there is general reliance on market mechanisms. Consumers will generally be well informed about responsiveness but poorly informed about health outcomes because of the asymmetry of knowledge between consumers and providers. They will be well informed about prices but only partially sensitive to such prices if they have health insurance (moral hazard). They will be well informed about the annual cost of health insurance but may be only partially sensitive to it if there are tax subsidies. They may contribute to equity via private charity but that will be subject to free rider problems. Although professional providers will be better informed than consumers about health outcomes there will still be

Table 2. **Subsystems with private health insurance and private providers**
Key actors in relation to objectives

Actors \ Objectives	Responsiveness	Health outcomes	Prices and unit costs	Level of health expenditure	Equity
Consumers	L	S	M	L	S
Professional providers	M	M	L		S
Provider managers	M	S	L		S
Insurance managers				L	
Government	S	S	S		S

Key: An "L" (for "largely") indicates that the actor concerned is well informed, appropriately incentivised and empowered to act in relation to the objective concerned. An "M" (for "moderately") indicates that these conditions are met partially. An "S" (for "slightly") indicates that these conditions are met very partially. An empty cell indicates the absence of one or more of these conditions.

much medical uncertainty. Providers may contribute to equity in a small way by price discrimination. Provider managers are likely to be much better informed about costs than about outcomes. Managers of indemnity insurance are likely to confine their interest and attention mainly to levels of premiums, risks and claims experience. The government may adopt a low profile, especially if the private health insurance subsystem coexists with a public health insurance subsystem. If the private subsystem is dominant, the government may seek to regulate outcomes and prices but it is likely to be handicapped by information deficiencies in doing so. Any regulation is likely to be pro-competitive. Meanwhile, tax subsidies to private health insurance may benefit the rich more than the poor.

Private subsystems are likely to achieve high levels of responsiveness and may provide good health outcomes for those who are insured. However, such systems usually have a history of rapid cost escalation because of moral hazard, fee for service incentives and, in many cases, tax subsidies. The combination of high quality of care (for the insured) and high health expenditure, in a system dominated by private arrangements, is illustrated by US experience. The US spends much more on health care per capita than would be expected for a country with its standard of living. There are scraps of evidence which suggest that in some respects it achieves slightly better results than other countries for its higher health expenditure per capita. An international comparison among a selection of OECD countries suggested that the US had the highest rate of survival among women, following a diagnosis of breast cancer, and the shortest waiting times for coronary artery bypass grafting (Anderson *et al.*, 2000).

Table 3 illustrates how key actors relate to objectives in subsystems financed mainly by social health insurance, with mainly private providers, or a mix of private and public providers, paid by fee for service. Because there is usually freedom of consumer choice in the market for services in such systems, their behaviour may resemble that of privately insured systems, in terms of service delivery. However, these systems differ from privately insured systems in certain important respects. First, with universal coverage funded by compulsory, income-related contributions, they can achieve much greater equity in relation to access to services and ability to pay than can private, voluntary arrangements. Secondly,

Table 3. **Subsystems with social health insurance and private or mixed providers**
Key actors in relation to objectives

Actors \ Objectives	Responsiveness	Health outcomes	Prices and unit costs	Level of health expenditure	Equity
Consumers	L	S	M	M	
Professional providers	M	M	L		
Provider managers	M	S	L		
Insurance managers				M	
Government	S	S	S	L	L

Key: An "L" (for "largely") indicates that the actor concerned is well informed, appropriately incentivised and empowered to act in relation to the objective concerned. An "M" (for "moderately") indicates that these conditions are met partially. An "S" (for "slightly") indicates that these conditions are met very partially. An empty cell indicates the absence of one or more of these conditions.

although traditionally they have not provided contributors with choice of insurer there is more awareness of the total annual cost of health insurance coupled with feelings of entitlement to benefits than in tax funded systems. Moreover, at least two countries, Germany and the Netherlands, have now introduced choice of sickness fund. Third, because such systems have all experienced strong upward pressure on publicly funded health expenditure, their governments have become heavily involved in determining (or regulating indirectly) the level of health expenditure via global budgeting, maintenance of cost sharing and "managed care" arrangements, such as direct contracting by insurers with providers. These systems have a reputation for being highly responsive – for example, they seldom have significant waiting times for elective surgery. Although, they tend to have persistent problems with cost containment, governments have been able to use their monopsony power to restrain the growth of fees and, hence, the growth of total health expenditure.

Table 4 illustrates how key actors relate to objectives in subsystems financed mainly by general taxation with public providers. In the pure form of these systems there is vertical integration between the financing and provision of care in the public sector. Hence, there are no independent third party insurance bodies, with consequent savings on administrative costs. Compared with the previous subsystems, these subsystems tend to be characterised by consumer disempowerment. In their pure form, these subsystems give little or no choice of provider and no choice of "insurer". Moreover, because financing is by general taxation and cost sharing is often minimal, there is attenuation of the sense of entitlement among beneficiaries and little or no awareness of prices and unit costs. As in the social health insurance model, the government can secure significant equity of access and in payment for care via universal coverage and income related tax payments. Also, these subsystems are noted for the ability they give to governments to contain costs. The government has monopsony power, can control expenditure through global budgets and will often pay providers by salary or capitation, reducing their incentives to increase the volume of care.

These subsystems may provide good quality medical care if providers are well trained and conscientious but they have a reputation for being unresponsive to consumers because there is lack of choice, lack of payment incentives for providers and rationing of care according to clinically-perceived "need" rather than according to consumer demand. These subsystems are essentially paternalistic. In a famous British phrase, patients become "grateful supplicants" rather than empowered consumers. That is supported by some of the evidence in Coulter and Cleary (Part III, Chapter 10 in this volume). Their Table 3 suggests that "respect for patient preferences" is greater in Germany, Switzerland and the US than in Sweden and the UK. In particular, whereas in Germany, Switzerland and the US, 10.0 per cent, 11.3 per cent and 12.5 per cent of patients, respectively, reported that "Doctors sometimes talked as if I wasn't there", the corresponding figure was 29.4 per cent in the UK. These are also the systems which tend to have long queues for elective surgery.

Table 4. **Subsystems with general taxation funding and "integrated" public providers**

Key actors in relation to objectives

Actors / Objectives	Responsiveness	Health outcomes	Prices and unit costs	Level of health expenditure	Equity
Consumers	S	S			
Professional providers	S	M			
Provider managers	S	S	M	L	
Insurance managers	n.a.	n.a.	n.a.	n.a.	n.a.
Government	S	S	S	L	L

n.a.: not applicable.

Key: An "L" (for "largely") indicates that the actor concerned is well informed, appropriately incentivised and empowered to act in relation to the objective concerned. An "M" (for "moderately") indicates that these conditions are met partially. An "S" (for "slightly") indicates that these conditions are met very partially. An empty cell indicates the absence of one or more of these conditions.

Countries dominated by these systems often have high levels of health status yet report per capita health expenditure below the expected level for OECD countries.

6.2. *Better alignment of information, empowerment and incentives with policy objectives*

A few general points may be drawn out in relation to the preceding comparison of systems and subsystems. First, all suffer from a lack of health outcome information. At the level of the individual patient/provider encounter, there is an asymmetry of clinical information across patients and professionals. At the population level, it is rather the case that there is symmetry of ignorance across all the key actors, consumers, professionals, managers and governors. That is to say, there is widespead uncertainty about the effectiveness of medical care at a community level, at least at the margin. Secondly, the dissemination of better measures of quality and outcomes is likely to be most effective if it reaches the hands of the right actors – those who are empowered and incentivised. For example, American consumers of health care are in a better position to make choices on the basis of performance data, which drive improvements in efficiency, than are British consumers. Similarly, governments which are in a position to control total health expenditure are in more need of performance indicators than are governments which leave the level of health expenditure to be determined mainly by the market. Third, there are well known drawbacks to all the major payment methods for professional providers, fee for service, capitation or salary. Mixed payment systems may be better. However, what may really be wanted is payment for results (Leatherman, Part V, Chapter 15 in this volume) That, in turn, would require progress to be made on solving the problem of the lack of health outcome information.

7. Some examples of actions in different types of health system

It may be useful to illustrate the generalisations made above with some examples of the use of performance measurement and improvement. An attempt is made to identify, below, case studies in relation to each of the main objectives of health policy set out above. These examples were not necessarily seen, by the actors concerned at the time, as circuits of a performance measurement/ improvement cycle but it appears that they can be portrayed in such terms, retrospectively. Although the examples below come from a mix of OECD countries, a disproportionate number come from the UK. That is not because UK experience is necessarily of greater interest to students of health policy than that of other OECD countries, but simply because the author had limited access to non-UK examples when this paper was written.

7.1. *Responsiveness*

One of the leading health policy problems in OECD health subsystems of the third type described above, is their length of their waiting times for elective surgery. Waiting for elective surgery may be interpreted as a lack of responsiveness, although some experts would argue that excess demand for surgery is inevitable in any system that has an efficient level of total health expenditure and, in the interests of equity of access, zero prices for surgery. They would argue that some systems hide this excess demand and others make it visible. Many countries dominated by the third type of subsystem have introduced measures to reduce waiting for surgery in recent years. Apart from increasing resources, these include: collecting better data on waiting times, publicising differences in waiting times on the Internet, enabling patients to exercise choice of provider, giving patients guarantees for maximum waiting periods, and giving physicians and hospitals better incentives to reduce waiting. However, often such measures have resulted in only temporary reductions in waiting times.

The UK has long collected national statistics on surgical waiting times at hospital level. These were not well known by the public even after they were analysed and published for public consumption first, independently, by the College for Health and later, from 1991 by the government, in booklet form, under the "Patient's Charter". Over the years, the government launched a number of initiatives aimed at reducing waiting times. These were targeted almost entirely at managers and providers. There were a series of major initiatives between 1986 and 1994. Extra resources were provided and targets were set for eliminating the longest waits, initially over two years and then over 18 months. On the face of it,

47

these initiatives met with success. Whereas at the beginning of the period, nearly 25 per cent of those on the waiting list for elective surgery were waiting more than 12 months, by 1998 only about 5 per cent were waiting over 12 months. However, the policy seems to have been achieved mainly by changing the shape of the distribution of waiting times rather than by reducing the average time waited by those admitted to surgical units. The latter remained remarkably stable, fluctuating around 15 weeks between 1989 and 1998. Presumably, some of the 75 per cent of patients waiting for less than a year must have had their waiting times prolonged. Moreover, when the National Audit Office conducted a survey of surgeons, 20 per cent said that they frequently treated patients in different order to their clinical priority in order to reduce their waiting list or to avoid patients waiting for more than the 18 month target (National Audit Office, 2001). There are perhaps two suggestions from this experience: that it is difficult to change the underlying problem of waiting in the English NHS; and that there is a risk that adherence by surgeons to responsiveness targets may be achieved at the expense of health outcomes for some patients.

7.2. Health outcomes

Measurement of health outcomes is technically the most intractable part of the performance measurement agenda. To the small extent that such measures are available, there are large differences between OECD countries in policies about openness in reporting them and, more generally, in the division of labour between regulation and self-regulation of clinical safety and effectiveness. That division of labour is undergoing some re-negotiation currently in a number of OECD countries.

One of the most open countries in relation to the reporting of health outcomes is the United States. US experience has been reviewed thoroughly in Marshall *et al.* (2000). For example, the public reporting of surgeon-specific coronary artery bypass grafting (CABG) mortality in New York was followed by a reduction in CABG mortality rates well in excess of the national average. However, similar outstanding results were obtained in northern New England where surgeon-specific mortality rates were also assembled, although for internal use rather than for publication.

On the whole, it seems that consumers have made relatively little use of health outcome data in the US. Reasons given by consumers for lack of interest in such information include difficulty in understanding the information, lack of trust in the data and lack of choice. Consumers seem to prefer anecdotal evidence about surgeon's and hospitals from family and friends.

Physicians are more receptive in relation to CABG mortality data. In New York, they found the information easy to read and considered the data to be accurate. 38 per cent considered it to have affected their referral patterns but many expressed concerns that it discouraged cardiac surgeons from operating on high-risk patients. In Pennsylvania there were similar reactions from physicians and surgeons. It is difficult to adjust mortality or morbidity data fully for the level of the sickness of the patient.

It is hospital managers who appear to make most use of publicly reported health outcome data in the competitive hospital market of the US. There was an exodus of low volume and high mortality surgeons following publication of the CABG mortality data in New York, probably as a result of hospital managers restricting the operating privileges of surgeons.

An OECD review of performance measurement and improvement activities in four European countries provides evidence of a range of relationships between the key actors in relation to the difficult task of improving the quality of clinical care (Or, 2002).

In the Netherlands, which has a health system mainly of the second type, among the three subsystems set out above, there is a strong emphasis on self-regulation by each of the health care professions via peer review (Klazinga, Part II, Chapter 6 in this volume). The general approach is one of continuous quality improvement which is team based and non-threatening to individual professionals. The Government has supported this process by setting up an Institute for Health Care Improvement (CBO) which helps the professions to develop guidelines and to monitor their clinical performance. There is also an external Health Care Inspectorate (IGZ) which verifies that quality improvement mechanisms are in place but does not report on the quality of care as such. Taken as a whole, the Dutch approach to regulation appears to enjoy a high level of ownership by the professions concerned but to display little openness so far as consumers, managers or governors are concerned.

In France, which has also a health system mainly of the second type, there are a variety of regulatory and self-regulatory institutions which are aimed at maintaining and improving quality of clinical care. Among these has been the preparation and publication of regulatory practice guidelines (RMOs) since 1993. These guidelines are aimed at improving health outcomes, avoiding dangerous medical practice and containing costs. They are disseminated by the major health insurance fund (CNAMTS) but are prepared by an independent body (ANAES) which has a mandate to improve the evidence base for medicine. Doctors were expected to comply with the guidelines and a system of financial penalties was set up for non-compliance.

A survey of the impact of 18 pharmaceutical RMOs introduced in 1994 and 1995 suggested that they modified the prescribing habits of about 25 per cent of doctors and had a minor effect in achieving cost reductions. These effects were sustained. There was no monitoring of quality effects. However the publication of subsequent RMOs in the therapeutic area seems to have had little effect. The system of imposing financial sanctions for non-compliance did not survive challenge in the courts. Although RMOs are still published in France, they are seen by doctors mainly as a cost containment device and seem to lack legitimacy. Perhaps this is an example of an externally imposed, "value for money" initiative, aimed at the medical profession, which achieves openness but not physician ownership (Or, 2002).

In Sweden, which has a health system mainly of the third type, a few "quality registers" were set up in the 1970s by the medical profession in certain hospitals and specialities to identify variations in the utilisation and outcomes of particular treatments with a view to supporting learning and improving clinical performance. By the early 1990s this approach had spread across many specialities and many hospitals and had secured financial support nationally from the National Board of Health and Welfare. Many significant improvements in health outcomes can be traced to the (now) national quality registers (Rehnqvist, Part II, Chapter 4 in this volume). This is a system of support for self- regulation which seems to combine both openness and ownership by the medical profession.

7.3. Efficiency

In the US health care market, efficiency is determined mainly by micro-economic behaviour. In the 1980s and 1990s, US employers, and, where they were given choice of plan, US consumers, reacting to a long history of rises in health insurance premiums above the rate of increase in the standard of living, voluntarily embraced cost containment by limiting consumer choice of provider to defined networks of providers with whom managed care organisations had negotiated favourable rates. These insurance organisations controlled costs, in turn, by contracting with, or employing, providers. Many physicians switched from fee for service to salary or capitation remuneration and were, in effect recruited as rationers of health care. The health expenditure share of GDP in the US stabilised in the 6 years between 1992 and 1998.

The rise in managed care and the cost containment it brought about seem to have been a temporary phenomenon. From 1997 health insurance premiums began to accelerate upwards again. There had been growing complaints from consumers about a decline in quality of care under managed care plans. In a tightening labour market, employers conceded less restrictive plans to employees (Reinhardt, 2001). Nevertheless, the option to manage care remains available if health care costs once again reach levels which are not tolerated by consumers or employers.

Although there have been important developments in pricing and costing of hospital services in many health systems of the second and third type, partly as a result of the trend towards purchaser/ provider separation in some systems, there seem to be few examples of the use of overall efficiency indicators in attempts to improve performance. That is probably because of the lack of sufficient health outcome and responsiveness data to allow for the calculation of efficiency measures of the kind outlined in the section on measurement, above.

However, as was mentioned above, the UK (which has a system mainly of the third type) developed a less ambitious measure of micro-determined efficiency for hospital and community health services in England – the ratio of: annual changes in a basket of activities, weighted by unit costs; to annual changes in real health expenditure. This index was used to set targets for annual gains in efficiency for health authorities and for hospitals from the early 1990s. There were significant gains in measured efficiency during the period of targeting. In the five years 1991/92 to 1996/97, cost weighted activity rose by 18 per cent compared with a rise in real expenditure of about 9.6 per cent. Consequently, measured efficiency rose by about 8 per cent. This was an improvement on earlier periods. For example, using the same measure, efficiency did not change in the five years preceding 1979/80. The improvements could be attributed mainly to a rise in the proportion of patients treated as day cases and a fall in inpatient length of stay. However, the emphasis on increasing activity faster than resources led to widespread complaints that physicians and managers were being forced to sacrifice quality of care. There was also suspicion of manipulation of the data – for example hospitals could re-classify some outpatient attendances as day cases. The targets were abandoned following the election of a new government in 1997.

In countries dominated by health subsystems of the second and third type, the dominant source of health expenditure is public. Hence, the bulk of the responsibility for setting the right level of health expenditure in these countries rests with their governments. In the 1970s and 1980s, if they had not done so earlier, most governments responsible for systems of these two types developed and applied instruments by which to control health expenditure. These developments were reported in earlier OECD work (OECD, 1992).

As was mentioned above, it is possible for governments either to overspend or to underspend on health services. What is the "right" level is a matter for the judgement of the government and the electorate.

On some occasions there have been sharp changes in the rate of growth of public spending on health in certain OECD countries. These "reveal" changes in government preferences for health expenditure – often associated with changes in governments themselves. Occasionally, governments make it explicit that judgements have changed. For example, after announcing in 2000 a very large increase in spending on the National Health Service (NHS), the UK government said, "In part the NHS is failing to deliver because over the years it has been underfunded" (Department of Health, 2000).

That announcement came after the publication of fresh international evidence suggesting that the UK had surprisingly low rates of survival among her citizens, following diagnoses of heart attacks and certain cancers, as well as the longest waiting times for elective surgery among a list of countries for which data had become available. It is tempting to see this as an example of the role that international comparisons of health outcomes and responsiveness can play in informing government decisions on levels of health expenditure.

7.4. *Equity*

Measurement of equity requires that sufficient data can be assembled on the distribution of health status, payment for health services and access to health services across the population. Most OECD countries have already taken major steps towards "payment according to ability to pay and treatment according to need" by suitable public funding of health services. Those that have further to go may be inhibited less by information deficiencies or by technical problems as by the lack of a political consensus, or the lack of the political will, to change. Also, achieving redistribution can take much time, as the example below suggests.

The pursuit of "territorial justice", or geographical equity of access, for hospital services in the English NHS provides an example of successive circuits of the performance measurement and improvement cycle over a prolonged period. When the NHS was set up in 1948, it inherited an unequal geographical distribution of hospital services. Early attempts to remedy that were partial and even somewhat misdirected and by the early 1970s little progress towards equity had been made (Griffiths, 1971). At about the same time, Cooper and Culyer (1970) published a statistical analysis which used, for the first time, regional mortality rates as an indicator of need. That helped to provide evidence that an "inverse care law" was at work. Areas which had high needs had few resources per capita and areas with low needs had high resources per capita. When a Labour Government was elected in 1974, the Health Minister asked for a review of policy on the geographical distribution of central funding of the NHS. The "Resource Allocation Working Party" proposed a formula for basing geographical funding on need, including mortality rates as one of its main elements (Department of Health, 1976). However, it was soon realised that the rate of redistribution of cash towards the targets set by the formula would have to be constrained by the undesirability of forcing actual cuts in resources on "losing" regions. By the time that the formula was revised in the late 1980s, only partial progress had been made towards basing actual regional funding on targets and it was not until the mid 1990s that targets had almost been achieved for districts. At that point, new thinking on equity suggested that the ultimate goal was equity of health status rather than equity of access. That suggested that there should be, in effect, positive discrimination in favour of deprived populations – at least to the extent that inequities are avoidable by improving the delivery of health care. Hence, a further circuit of the performance measurement and improvement cycle in pursuit of greater equity of health is now in prospect, over 50 years after the founding of the NHS.

8.   Costs of activities to measure and improve performance

It should not be forgotten that measuring and improving performance are activities which carry costs. Apart from the usual costs of collecting and analysing data, it is necessary to take account of the time that professional staff must take in keeping records and in participating in review meetings and in research. One of the reasons professional staff sometimes give for low morale or for quitting their posts, is excessive administrative work which takes them away from their patients.

9.   Conclusion

It is possible to draw no more than tentative conclusions from the material presented above.

There is potential to make demonstrable improvements to the performance of health systems when information, incentives and action are all aligned with appropriate policy objectives. Many improvements in health outcomes in Sweden can be traced to quality registers. Cost containment in the US in recent years was attributable to the spread of managed care in a well-informed private health insurance market that offered choice of insurer, including insurers that restricted choice of provider. The steady progress made towards geographical equity in the UK shows that a combination of appropriate measurement and analysis associated with the consistent application of political will over time can bring about substantial redistribution of resources.

At the same time, there is evidence to suggest that when incentives are not aligned with policy goals, performance improvement may be lacking, despite improvements in information. It is hard to change the characteristic behaviour or "signature" of health systems. The UK has better waiting times data than many other countries. However, the remarkable stability of its average waiting time for elective surgery, despite a series of waiting times "initiatives" over several decades, suggests that information may be necessary but not sufficient to bring about improvements in performance. The relatively small impact that RMOs (regulatory practice guidelines) made on cost containment in France may provide another such example.

Also, it is easy to glimpse examples of perverse effects in the application of incomplete performance measures, especially if they are linked to strong incentives, such as mandatory targets. Concern over the effect on treatment of high-risk patients from public reporting of surgeon-specific CABG mortality rates in the US is a case in point. Concern about the effect on clinical priorities of targeting waiting times at no longer than 18 months in the UK is another such case. Concern about the effect of targeting an efficiency measure which included volume of care but not its quality in the UK is yet another. In all these cases, the problem was one of a perceived distortion of priorities brought about by combining strong incentives or regulations with incomplete measurement of performance.

The measurement of health outcomes remains the central difficulty. Compared with this, the measurement of responsiveness, cost and equity remain comparatively straightforward. Linked to that is the apparent requirement for a continuation of self-regulation as a key institution in relation to performance measurement and performance improvement. It seems clear that self-regulation, particularly monitoring of the safety and effectiveness of routine care, is a difficult task which requires government support. The issues that then arise include the ownership of the results by the professions concerned, and the openness and accessibility of the results to those to whom the professions should be accountable. Managers and governors too, need effectiveness data if they are to act appropriately. It seems that with the CBO, the Netherlands has achieved ownership without openness and that in its RMOs, France has achieved some openness without ownership. Perhaps Sweden's experience with quality registers, which seem to combine ownership with accountability, has lessons for other OECD countries.

It remains important to subject performance measurement and improvement activities to critical review *ex ante* and *ex post*. There are likely to be diminishing returns to such activity, as to any other, and the aim should be to pursue performance measurement and improvement activities only up to the point that they remain cost effective.

Finally, given the remaining gaps in evidence and in our understanding of the effectiveness of the institutions of health care, there seems to be a strong case for further work at an international level to advance the performance measurement and improvement agenda.

REFERENCES

ANDERSON, G.F. *et al.* (2000),
"Health spending and outcomes: trends in OECD countries, 1960-1998", *Health Affairs*, Vol. 19, No. 3, pp. 150-157.

COOPER, M.H. and CULYER, A.J. (1970),
"An economic assessment of some aspects of the operation of the National Health Service", *Health Services Financing*, British Medical Association, pp. 187-250.

CULYER, A.J. and WAGSTAFF, A. (1993),
"Equity in health and health care", *Journal of Health Economics*, Vol. 12, pp. 431-457.

DAVIS, P. *et al.* (2001),
"Adverse events regional feasibility study: indicative findings", NZ *Medical Journal*, 11 May, pp. 203-205.

DEPARTMENT OF HEALTH (1976),
"Sharing resources for health in England", Report of the Resource Allocation Working Party.

DEPARTMENT OF HEALTH (2000),
The NHS Plan. A *plan for investment*: A *plan for reform*.

DONELAN, K. *et al.* (1999),
"The cost of health system change: public discontent in five nations", *Health Affairs*, Vol. 18, No. 3, May/June.

GIUFFRIDA, A. (1999),
"Measuring quality of care with routine data: avoiding confusion between performance indicators and health outcomes", *British Medical Journal*, Vol. 319, pp. 94-98.

GRIFFITHS, D.A.T. (1971),
"Inequalities and management in the NHS", *The Hospital*, July.

HSIAO, W. (2000),
"What should macroeconomists know about health care policy? A primer", IMF Working Paper WP/00/136, International Monetary Fund.

HURST, J. and JEE-HUGHES, M. (2001),
"Performance measurement and performance management in OECD health systems", Labour Market and Social Policy Occasional Papers No. 47, OECD, Paris.

HURTADO, M.P. *et al.* (eds) (2000),
"Envisioning the National Health Care Quality Report", Committee on the National Quality Report on Health Care Delivery, Institute of Medicine, Washington, D.C.

KOHN, L.T. *et al.* (eds) (2000),
To Err is Human, Committee on Quality of Health Care in America, Institute of Medicine, Washington D.C.

MARSHALL, M.N. *et al.* (2000),
"The public release of performance data. What do we expect to gain? A review of the evidence", JAMA, Vol. 283, pp. 1866-1874.

MURRAY, C.J.L. and FRENK, J. (2000),
"A framework for assessing the performance of health systems", *Bulletin of the World Health Organisation*, Vol. 78, No. 6.

NATIONAL AUDIT OFFICE (2001),
"Inpatient and outpatient waiting in the NHS", Report by the Comptroller and Auditor General, HC 221, July

NUTLEY, S. and SMITH, P.C. (1998),
"League tables for performance improvement in health care", J. *of Health Serv. Res. Policy*, Vol. 3, No. 1, January.

OECD (1992),
The Reform of Health Care: a comparative analysis of seven OECD countries, Health Policy Studies, No. 2, Paris.

OECD (2000),
A *System of Health Accounts*, Version 1.0, Paris.

OR, Z. (2000),
"Exploring the effects of health care on mortality across OECD countries", Labour Market and Social Policy Occasional Papers No. 46, OECD, Paris.

OR, Z. (2002),
"Improving the performance of health systems: from measures to action. A review of experiences in four OECD countries", Labour Market and Social Policy Occasional Papers, OECD.

REINHARDT, U.E. (2001),
"The United States health-care system: recent history and prospects", paper presented to the Commonwealth Fund's 2001 International Symposium on Health Care Policy, Washington DC, October 9-11.

TECH RESEARCH NETWORK (2001),
"Technological change around the world", Health Affairs, Vol. 20, No. 3, pp. 25-42, May/June.

VINCENT, C. et al. (2001),
"Adverse events in British hospitals: preliminary, retrospective record review", British Medical Journal, Vol. 322, pp. 517-519.

VAN DOORSLAER, E. et al. (1999),
"Equity in the finance of health care: some further international comparisons", Journal of Health Economics, Vol. 18, pp. 263-290.

VAN DOORSLAER, et al. (2000),
"Equity in the delivery of health care in Europe and the US", Journal of Health Economics, Vol. 19, pp. 553-583.

WILSON, R.M. et al. (1995),
"The quality in Australian healthcare study", Med J. Aust, Vol. 163, pp. 458-471.

WORLD HEALTH ORGANISATION (2000),
The World Health Report, 2000.

Part II

PERFORMANCE MEASUREMENT
AND PERFORMANCE MANAGEMENT
FROM THE PERSPECTIVE OF VARIOUS ACTORS:
A REVIEW OF EXPERIENCES IN SELECTED COUNTRIES

Chapter 3

IMPROVING VALUE FOR MONEY IN THE UNITED KINGDOM NATIONAL HEALTH SERVICE: PERFORMANCE MEASUREMENT AND IMPROVEMENT IN A CENTRALISED SYSTEM

by

Clive H. Smee[*]

Abstract

This paper charts the development of performance measures in health care in England and their current use in managing the NHS. The last 10 years have seen a shift from measures of activities and costs, to measures of outputs and outcomes and from a focus on efficiency to a "balanced scorecard" approach to monitoring and measuring performance. It has also been recognised that performance measures are only one element of a performance management system. The current framework for assessing NHS performance, "The Performance Assessment Framework (PAF)" is complemented by mechanisms for defining standards and targets (the NHS Plan, National Service Frameworks and National Institute for Clinical Excellence), by systems of incentives (including NHS Performance Ratings, a system of "earned autonomy" and a new NHS Performance Fund), and by services to monitor and support behavioural change (clinical governance, a Commission for Health Improvement and a Modernisation Agency). The paper reflects on what has been learnt from the NHS's experience with performance measurement and performance improvement to date. It ends with some thoughts about future developments.

Introduction

When the OECD Secretariat reviewed the British health care system in 1994 it noted that the National Health Service (NHS) "was and is a remarkably cost-effective institution" (OECD, 1994). When the OECD revisited the NHS in 2000 the plaudits for cost-effectiveness were muted. Instead the focus was on poor health outcomes and over-tight budget constraints (OECD, 2000). The explanation for this change in assessment may lie partly in rising national and international expectations. But equally important was an improvement in comparative measures of health outcomes: it could now be seen that excessive waiting times, long the Achilles heel of the NHS, were complemented by poor cancer survival rates and other indicators of clinical outcomes. The change in the OECD's views is a good illustration of the importance of developing appropriate and well balanced performance measures. As this paper will make clear, the UK Government has been aware for some time of the vital role of an adequate performance information framework for holding the NHS to account against its objectives, and for promoting improved performance.

---

[*] Chief Economic Adviser, Department of Health, UK. The views expressed here are those of the author only and should not be taken to represent the views of the UK Department of Health or government. I am grateful to Steve Dunn, Nick Hicks, Jeremy Hurst, Rob Shaw, Nick York, Simon Peck and Giles Wilmore for helpful comments.

It is impossible to make improvement without measurement, formal or informal. This paper charts the development of performance measures in health care in England[1] and their current use in managing the NHS. The next three sections give a brief description of the organisation of the NHS, a summary of the UK Government's overall approach to performance management of the public sector and a short history of the evolution of performance indicators within the NHS. The paper then goes on to discuss current approaches to performance measurement and management. It describes how a new framework for assessing NHS performance, the Performance Assessment Framework (PAF) is complemented by new mechanisms for defining standards and targets (the NHS Plan, National Service Frameworks and the National Institute for Clinical Excellence), by new systems of incentives (including NHS Performance Ratings, a system of "earned autonomy" and a new NHS Performance Fund), and by new services to monitor and support behavioural change (clinical governance, a Commission for Health Improvement and a Modernisation Agency). This leads into some reflections on what has been learnt from the NHS's experience with performance measurement and performance improvement to date.

1. The government's role in the financing and delivery of health services

To make the later discussion more intelligible it may be helpful to briefly describe the financing and organisation of the National Health Service.

First funding: 85 per cent of total health expenditure in the UK is publicly funded through the NHS. The NHS is funded primarily from general (central) taxation, with a residual element from National Insurance contributions. Central government budget-setting arrangements determine the size of NHS funding, the annual rate of increase and allocations between major service areas and regions.

The NHS in England is administered by the Department of Health through its Regional Offices and Health Authorities. Primary care is provided by GPs who act as gatekeepers and are formed into Primary Care Groups (or Primary Care Trusts) with increasing influence or control over the health care budgets for their enrolled populations. Most GPs are technically self-employed but are paid directly by the government through a combination of methods: capitation, fee for service and allowance. Secondary and tertiary care is provided mainly through publicly owned semi-autonomous, self-governing hospitals known as NHS Trusts, which contract with groups of commissioners or purchasers on a long-term basis. District Health Authorities were formerly the major purchasers but these responsibilities are currently being transferred to Primary Care Groups and Trusts.[2]

The UK Government steers the delivery of health services through the development of policies that are enshrined in legislation and regulations. The Department of Health is held to account through a Delivery Contract and Performance Service Agreement with central departments (the Prime Minister's Office and the Finance Ministry). Through its Regional Offices the Department holds Health Authorities accountable for local services and the delivery of Local Action Plans. In turn health authorities draw up performance agreements with their Primary Care Trusts/Groups. NHS Trusts are currently held to account by Regional Offices but this responsibility will move to health authorities as the number of the latter shrinks from close to 100 to around 30 by April 2002 (Department of Health, 2001a; see Figure 1).

Since 1998 the government's approach to improving performance in the NHS has been broadly similar to that adopted across the public sector (Cabinet Office, 1999). For each government department the approach is characterised by:

- Public Service Agreements setting out the aims of the Department or policy area, supporting objectives and related performance targets;

- Service Delivery Agreements which specify how these targets will be achieved and who is accountable;

- Rigorous performance measurement methods to monitor progress;

- Reinforcement/incentive mechanisms offering positive consequences for success and negative consequences for failure.

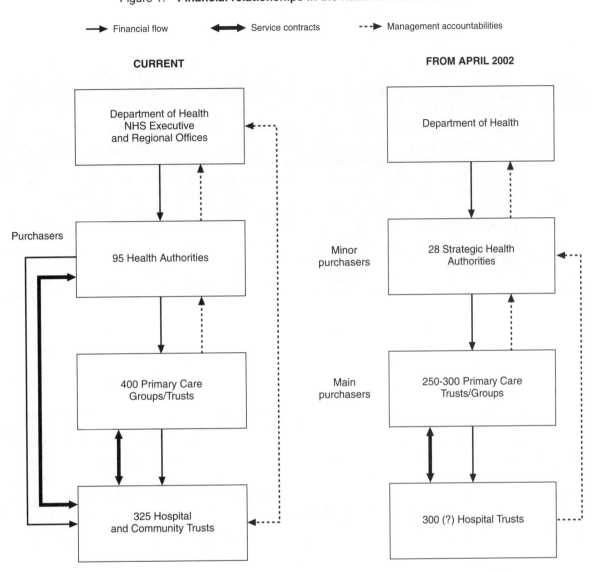

Figure 1. **Financial relationships in the National Health Service**

These business planning arrangements are now integral to the allocation of three yearly budgets to each public sector department. The trend is towards reducing the number of targets and to specifying them in terms of outcomes (National Audit Office, 2001a).

2. The development of performance measures in the National Health Service

Current approaches to performance measurement in the NHS are the product of a long period of learning. The use of national sets of performance indicators can be traced back at least to the NHS Performance Indicators Initiative of 1981. Then the emphasis was on internal control by local managers, not on public accountability or on performance management by the centre. The indicators were drawn from routine administrative data sets and focused almost entirely on activities and costs. There was little or no attention to outcomes or indeed to measures of efficiency. Some of the indicators generated unintended behaviours later documented by researchers: tunnel vision, sub-optimisation, myopia, misrepresentation and gaming (Goddard and Smith, 2001). But others were undoubtedly helpful to health districts and later (when renamed Health Service Indicators), to hospitals and other providers.

However, while the 1980s saw the adoption of a new managerial approach to the NHS the Department of Health found the indicators of limited use in assessing the performance of Regional Health Authorities. They also provided very limited accountability to the Treasury, Parliament and the public. The sheer number of indicators (by the late 1980s there were several hundred) taxed management understanding and precluded the making of simple comparisons or the drawing of general conclusions. The focus on activities and costs also reduced their interest to the public and to politicians.

There were two exceptions to these generalisations. First, by weighting individual activities by national unit costs and aggregating across the country, it was possible to produce a cost-weighted activity index. Relating this index to expenditure produced a crude measure of trends in technical efficiency. Once such a measure had been developed by the Department's economists in the 1980s, it could be used to track efficiency back to the mid-1970s; to demonstrate to the Treasury that the NHS was steadily making better use of public funds; and to set increasingly demanding efficiency targets as part of the annual public expenditure round.

The other area where aggregation facilitated accountability was for the various measures of waiting times that went into a "Patient's Charter" announced in 1991 (Department of Health, 1991). The Charter included the first set of performance indicators specifically aimed at informing the public about the performance of their local health service. In addition to waiting times they also included data relating to vaccination and immunisation rates and cervical cytology screening.

The Conservative Government's "internal market" reforms announced in 1989 (Her Majesty's Stationery Office, 1989) ostensibly introduced a major element of decentralisation into the NHS, but they also gave the Department (or more precisely its executive arm, the NHS Management Executive) new regulatory and performance management responsibilities. By the early 1990s it was clear to the Executive that it lacked the information tools to effectively manage Regional Health Authorities. It had too much data and too little useful information. Those indicators that had been summarised and turned into targets – notably the cost-weighted activity indicator and various waiting times measures – shed light on only limited aspects of health service performance. Moreover the cost-weighted activity indicator and the targets related to it gave all levels of the health service strong incentives to reduce or to shift costs regardless of the impact on the quality of care or on the performance of the whole health care system.

Responding to these concerns, in 1992 the Executive set up a group "to consider what measures of quality, effectiveness and health outcomes and patient satisfaction can be used as systematic measures of NHS performance for the national accountability process", including public expenditure negotiations (NHS Management Executice, 1993). The group was specifically asked to identify a small number of indicators, "around six" that could inform future performance contracts with Regional Health Authorities. In two reports in 1993 the group identified a set of summary indicators that could be used to monitor progress under the Management Executive's then key strategies: public health, community care, effective purchasing, the Patient's Charter, clinical quality, strengthening the scientific base, and giving choice and influence to health service users.

In subsequent years the work on developing summary indicators of performance proceeded at different speeds as the various policy groups tested their proposals with the professions and other stakeholders. Doubts about data quality and the appropriateness of the indicators and worries about professional and management reactions led to a strong emphasis on using the indicators to raise questions rather than to measure or judge performance. In the search for providing the centre with a more balanced set of high level indicators further working groups identified additional potential indicators, most notably in relation to primary care (NHS Management Executive, 1995).

One of the incidental benefits of this slow developmental process was that it sharpened up thinking about policy objectives. For example, the process of identifying performance indicators for primary care revealed that the GP terms of service included no particular requirements to meet patients' expectations or to provide them with services that they found satisfactory. Another important if somewhat obvious conclusion drawn from the same exercise was that ideally measures of efficiency should look at the resources used to achieve health service objectives, specified in terms of outcomes, not at the cost of specific activities that happened to be easy to measure.

By 1997 there were several new sets of indicators under development but their relationships with each other were unclear and none was being published or used for performance management purposes. The election of the Labour Government with a manifesto commitment to change the focus of performance management away from activity and efficiency and towards quality of outcome, provided the spur to develop a conceptual framework to pull together the proliferating indicator sets. Borrowing from the thinking behind the "balanced score card" approach to measuring private sector performance (Kaplan and Norton, 1992) and from the attempts of US employers to systematically compare the performance of American health plans (the Health Plan Employer Data and Information Set – HEDIS),[3] an attempt was made to identify the aspects of the health service that were given the most importance by patients, the public and other stakeholders. The objective was to channel indicators, monitoring and management towards those aspects of performance that most resonated with the users and funders of the NHS. The criteria used to select the key performance areas are at Annex A.

In the summer of 1997 Ministers agreed that the new performance framework should cover six areas:

- Health improvement (*i.e.* improvement of health status regardless of cause);
- Fair access;
- Effective delivery of appropriate healthcare;
- Efficiency;
- Patient/carer experience; and
- Health outcomes of NHS care.

Work began immediately to populate the areas with high level indicators. The selection criteria drew on the experience of the previous 15 years and paid particular attention to minimising adverse behavioural effects. A first set of high level indicators was selected by the late summer. Reflecting the limited number of relevant data sets to choose from, this selection proved surprisingly robust with many of the indicators surviving extensive consultation and field testing with the NHS.

The Performance Assessment Framework was announced in November 1997 in the new Government's first major policy statement, "The New NHS: Modern, Dependable". Proposals for the nature and content of the Framework were issued for consultation in January 1998 (NHS Executive, 1998). The first set of High Level Performance Indicators was published in June 1999 (NHS Executive, 1999). In July 2000 a second set of indicators was published which reflected more closely key Government priorities for health (NHS Executive, 2000). These are illustrated at Annex B: they have been used to compare the performance of the 99 health authorities. The first two sets of indicators were based on what data were available. A further consultation document was issued in May 2001 under the title NHS *Performance Indicators: A Consultation* (see Department of Health, 2001*b*) with the particular objective of seeking comments on what new data should be collected to create an indicator set more closely aligned to the policy priorities in the 10 year NHS Plan, published the previous summer (Department of Health, 2000*a*). To encourage local ownership and use the consultation will be an annual exercise.

The latest consultation document explicitly recognises that performance indicators are required to serve a variety of functions. While central management and accountability to the public can both be facilitated by having a relatively small number of "headline" performance indicators to capture the all round performance of each NHS organisation, other purposes require a different and/or wider range of indicators. For example, for benchmarking purposes NHS organisations and clinicians may wish to take account of a wide range of background and supporting information and to compare performance on more detailed indicators than would warrant wider dissemination for public accountability or central management purposes. Recognising that performance indicators should be "fit for purpose" the Department of Health has agreed a number of key principles for developing and using performance indicators (see Annex C).

Looking back on this short history, one noticeable feature is how long it took to move from awareness of the distorting effects of focusing public accountability and performance management on a partial measure of efficiency (and to a lesser extent waiting times) to the development of a more rounded set of outcome-based performance measures adequately reflecting the objectives of the health service. Factors that contributed to the delay included the lack of incentives to develop an effective performance management system while performance was expected to be driven by the internal market; worries about resistance from clinicians if clinical indicators were introduced without lengthy consultation; the research community's wish to provide an evidence-base for any new performance indicators; and concerns about raising public expectations to unaffordable levels if patients were systematically surveyed on their experiences (Smee, 2000).

3. Integrating performance measurement into performance improvement

The Performance Assessment Framework supplies a major element of the infrastructure for effective performance management. It provides a framework for capturing the past performance of NHS organisations in a rounded and balanced way. It provides a framework for monitoring how the performance of those organisations will change in the future. It also provides a tool for making comparisons between health authorities, Primary Care Groups and Primary Care Trusts and NHS Trusts. How well it performs these roles will depend, first on whether the areas within the framework are a good reflection of stakeholders' views on what is important about the NHS and second, on whether it is possible to populate the areas with relevant and robust indicators. Widespread consultation suggests that the first of these conditions has so far broadly been met, though changing policy concerns/objectives are likely to require the occasional adjustment of area definitions. (For example, the performance rating system published in 2001 – and discussed later – gives more emphasis to staff issues. Under the PAF it is also proposed to create a seventh domain for hospitals and other providers called "Capacity and Capability", to cover infrastructure issues such as staffing, IT, etc.) On the second condition, there is clearly much more to be done, particularly as relevance and robustness are very sensitive to purpose.

But monitoring, comparing and assessing performance will not by itself improve performance. Through a number of policy initiatives announced in The New NHS (1997) and in The NHS Plan (2000) the government has recognised that performance improvement requires a range of other tools in addition to a sound system of performance assessment. In particular it requires:

- Mechanisms for defining standards and targets so that poor performance is clearly identified;
- Incentives to change behaviour to overcome natural conservatism;
- Support to behavioural change to help those who may want to change but do not know how.

The recent initiatives to address these issues are worth setting out in a little more detail.

3.1. Mechanisms for defining standards and targets

The NHS Plan sets out a range of targets for the NHS over the next 10 years relating to all the areas in the Performance Assessment Framework, *i.e.* health improvement, health outcomes of NHS care, effective care delivery, equity of access, patient/carer experience and efficiency. The key targets are reflected in a Delivery Contract with the Prime Minister's office and in a Public Service Agreement with the Treasury. Current examples include: *a*) starting with children under one year, by 2010 to reduce by at least 10 per cent the gap in mortality between manual groups and the population as a whole; *b*) reduce the maximum wait for an outpatient appointment to 3 months and for an in-patient appointment to 6 months by the end of 2005; *c*) guaranteed access to a primary care professional within 24 hours and to a primary care doctor within 48 hours by 2004. The clinical targets are based on a growing number of National Service Frameworks (NSFs) which set out standards of care, milestones and goals for major disease areas and patient groups. Those published or in preparation cover cancer, coronary heart disease (CHD), mental health, diabetes, renal services, older people, children and long-term conditions. Examples of the CHD standards and goals are: *a*) people thought to be suffering from heart attack should receive thrombolysis within 60 minutes of calling for professional help; *b*) everyone meeting the NSF criteria for angiography and revascularisation is identified and treated within 3 months to the standard set out in the NSF (Department of Health, 2000*b*). More detailed guidance on the use of drugs and other technologies and on clinical guidelines is provided by the National Institute for Clinical Excellence (NICE). Local health communities are expected to deliver on these national standards and targets and on their own targets through local planning mechanisms. The purpose of all these mechanisms for defining standards and targets is both to motivate, through setting compelling and stretching aspirations for the future, and to provide clear yardsticks against which current performance can be compared.

3.2. Incentives to change behaviour

Having ended the previous government's flirtation with market forces the present government sought other mechanisms to encourage health service organisations to continually search for ways of improving services. New initiatives have been announced in two stages.

The first set of reforms announced in 1997 removed financial and information barriers to the more efficient deployment of resources. Virtually all budgets, for primary care, secondary care and tertiary care, are being unified under Primary Care Groups and Primary Care Trusts giving them freedom to move resources between different services and service providers. Primary Care Groups/Trusts and NHS Trusts (hospitals) have also been given greater freedom to retain and redeploy surpluses. Information barriers to identifying the scope for doing things more efficiently or to a higher quality are being reduced by the development and publication of treatment reference costs for each provider (based on the UK equivalent of diagnostic related groups – DRGs; see Department of Health, NHS Executive, 2000) and encouragement to increasingly sophisticated benchmarking.

The initiatives announced in the 2000 NHS Plan went a stage further and offered positive incentives for improvement and innovation. They built on research confirming that NHS managers, clinicians and staff are motivated by many things in addition to money, including reputation and scope for autonomy. This is reflected in four policies that are currently under development.

i) A system of NHS performance ratings

In September 2001, all non-specialist acute NHS Hospital Trusts (general hospitals) were rated and awarded three, two, one or zero stars on the basis of their performance during 2000/01 (Department of Health, 2001c). The NHS Performance Ratings system will be further developed for 2002 and beyond to cover other NHS bodies, such as specialist NHS Trusts and Primary Care Trusts. In this initial year hospitals have been classified on the basis of first, their success in delivering key national targets and second, their performance in terms of a balanced scorecard of measures covering patient, clinical and staff issues. (The initial measures are at Annex D.) The "balanced scorecard" is an extension and re-presentation of the Performance Assessment Framework to serve the specific purpose of rating providers. It is extended to include the staff dimension which has increasingly been recognised as key to improvements. It is re-presented to focus more clearly on the three perspectives of patients, staff and clinicians. In the longer term it is planned to issue the annual Performance Ratings and PAF performance indicators at the same time, with the former being a subset of the latter and used to rank NHS bodies against areas of performance the government deems most crucial.

The intention of the performance rating system is to improve public accountability and to highlight good and poor performance in a way that provides incentives to continually improve for all NHS organisations, regardless of their starting point. In this first year 20 per cent of hospitals have been classified as "three stars", 60 per cent have been classified as "two stars", 13 per cent as "one star" and 7 per cent as "zero stars". The challenges involved in establishing a performance rating system that is simple and easy to explain, fair in operation, reasonably stable and specific about what has to be done to improve status, are discussed later.

ii) Earned autonomy

The performance ratings bring not only kudos or shame but also larger or smaller operational freedoms. The best performing hospitals – those with three stars – benefit from:

- automatic access to a National Performance Fund (see below);

- less frequent monitoring by the centre and central agencies;
- greater freedom to develop their own investment programmes and to decide the local organisation of services;
- being used as pilot sites for new initiatives;
- support in creating new spin-out business ventures;
- opportunities to shape national policy.

The best performers will be able to propose further freedoms. The purpose of these freedoms is to stimulate local innovation as well as to reduce the bureaucratic burden on NHS organisations. The government is committed to devolving responsibility and decision making away from the centre where NHS organisations have demonstrated they can use this freedom to perform to a high standard.

The poorest performers (those with zero stars) are not only denied these freedoms, but their managers are placed on "probation", with the prospect of dismissal if improvement plans are not developed immediately.

iii)   The NHS Performance Fund

A third new element is a Performance Fund to provide resources for locally developed and designed incentive schemes across each local health service. It is for incentivising staff, especially those involved in delivering care, to develop services in ways which lead to real and sustained improvements in care. It is not intended to reward staff for the jobs that they are already doing. Local incentive schemes are therefore expected to set challenging objectives, encourage whole system working, strengthen innovation and remove barriers to change. Resources for the Fund, which will rise to £500m in year three (2003/04) are being shared equitably across every NHS organisation. Organisations are expected to hold back 60 per cent of the funds against evidence of improvements in staff performance. Local health organisations will have as much autonomy as possible in the use of the funds but the degree of freedom will vary according to their performance rating. Three star Trusts, for example, are not required to sign off their plans for the use of the Fund with anyone else, while two star and one star Trusts need the agreement of Regional Offices or the Modernisation Agency (the latter is discussed below). The handful of Trusts with zero stars will have their share of the Performance Fund deployed by the Modernisation Agency. Examples of good practice are to be shared through the internet and other dissemination mechanisms.

iv)   New contracts for hospital doctors and general practitioners

There is little point in introducing supplementary performance bonus systems if the basic employment contracts for clinicians do not align their incentives with national service objectives. Negotiations are therefore underway aimed at agreeing new contracts for both hospital doctors and general practitioners. For hospital doctors the government's aims include linking earnings more closely to the delivery of service objectives and encouraging greater commitment to the National Health Service. For general practitioners the aims include expanding the coverage of Personal Medical Services (PMS) contracts – which pay GPs on the basis of meeting set quality standards and the particular needs of their local populations – and revising the standard national contract to reflect the new emphasis on quality and improved outcomes.

3.3. Support to behavioural change

As with strengthening incentives, the government's initiatives to provide expert support to spread best practice and assist change locally have come in two stages. The first stage began in 1997 with announcement of the introduction of clinical governance and the establishment of the Commission for Health Improvement. These were responses to a number of medical scandals and to evidence that the quality of care varied greatly between NHS organisations. To tackle these shortcomings a new system for quality assuring clinical decisions was introduced, called clinical governance, and was backed by laying a statutory duty of quality on Chief Executives. The new Commission for Health Improvement was to provide independent scrutiny of local efforts to improve quality, and to help address any serious problems. It was required to inspect all Trusts, Health Authorities and Primary Care Groups/Trusts every four years. More recently it has been given a critical role in the assessment of Trust performance ratings.

The second stage was announced in the 2000 NHS Plan in the form of a Modernisation Agency. The new Agency encompasses and builds on a range of earlier initiatives and mechanisms aimed at disseminating best practice in service delivery, facilitating clinical collaborations and taking forward support to clinical governance. It aims to strengthen leadership across the NHS and to provide the Service with a centre of excellence on how knowledge and know-how about best practice can be spread. It will undertake diagnostic work and support organisations needing help to improve their performance. Its range of activities extends from demand management at the primary care level, through reducing delays in access to secondary care and streamlining care within the hospital sector, to developing and applying clear national protocols for care pathways. It will work with managers to avoid organisations being designated as under-performing, as indicated by the award of one or zero stars. Once organisations have been so designated the Agency will work with them to improve their performance and status.

4. Some reflections

What are some of the more important lessons that have been learned about the development of performance measures in a centralised health care system? What challenges need to be tackled if those measures are to be used to improve performance? These are the questions to which we now turn.

4.1. *Lessons about performance measurement*

Some of the more important lessons can be summarised as follows:

i) *Developing good performance indicators is a complex and resource intensive task*

Those in England who began the search for high level indicators in the early 1990s had no idea how long and complicated the process would prove. And the end of the process is still not in sight! Identifying what is important to different stakeholders, selecting measures, identifying and evaluating data sources, launching new surveys and consulting at all stages of the process, invariably takes far more time and resources than expected: or it certainly has in Britain. The rapid growth in research evidence on the design and use of performance measures suggests that the process will not become simpler in the future. The complexities, delays and resource implications need to be properly planned for.

ii) *Start using the data to hand, do not wait for the ideal indicators to be developed*

Whether the purposes is accountability or improved performance, progress will be more rapid if a start is made with the imperfect data to hand. Providing the direction of travel is made clear, using deficient data will stimulate the demand for better indicators, as other countries have also discovered.[4] Waiting for perfect indicators will aid the procrastinators who are sceptical or frightened by measurement and comparison. However, adapting the indicators to hand should not become an excuse for postponing the search for ideal measures. Relevant and high quality measures are essential if the interest of patients and clinicians is to be gained and maintained. In Britain the process of developing improved indicators has now been put on a systematic basis with a commitment to an annual public consultation on what performance information should be collected and published (Department of Health, 2001*b*).

iii) *Different stakeholders require different data sets*

Pulling performance measures together into a single framework such as the Performance Assessment Framework has major benefits in terms of understanding, consistency and simplicity. However, it should not be allowed to become a straitjacket. Different stakeholders in different parts of the health system will have different interests and different objectives. It is unrealistic to expect to identify sets of indicators that will be equally effective at informing the public, incentivising health service managers and attracting the ownership of clinicians. Attempts to do so, encouraged by resource constraints, may simply generate lack of recognition and ownership by all the key stakeholders.

iv) *Parsimony is preferable to comprehensiveness*

For high level performance monitoring and for accountability to the public it is better to strive for a small but balanced number of composite or sentinel indicators than to attempt to cover all aspects of performance. The initial NHS Performance Ratings for hospitals use 21 indicators. So long as the high-level indicators are well balanced, covering quality and efficiency, the distortions risked by averaging or incomplete coverage are likely to be small in cost relative to the paralysis and incomprehension produced by large sets of measures. Unfortunately, there are usually far more pressures for expanding sets of performance indicators, than for weeding and prioritising them. The conflicting pressures for more indicators from those who want to make detailed comparisons and for fewer indicators from those who want simple, clear overall pictures can be reconciled through developing different sets of indicators for different purposes, perhaps in hierarchical form. In the NHS one distinction is between "headline" and "benchmarking" indicators. Other organisations distinguish between indicators for "strategy", "management" and "peer comparison", purposes. Software tools can help in drilling down from summary measures to the detailed components.

v) *Think "outcomes" but use "output" and "process" indicators as stepping stones or proxies*

In designing performance measures the focus should always be on desired outcomes. How far it will be feasible to use outcome measures will depend on the purpose – *e.g.* it will be much easier for planning than for accountability purposes – on the organisational unit – *e.g.* it will be easier for large units than for small – and on the available data. Even where the purpose is accountability and the unit is small outcome measures should be used if possible, notably for assessing patient/carer experiences. In other areas such as clinical outcomes it may be necessary to identify output or process indicators that are proxies or predictors of outcomes; for example, for heart attacks re-perfusion rates may be a better guide to performance than mortality. Here there should if possible be good evidence of the link between the proxy measures and the desired outcomes. In the UK the National Service Frameworks for particular disease areas attempt to provide this linkage and rationale.

Data deficiencies are the main reason why the NHS Performance Rating System has initially relied heavily on process measures. From 2002 direct measures of patient and staff views and experiences will be available to supplant (or supplement) the current proxies.

vi) *Governments initially focus on measuring the performance of big planning or funding units while the public, patients and users are more interested in the performance of "small" providers and on care for particular conditions*

Reflecting concerns about national accountability, performance measurement in England initially focused on regional and district health authorities. But the public and patients are interested in the performance of individual providers such as hospitals and primary care practices and in the care they will receive for particular conditions like cancer and diabetes. There is also evidence from the US and UK that it is providers and clinicians not planners and purchasers whose behaviours is most likely to be influenced by the publication of performance indicators (Marshall *et al.*, 2000). The message is clear: if performance indicators are to be published either to promote local accountability or to change behaviours, they need to relate to individual providers and/or specific conditions. Indicators that relate to conditions are most likely to attract clinician interest and ownership. They may also focus attention on care pathways rather than on particular organisational forms.

The first set of NHS Performance Ratings reflect this learning – they focus entirely on providers. As a wider range of clinical indicators become available it should also be possible to compare performance by condition.

vii) The effectiveness of performance measures depends critically on presentation

Poorly presented performance indicators can be and will be ignored whether their purpose is accountability or improving performance. The investment and skills required to present performance indicators in ways that are comprehensible to their audiences and stimulate changes in behaviour are invariably underestimated. These presentational investments may need to be complemented by programmes aimed at educating the public and providers in interpreting the new performance indicators. In England, for example software programmes have been developed to help hospitals to understand their comparative clinical performance and to trace the causes. Where the objective is to inform the public, recent developments in the UK suggest that media based private organisations (for example "Dr Foster"[5]) may have a comparative advantage over public bureaucracies in stimulating interest in performance measures. Such competitive pressures can stimulate the public sector to raise its game. Imaginative approaches are also required to summarise performance measures: "spider diagrams" have been found to be particularly helpful (see Annex E).

The development of the NHS Performance Ratings system may have other lessons. One is that a balance has to be struck between stimulating behavioural change and demotivating providers and/or alarming patients. The NHS Plan proposed that the performance of all parts of the NHS should be publicly classified under a "traffic lights" system as "red", "yellow", or "green". Public consultation indicated that labelling hospitals as "red" might affect public confidence by suggesting they were dangerous, rather than that the overall patient experience was poor. A star system was judged to be less open to misinterpretation.[6] A second lesson is that in-depth assessment of clinical quality can substantially add to the impact of high level performance indicators, particularly when the assessments are carried out by an independent body. The 2000/1 NHS Performance Ratings took account of the first tranche of inspections by the independent Commission for Health Improvement. In consequence four hospitals were re-classified. The role of the Commission is expected to become even more important in the future.

4.2. Challenges in using performance measures to improve performance

The UK's experience in explicitly *using* performance measures to improve or manage NHS performance is much more limited than its experience in *developing* such measures. At this stage it may be more appropriate to talk about the challenges that have been identified rather than the lessons that have been learnt! The general objective is clear: to identify ways in which performance measurement systems can be designed and implemented to maximise the favourable impact whilst minimising the adverse consequences. Some of the major challenges in trying to put this into practice are summarised below:

i) How effective are performance targets in improving performance?

There is general agreement that setting performance targets can concentrate resources and energy on particular objectives. But in systems where there are multiple objectives the issue is whether focusing on one or some may be at the cost of slower progress towards others, seen as equally desirable, and/or may stimulate game playing and other inefficient consequences. In health care a further difficulty is disentangling the impact of performance targets from numerous other mechanisms aimed at promoting improved performance.

In Britain hard evidence on the impact of performance targets in health care is still limited. There is evidence that the setting of waiting times targets is associated with improved waiting times performance (Gravelle *et al.*, 2000). But there is also evidence that they can lead to misrepresentation and distortion of clinical priorities (National Audit Office, 2001*b*). The form of the targets can be of critical importance: for example, in relation to waiting, targets for waiting times will usually be more appropriate than targets for the length of waiting lists. A few years ago an attempt to assess the impact of health status targets (as part of a programme known as "The Health of the Nation"), came up with inconclusive results (Department of Health, 1998). In some other health systems, notably the US

Veterans Health Administration (VHA), the setting of targets has been associated with measurable improvements in quality[7] But in the case of the VHA, as with nearly all other target setting exercises a range of additional mechanisms aimed at performance enhancement were introduced at the same time.

The aspect of health care in England that has been subject to consistent performance targets longer than any other is efficiency in the hospital and community health sector. In this sector an efficiency index has been calculated back to the mid-1970s.[8] From around 1992 up to 2000 the Department set an annual efficiency target that was measured in roughly the same way. There has been no formal evaluation of the impact of converting the efficiency index into an efficiency target but eyeballing the data does not suggest there was any sustained break in the trend after 1990. However for most of the period the measure of efficiency was crude (e.g. there was no case-mix adjustment) and there may have been other factors, such as changes in the form of technological change, that reduced the scope for further efficiency improvements. An evaluation of the differential efficiency targets applied to NHS hospitals at the end of the 1990s concluded that they had no identifiable effect on relative performance (Jacobs and Dawson, 2001). What is clear is that the targets led to increasing reports of gaming and misrepresentation and concern that quality of care was at risk. Fears of the target's distortionary effects prompted adoption of the balanced score card approach to performance measurement discussed earlier (the PAF and the NHS Performance Ratings system) and a search for an improved measure of efficiency.

The evaluation of hospital efficiency targets at the end of the 1990s points up another important, if obvious, conclusion: if providers are to respond to targets they have to believe they will remain in existence long enough to be monitored and for rewards or penalties to be brought into play. A degree of stability is therefore essential. In the late 1990s the precise definition of hospital efficiency changed so frequently that central monitoring was effectively abandoned. It is perhaps not surprising that the targets had no identifiable effect on performance.

The NHS Performance Ratings take account of these lessons. The test of their effectiveness will be whether services for patients do improve.

ii) *Strengthening performance through top-down management or decentralised benchmarking?*

In Britain it is believed that good performance measures can improve performance both through strengthening top-down management and through facilitating benchmarking between NHS organisations. But in practice it has proved difficult to move forward equally rapidly on both fronts. The requirements of the government's approach to public sector business planning have so far taken precedence, leaving benchmarking generally lagging. Some argue benchmarks that demonstrate what is possible may be more motivating to local managers and clinicians than targets that show what is desirable. There is increasing experience of the use of performance measures for both purposes, but there appears to be little hard evidence on which use is likely to be most effective in which circumstances. What is clear from the British experience is that in the NHS benchmarking will remain a minority activity unless it is strongly supported, and possibly mandated, by the centre. With this in mind the Department has been developing a benchmarking database with web-based access aimed at serving clearly defined purposes, such as assisting Primary Care Trusts in their commissioning role. It has also been encouraging benchmarking by professional societies.

A few professional groups (i.e. Royal Colleges) have long worked on their own clinical benchmarking systems but it has taken highly publicised examples of clinician failure (e.g. Bristol) to persuade the organisers to make the activities mandatory and public. Clinical databases developed from audit projects now hold out the prospect of a major step forward in the monitoring and comparison of clinical quality across hospitals and clinical teams. For example, by 2003 the Myocardial Infarction National Audit Project (MINAP) developed by the Royal College of Physicians and British Cardiac Society to support implementation of the cardiac NSF is expected to deliver a range of sophisticated and detailed clinical indicators for heart attacks. Clinicians are likely to regard such indicators as more relevant and useful than the administrative data collected by the centre. This should encourage local ownership and local action.

iii) Balancing central targets and local autonomy

A good system of performance measures can arguably be used either to strengthen centralisation or to encourage decentralisation. In the NHS there is no doubt that overall the increasing range and sophistication of performance measures has so far assisted centralising tendencies. One reason is that the new indicators have drawn attention to what are seen as unacceptable variations in performance between regions, NHS organisations and individual clinicians. The development of a systematic performance framework, the Performance Assessment Framework, in part reflected a wish to tackle these variations. Setting central targets and standards is seen as the first step in equalising performance upwards. However, there are concerns that too many central targets will displace local initiatives, professional motivation and the addressing of local needs. The heart of the debate is over two issues:

- How much variation in health care should there be in a national health system;
- How can national programmes and local discretion be combined to promote the fastest and most sustained improvement in health care.

Both issues are judgement calls. The first is primarily an issue of values. The second should be informed by evidence. The Government's view is that the current variation in health care is unacceptable (as often is the mean level of performance). It also believes that rapid modernisation requires a national framework of objectives, targets, incentives and support mechanisms. Having now established that framework through the steps discussed earlier the government believes it is time to encourage decentralisation and the exercise of creativity by front-line health service staff (Department of Health, 2001*a*). "Checking" and "trusting" should continue to be kept in balance but with a strong checking framework in places the emphasis can shift towards trusting (Davies *et al.*, 2001).

Looking to the future it is interesting to speculate on whether some of the responsibilities for "checking" could be moved out of the centre to other agencies. Arguably the dominant role of the centre in performance management in England reflects the inability or failure of others groups including the professions, patients and the public to demand and enforce high standards of care. If informed patients were willing and able to act as partners with health care workers, and if professional associations were willing to identify and enforce a high standard of care this would help to spread performance management much more widely, taking some of the pressure off the centre. But these "ifs" assume it will prove possible to ameliorate health care's classic information asymmetry and principal-agent problems.

iv) What combination of financial and non-financial incentives should back up performance measures?

One of the most important recent changes in performance management in England has been making the rewards and penalties attached to performance on specific measures both sharper and more transparent. The performance management system announced in the NHS Plan places the main emphasis on non-financial incentives, particularly the publicity engendered by performance ratings and the freedoms of "earned autonomy". While performance will affect ease of access to additional funds there are no immediate proposals to tie organisational performance directly to financial rewards or penalties. However, through the expansion of Personal Medical Services contracts and a new national contract for GPs and through a new contract for hospital doctors there will be a major strengthening of the links between individual financial rewards and personal contributions to the quality, delivery and improvement of local health services.

It is too early to judge how effective this combination of incentives will prove to be. The economic literature provides good evidence on what forms of incentives encourage activity and there is some evidence on how payment systems can discourage improvements in the quality of care. But the evidence is sparse on what forms of incentives, financial or otherwise, will promote improvements in the *quality* of care (Reinhardt, 2001). For example, attempts by US employers to attach financial sanctions to health plans failing to deliver quality appear to have had little or no effect. It is not clear whether this is because the size of the incentives was insufficiently large or because health plans have too few levers over health care providers. Overall the US experience (particularly the New York CABG surgery mortality reporting programme) (Chassin *et al.*, 1996) and the responses to the publication of hospital mortality data in England suggests that public exposure of poor outcomes is the most effective stimulant to improving the quality of care that has yet been identified. On the other hand Scottish experience suggests that publication alone will not necessarily provoke providers to significantly change behaviours (Mannion and Goddard, 2001).

v) What aspects of performance should be rewarded?

Performance measures that are perfectly adequate for general monitoring purposes and for raising questions will more often than not be an unsuitable basis for allocating rewards and penalties. In England the first set of high level performance indicators were developed for raising questions – to be "can openers" – at health authority level. Few were found to be suitable to enter into an assessment of hospital performance that carried rewards and penalties.

Reasons why relatively few of the high level performance indicators were used in the 2000/1 performance rating of general hospitals included:

- The indicators of health status (or "health improvement") and of health inequalities were seen as only partially influenceable by hospitals, *inter alia*, because they were highly linked to socio-economic factors, and as more relevant to health authorities;

- Many indicators of the effectiveness and outcomes of NHS care were seen as the responsibility of other health care institutions (*e.g.* primary care) or requiring co-operation between hospitals and other providers, including social services;

- Some indicators of the clinical outcomes of acute care were judged to be insufficiently robust – because of lack of adjustment for casemix and other confounding factors – to be used to assess hospital performance (though again they might be quite adequate for assessing performance in larger populations such as health authorities);

- For the performance rating system to have bite as an incentive it had to have many fewer indicators than the PAF.

A benefit of attempting to use indicators to inform judgements, not just to raise questions, is that it highlights how much investment is needed in new clinical indicators and in patient and staff surveys.

In addition to tackling attribution issues, developing composite performance ratings for hospitals or other providers requires the addressing of a number of other important issues, including:

- How far should rewards and sanctions be attached to absolute levels of performance or to rates of improvement?

- Should organisations that inherit low absolute levels of performance be penalised even if they are improving rapidly?

- How should the different aspects of performance be weighted and whose values should determine the weights?

- How complex and how transparent should be the process of arriving at overall classifications?

All these questions were addressed in establishing the NHS Performance Ratings system. There are no easy answers but how these questions are tackled will determine the perceived fairness of the system of assessment and reward – and probably its long-term survival.

vi) How many aspects of performance can be changed at the same time?

Once the decision has been made to link performance measures to rewards and sanctions there is a strong temptation to try and tie in as many aspects of performance as possible. Unless there is a separate incentive system for each performance indicator applying multiple indicators will lead to two problems. First, the measured organisation may conclude that it is so difficult to gain the rewards or to avoid the sanctions that it is not worth the effort. Second, the performance assessor may find it increasingly difficult to judge what is good or poor performance and to justify the judgement. If, for example, there are 50 indicators why is success on 40 of them judged good, but success on only 35 is seen as failure? The problems associated with laying on too many conditions have been well illustrated in the international aid field. The IMFs' recent conclusion that parsimony and focus must be the watch words in setting conditions on the provision of aid may well also apply to schemes to incentivise improvements in health care performance (Goldstein, 2001).

For these kinds of reasons the NHS performance ratings system has less than half the number of indicators that are in the Performance Assessment Framework.

vii) *What are the infrastructure and skill requirements?*

It has already been noted that actively using performance measures to improve performance requires a major investment in the quality, relevance and reliability of data sets: data adequate for raising questions may not be able to bear the burden of informing judgements. In turn this will almost certainly necessitate major investments in information technology. But better data and IT are not in themselves sufficient. To use the new data effectively people need the skills and ability to analyse and understand it. Analytical skills have always been in short supply in the NHS and those available have tended to be brigaded at the centre in the Department of Health. If benchmarking and the search for continuous improvement are to become local ways of life there will need to be a major investment in building up local analytical capacity. The further down is decision making devolved the larger the number of units requiring an enhancement in analytical capacity.

New analytical skills will only be deployed effectively if managers and clinicians understand their value and importance. This in turn has implications for the training of NHS management trainees and future leaders. It may also have consequences for the size of the management cadre. Despite strong centralising tendencies, by international standards the NHS appears to be relatively lightly managed.

viii) *How can we learn more quickly?*

The concept of performance management enshrined in recent NHS reforms has been defined as "a set of managerial instruments designed to secure optimal performance of the health care system over time, in line with policy objectives" (Smith, 2001). As already noted, in addition to a new performance information system (the PAF), these instruments have included a national delivery contract, National Service Frameworks, the National Institute for Clinical Excellence, the Commission for Health Improvement, a NHS Performance Rating System, a system of "earned autonomy", a Performance Fund and a Modernisation Agency. All in one way or another are concerned with sharpening standards and guidance, improving monitoring, strengthening incentives or improving responses to poor performance. Critics have noted that some of these elements are supported by managerial theory or practice but others are untested. They also note that currently there is little knowledge on how to strike the best balance between them: for example, which organisation will respond best to "carrots and sticks" and which to "maps and compasses"? But they agree that together the elements amount to a programme of strategic management of organisational behaviour that in its ambition and comprehensiveness is probably unique in health care.

To ensure that the new instruments contribute to knowledge and that they adapt and learn, the Department is supporting a developing programme of monitoring and evaluation. For example, all providers are required to report publicly on their use of the Performance Fund and a sample of plans are to be evaluated. Again the collaborative programmes of the Modernisation Agency are being formally evaluated; and its work aimed at turning round poorly performing hospitals will also be the subject of careful piloting, to establish what works. Through the NHS Service Delivery and Organisation R and D Programme and the Department's own research programme there will be a co-ordinated approach to assessing the overall impact and coherence of the different instruments of performance management. But for many the best guide to the overall success of this strategic approach to changing organisational behaviour will be the delivery of the NHS Plan.

71

5. The Future

Developing useful performance measures and successfully applying them to improve health performance is a long and arduous road. There are no quick fixes but lessons for the future can and are being learnt. In relation to performance measurement it can be expected that policy makers in England will focus more heavily on identifying patient and clinician concerns and developing measures of outcomes that are directly relevant to each of these groups. To gain ownership there will be regular consultation with the wide range of stakeholders about the most appropriate measures. To encourage awareness and behavioural change media skills will be used to make the presentation of the results more attractive and understandable.

To make performance measures more effective as a tool for improving performance there are likely to be at least two parallel developments. First, for national and local accountability purposes there will be attention to a smaller number of targets aligned more closely with key policies and hopefully showing greater stability through time. Second, there will be more emphasis on promoting self-comparison and benchmarking, particularly by clinicians and drawing on performance indicators that are increasingly developed by and with clinicians and patients. To ensure that both developments are fully exploited it will be necessary to substantially expand investments and skills in information, IT and analysis at every level of the National Health Service. It will also be necessary to closely evaluate and learn from experience with the range of other tools that have been introduced to complement performance assessment: *i.e.* standard setting, incentives, and support and coaching mechanisms. Given the large number of these tools it will be important to rapidly discard those that prove ineffective (or generate large perverse incentives). The rest will need careful co-ordination to ensure that they support each other in promoting better patient care.

NOTES

1. This paper focuses on England and does not attempt to cover the experiences of Wales, Scotland or Northern Ireland.

2. These organisational changes were announced in: Department of Health (1997), *The New NHS: Modern, Dependable*, The Stationery Office, London (*www.doh.gov.uk/nnhsind.htm*).

3. HEDIS is sponsored, supported and maintained by the National Committee for Quality Assurance (NCQA), the organisation responsible for accrediting US managed care organisations.

4. For example, for the Australian experience see: Corden, S. and Luxmoore, J. (2000), "Managing Performance for Better Results", in Bloom, A. (ed.), *Health Reform in Australia and New Zealand*, Oxford University Press.

5. Dr Foster has produced a number of reports comparing the performance of hospitals and consultants that have been widely distributed through national newspapers.

6. The change also made it easier to incorporate the four categories (not three) that emerged as the natural way of clustering.

7. Personal communication from Dr Jonathan B. Perlin, Chief Quality and Performance Officer, Veterans Health Administration, October 2001.

8. The index is described in, for example: Department of Health (2000c), "The Government's Expenditure Plans 2000-2001", The Stationery Office, London (*www.doh.gov.uk/dohreport/report2000/dr2000.html*).

REFERENCES

CABINET OFFICE (1999),
>   *Performance Management – Civil Service Reform – A Report to the Meeting of Permanent Heads of Departments*, Sunningdale, London.

CHASSIN, M., HANNAN, E. and DEBUONO, B. (1996),
>   "Benefits and hazards of reporting medical outcomes publicly", *The New England Journal of Medicine*, No. 234, 8th February, pp. 394-398.

CORDEN, S. and LUXMOORE, J. (2000),
>   "Managing performance for better results", in Bloom, A. (ed.), *Health Reform in Australia and New Zealand*, Oxford University Press.

DAVIES, H., MANNION, R. and MARSHALL, M. (2001),
>   "Treading a third way for quality in health care", *Public Money and Management*, Vol.21, No.2, April-June, pp. 6-7.

DEPARTMENT OF HEALTH (1991),
>   *The Patient's Charter*, London.

DEPARTMENT OF HEALTH (1997),
>   *The New NHS: Modern, Dependable*, The Stationery Office, London (*www.doh.gov.uk/nnhsind.htm*).

DEPARTMENT OF HEALTH (1998),
>   *The Health of the Nation – A Policy Assessed*, The Stationery Office, London (*www.doh.gov.uk/ohn/natass.htm*).

DEPARTMENT OF HEALTH (2000a),
>   *The NHS Plan: A Plan for Investment, A Plan for Reform*, Stationery Office, London (*www.nhs.uk/nationalplan*).

DEPARTMENT OF HEALTH (2000b),
>   *The National Service Framework for Coronary Heart Disease: Modern Standards and Service Models*, Department of Health, London (*www.doh.gov.uk/nsf/coronary.htm*).

DEPARTMENT OF HEALTH (2000c),
>   *The Government's Expenditure Plans 2000-2001*, The Stationery Office, London (*www.doh.gov.uk/dohreport/report2000/dr2000.html*).

DEPARTMENT OF HEALTH (2001a),
>   *Shifting the Balance of Power within the NHS: Securing Delivery*, London (*www.doh.gov.uk/shiftingthebalance*).

DEPARTMENT OF HEALTH (2001b),
>   *NHS Performance Indicators: A Consultation*, Department of Health, London (*www.doh.gov.uk/piconsultation*).

DEPARTMENT OF HEALTH (2001c),
>   *NHS Performance Ratings – Acute Trusts 2000/01*, Department of Health, London (*www.doh.gov.uk/performanceratings*).

DEPARTMENT OF HEALTH, NHS Executive (2000),
>   *The New NHS 1999 Reference Costs*, Department of Health, Leeds (*www.doh.gov.uk/nhsexec/refcosts/refcosts99.htm*).

GODDARD, M. and SMITH, P. (2001),
>   "Performance Measurement in the New NHS", *Health Policy Matters*, No. 3, pp. 1-8.

GOLDSTEIN, M. (2001),
>   "IMF structural conditionality: How much is too much?", Institute for International Economics Working Paper, Washington D.C.

GRAVELLE, H., SMITH, P. and XAVIER, A. (2000),
>   *The Impact of Performance Measurement in the NHS. Report 2: Empirical Analysis of Waiting Times and Waiting Lists*, Report for the Department of Health, York.

HER MAJESTY'S STATIONERY OFFICE (1989),
>   *Working for Patients*, London.

JACOBS, R. and DAWSON, D. (2001),
>   "Hospital efficiency and target-setting", unpublished paper from University of York.

KAPLAN, R. and NORTON, D. (1992),
"The balanced scorecard – measures that drive performance", *Harvard Business Review*, Jan.-Feb., pp. 71-79.

MANNION, R. and GODDARD, M. (2001),
"Impact of published clinical outcomes data: case study in NHS hospital trusts", *British Medical Journal*, No. 323, pp. 260-263.

MARSHALL, M., SHEKELL, E.P., LEATHERMAN, S. and BROOK, R. (2000),
"What do we expect to gain from the public release of performance data? A review of the evidence", *Journal of American Medical Association*, Vol. 283, No. 14, pp. 1866-1874.

NATIONAL AUDIT OFFICE (2001*a*),
Measuring the Performance of Government Departments, The Stationery Office, London.

NATIONAL AUDIT OFFICE (2001*b*),
Department of Health: In-patient and out-patient waiting in the NHS, The Stationery Office, London.

NHS MANAGEMENT EXECUTIVE (1993),
"Indicators of Effectiveness and Quality that could inform consideration of NHS Performance in 1994/5 and 1995/6", Two Reports from the Working Group on Quality and Effectiveness Measures, Unpublished, London.

NHS MANAGEMENT EXECUTIVE (1995),
"Report of the Sub-group on Primary Care Effectiveness and Efficiency", Unpublished, London.

NHS EXECUTIVE (1998),
"The New NHS Modern and Dependable: A National Framework for Assessing Performance", Consultation Document, Department of Health, London (*www.doh.gov.uk/newnhs/consult.htm*)

NHS EXECUTIVE (1999),
Quality and Performance in the NHS: *High Level Performance Indicators*, Department of Health, London (*www.doh.gov.uk/indicat/nhshlpi.htm*)

NHS EXECUTIVE (2000),
Quality and Performance in the NHS: NHS *Performance Indicators*, Department of Health, London (*www.doh.gov.uk/nhsperformanceindicators/index.htm*)

OECD (1994),
OECD *Economic Surveys*: *United Kingdom*, Paris.

OECD (2000),
OECD *Economic Surveys*: *United Kingdom*, Paris.

REINHARDT, U. (2001),
"Structuring Financial Flows in Health Care to Support High Quality Health Care", Paper presented to The Commonwealth Fund Symposium on Improving Quality of Health Care in the US and the UK, Unpublished, Pennyhill Park, Bagshot.

SMEE, C. (2000),
"The Performance Assessment Framework: Where did it come from and where is it going?", *Health Care* UK, King's Fund, London, Spring.

SMITH, P. (2001),
"Performance Management in British Health Care: Will it Deliver?", Unpublished paper presented to The Commonwealth Fund International Symposium, Washington D.C., October.

Annex A

CRITERIA USED TO SELECT THE KEY DOMAINS
OF THE PERFORMANCE ASSESSMENT FRAMEWORK

Consideration was given to various approaches to identifying the key domains of health service performance. The approach adopted required the areas to:

- Reflect the purposes of the NHS;
- Be easily understood as a concept;
- Focus on the perspectives of most importance for stakeholders, including those of users, carers, professionals and the public;
- Be small in number;
- Be as mutually exclusive as categories as possible;
- Reflect a rounded approach to the NHS's performance
- Be flexible in interpretation, to allow incorporation of changing policy objectives.

Annex B

LIST OF HIGH LEVEL PERFORMANCE INDICATORS
IN THE PERFORMANCE ASSESSMENT FRAMEWORK (JULY 2000)

Area	Indicators
1. Health improvement	Deaths from all causes (ages 15-64) Deaths from all causes (ages 65-74) Deaths from cancer Deaths from circulatory diseases Suicide rates Deaths from accident Serious injury from accidents

Detailed example:

Suicide rates. Suicides are a significant cause of early death and are responsible each year for nearly half a million years of life lost in those aged under 75 years. In England, on average, more than one person dies every two hours as a result of suicide. This is a priority area in *Our Healthier Nation*, and this indicator is also in the *Mental Health National Service Framework*. The target is to reduce the death rate from suicide and undetermined injury by at least a fifth by 2010 – saving up to 4 000 lives in total. The data presented here pre-dates the start of the OHN strategy.

Area	Indicators
2. Fair access	In-patient waiting list Adult dental registrations Early detection of cancer Cancer waiting times Number of GPs GP practice availability Elective surgery rates Surgery rates – Coronary heart disease

Detailed example:

Early detection of cancer. This indicator combines cervical and breast screening coverage. Cervical pre-cancer is readily diagnosed and there is successful treatment for pre-invasive and early state invasive disease. The Forrest Working Group concluded that screening by mammography among women aged 50-64 could reduce deaths from breast cancer.

Area	Indicators
3. Effective Delivery of Appropriate Health Care	Childhood immunisations Inappropriately used surgery Acute care management Chronic care management Mental health in primary care Cost effective prescribing Returning home following treatment for a stroke Returning home following treatment for a fractured hip

Detailed example:

Childhood immunisations. By age 2 children should be immunised against diphtheria, tetanus, polio, pertussis, measles, mumps, rubella and meningitis. This indicator combines coverage rates for MMR (mumps, measles, rubella) and diphtheria and takes this as representative of the whole list.

Area	Indicators
4. Efficiency	Day case rate Length of stay Maternity unit costs Mental health unit costs Generic prescribing

Detailed example:

Generic prescribing. Considerable cost savings have been achieved by promoting the prescribing of generic products, as some branded products can cost the NHS substantially more than the generic version. Also, prescribing a drug by its generic name is recognised as good prescribing practice. Generic manufacturers must satisfy the Medicines Control Agency that their products are of a similar quality to branded products before a license is granted.

Area	Indicators
5. Patient/Carer experience of the NHS	Patients who wait less 2 hours for emergency admission (through A&E) Cancelled operations Delayed discharges First outpatient appointments for which patient did not attend Outpatient seen within 13 weeks of GP referral Number of those on waiting list waiting 18 months or more Patients satisfaction

Detailed example:

Delayed discharge. Most episodes of care involve several members of NHS staff. Treatment or care over time often includes different NHS organisations and other agencies. The ways in which staff and organisations communicate and co-ordinate within and among themselves are important components of the patient experience. Hospital discharge marks the boundary between the responsibility of the acute, continuing and community health services of the NHS and Local Authorities. Delayed discharge may be the result of poor communication between the relevant care organisations. This indicator is an interface indicator with the PSS *Performance Assessment Framework* Interface indicator.

Area	Indicators
6. Health outcomes of NHS healthcare	Conceptions below age 18 Decayed, missing or filled teeth in five year old children Re-admission to hospital following discharge Emergency admission of older people Emergency psychiatric re-admission Stillbirths and infant deaths Breast cancer survival Cervical cancer survival Lung cancer survival Colon cancer survival Deaths in hospital following surgery (emergency admissions) Deaths in hospital (following surgery (non-emergency admissions) Deaths in hospital following heart attack (ages 35-74) Deaths in hospital following a fractured hip

Detailed example:

Deaths in hospital following surgery (emergency and non-emergency). The purpose of monitoring deaths occurring in hospital within 30 days of surgery is to help prevent (or reduce to a minimum) potentially avoidable deaths. Since the number of such deaths is related to the total number of hospital stays of people undergoing surgery, the data are expressed per 100 000 such stays. The figures include people of all ages, and relate to hospital admissions in the year ending 31 March 1999. Information is provided for England, Health Authorities and NHS Hospital Trusts in England who carried out at least 200 operations in 1998/99. The risk of dying after surgery will depend in part on whether the surgery was pre-planned or an emergency response to an acute condition. For this reason, the information is provided separately for emergency and non-emergency admissions. Deaths occurring within 30 days of surgery but after a patient has been discharged from hospital, are not included as the data are not available. It is estimated that these account for about 6 per cent of all deaths within 30 days of surgery. Deaths following readmission to hospital after a period outside hospital, for problems arising from previous surgery, are also missing from the indicator. The death rates may vary between Trusts due to the variation in the complexity of procedures carried out. For example, the major cardiac centres may have high death rates due to the complexity of the operations carried out.

Annex C

PRINCIPLES OF DEVELOPING AND USING PERFORMANCE INDICATORS

The approach suggested below reflects the emerging consensus in the UK central government on the principles of performance management and a strategic approach to performance indicators.

Principles

The NHS Performance Assessment Framework (PAF) and supporting indicators should support:

- the *vision* for the NHS set out in the NHS Plan;
- national and local objectives;
- *leadership and performance management* at all levels in the NHS.

The NHS PAF and supporting indicators should enable:

- the public to understand the performance of the NHS;
- challenging *targets* to be set, based on robust performance indicators and in SMART form;
- these targets to be *communicated and owned* across the NHS, especially by clinicians and managers;
- *monitoring and review*.

The NHS PAF should become the *one prime system* for key performance information; over time, other existing systems should converge.

The NHS PAF should facilitate *continuous improvement* in the NHS and so be part of quality improving strategies at national and local levels.

Performance indicators and targets should help clinicians and managers focus on *priorities for change*.

Performance information should only be collected where *it is needed for clinical or managerial decision-making*, or monitoring for *accountability*.

The NHS PAF should be *integrated across all areas of* NHS – including primary care and interfaces with organisations outside the NHS, especially social services. Interface indicators should be in areas where health and social services are jointly accountable and cannot make improvements individually.

It should be clear how *clinical or managerial decisions at the front-line* will influence higher level or aggregate performance indicators.

PAF and *external scrutiny* such as audit/inspection and research should be complementary, and be seen by clinicians and managers as forming an integrated system, relevant to their needs at local level, as well as providing accountability.

The performance assessment framework and indicators should be subject to *continuous improvement* in the light of experience, and as priorities change.

Use of performance indicators in the PAF

Performance indicators can be used for a number of purposes. T*he characteristics of performance indicators used for some purposes can make them inappropriate for others*.

Performance information should be appropriate for the purposes for which it is collected; the purposes should be clear, and the reliability of the underlying data must be adequate for the use to which they will be put.

Key choices will need to be made about the prime purpose of the PAF before selecting performance indicators for inclusion.

If performance indicators are used to *compare* performance between similar bodies, they need to:

- be clearly defined;
- have definitions which are consistently applied;

- allow local circumstances to be taken into account (*e.g.* socio-economic factors and case mix);
- identify good and poor performance which the organisations being measured can influence.

If performance indicators are used to *track changes* in performance over time, they need to:

- have stable definitions;
- be valid irrespective of (changing) models of service delivery;
- enable the impact of changes in local circumstances to be understood;
- enable clinicians and managers to understand how their decisions have affected performance.

If performance indicators are to be used to set targets that are:

Specific

Measurable

Achievable

Relevant

Time-limited

They need to be:

- related to the organisation's objectives, including applicable national objectives;
- seen to be reasonable by those who will be held to account for achieving them;
- monitored through the organisation's accountability systems.

If *resources are to be allocated* based on performance indicators, they need to:

- be based on robust financial data, linked to financial accounts;
- show how performance and cost are related;
- cover a full range of services;
- allow local circumstances to be taken properly into account;
- be seen to be fair by those (not) receiving the resources.

If performance indicators are to be used for *in-year management*, they need to:

- be aligned with the organisation's priorities and responsibilities;
- be timely; many will need to be collected and presented in near real-time, but not be an additional burden on clinicians and managers;
- enable clinicians and managers to predict how their decisions will change performance;
- have definitions which are accepted by those who will use them.

If performance indicators are to be used to drive *continuous improvement* in:

- *quality/effectiveness*, they need to:
  - genuinely measure aspects of quality;
  - reflect a clear link between outputs and outcomes, or between processes and patient-experienced quality;
  - be linked to follow-up by line management and independent scrutineers and strategies for quality improvement.
- *efficiency*, they need to:
  - reflect a clear link between inputs and outputs;
  - be based on robust financial data, linked to financial accounts and with consistent allocation of overheads;
  - be based on robust and consistently defined activity data;
  - provide the basis for follow-up by line management and independent scrutineers.

If performance indicators are used for *accountability*, they need to:

  - be aligned with the responsibilities of the bodies being held to account;
  - link with the bodies' processes for clinical and corporate governance;
  - be seen to be fair by all key stakeholders, including the public and the bodies being held to account;
  - be subject to independent public scrutiny.

Continuous improvement of the PAF

If the PAF is to retain credibility, it needs to change in line with learning from:

- "what works" in improving services, including lessons from national research and local inspections and audits;
- changes in clinical practice;
- changes in behaviour (both expected and unexpected), including the impact of perverse incentives;

what managers and clinicians actually use for decision-making.

Annex D

NHS PERFORMANCE RATINGS
MEASURES USED TO CLASSIFY GENERAL HOSPITALS 2000/01

Key targets

- Reduction in In-patient Waiting Lists

- Reduction in Out-patient Waiting Lists

- No patients waiting more than 18 months

- Fewer patients waiting on trolleys for more than 12 hours

- Less than 1 per cent of operations cancelled on the day

- No patients with suspected breast cancer waiting more than 2 weeks to be seen in hospital

- Commitment to improve the working lives of staff

- Hospital cleanliness

- Satisfactory financial position

- No critical report from the Commission for Health Improvement

Balanced scorecard

Patient focus

- percentage of patients waiting less than 6 months for treatment

- percentage of out-patients seen within 13 weeks

- percentage of patients in A&E who wait more than 4 hours on a trolley before admission

- percentage of complaints resolved within 4 weeks

Clinical focus

- Low risk of clinical negligence

- Emergency re-admission rates

- Deaths in hospital within 30 days of surgery for patients admitted on an unplanned basis

Staff focus

- Sickness/absence rate for directly employed NHS staff

- Rates of vacancies for key staff groups

- Compliance with new deal on junior doctors' hours (working a maximum 56 hours a week)

Annex E

SUMMARISING PERFORMANCE ASSESSMENT FRAMEWORK:
TWO HEALTH AUTHORITY ILLUSTRATIONS

Diagram 1. **Performance assessment framework: summary presentations for West Surrey Health Authority**

Domain values standardised by range in base year

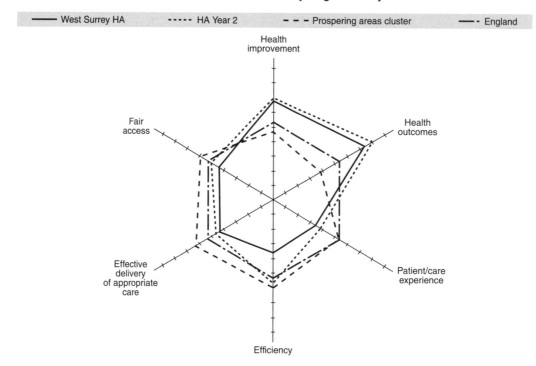

Adjusted domain values

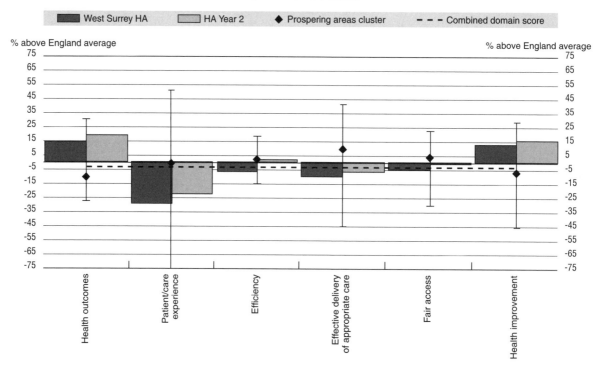

Diagram 2. **Performance assessment framework:
summary presentations for Manchester Health Authority**

Domain values standardised by range in base year

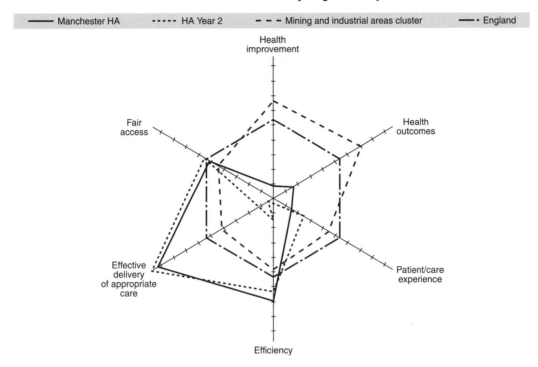

Adjusted domain values

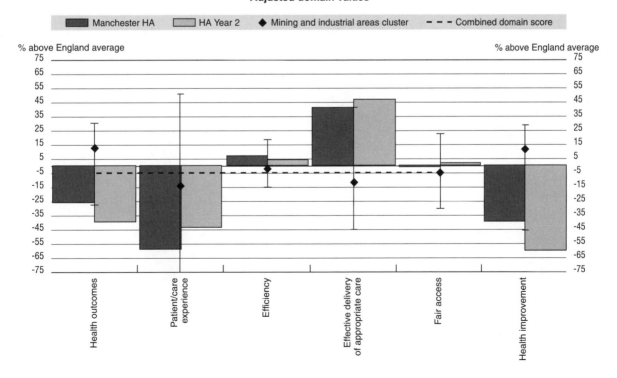

Chapter 4

IMPROVING ACCOUNTABILITY IN A DECENTRALISED SYSTEM: A SWEDISH PERSPECTIVE

by

*Nina Rehnqvist**

Abstract

Swedish health care is publicly financed through local county taxes. Care is delivered either by institutions run by the county councils or, increasingly, by private organisations, often owned by the county councils. The National Board of Health and Welfare is independent from the Ministry of Health and is non-political. It has two tasks: to issue guidelines on evidence-based medicine and good practice; and to undertake surveillance of institutions and personnel providing health care.

Swedish legislation states that health care services shall be of good quality and given on equal terms to all people. This is enshrined in the 1997 Code of Statutes of the National Board of Health and Welfare: "Continuous and systematic quality assurance and improvement shall be implemented in all medical and dental services." From 1998 a similar regulation concerning the care of the elderly has been in effect.

The philosophy underlying the Board's work has been to promote professional and institutional self-evaluation. However, the Code also requires that institutions should present material for benchmarking and comparisons. For almost 50 conditions such comparative material is available on a national level through a system of quality registers. In addition, national clinical guidelines have been prepared for about ten major clinical conditions comprising about 70 per cent of disease burden.

Follow up legislation to the Code of Statutes is planned. The intention is that data from a patient, professional and organisational perspective will have to be openly reported on an annual basis, with the objective of thereby strengthening the surveillance function.

This paper summarizes the Swedish experience in promoting greater accountability in health care. It first describes briefly the Swedish health care system, and then the system of quality registers started in 1979. The process of developing clinical guidelines, and its relationship to quality registers, is outlined in Section 3. The paper concludes with an assessment of progress to date.

1. The Swedish health care system

Good health and equal access to health services for everyone are the goals of the Swedish health care system. A fundamental principle underlying Swedish health care is that it is a public sector responsibility to provide and finance health services for the entire population. Responsibility for these services rests primarily with the 21 county councils, which levy local payroll taxes varying from 9.4 to 10.7 per cent to finance health care. They also deliver most of the services provided. Thus it is in the

---

* Deputy General Director, National Board of Health and Welfare.

Acknowledgements: Special thanks go to Marie Lawrence for helping to prepare this manuscript. Assistance from Lennart Rinder, Bo Lindblom, Ingemar Eckerlund, Lars Steen is also gratefully acknowledged.

Figure 1. **Organisation of health services and long-term care
at the regional and local level in Sweden**

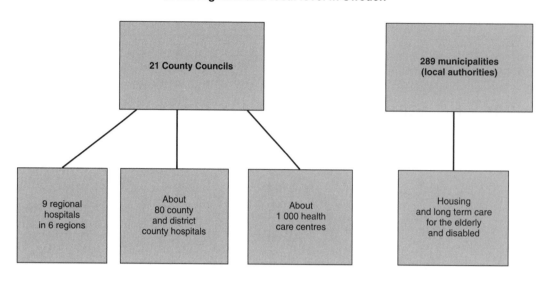

first instance local politicians who are responsible for organizing health care in Sweden. Two distinctive characteristics of the Swedish system are therefore that it is decentralised and that it is run on democratic principles (Figure 1).

In most counties there is a split between the purchasers and providers of health care. Although institutions providing health care services are mainly owned and run by the county councils, private enterprises are becoming more frequent, especially in primary care and in care for the elderly. At present the privatisation of hospitals taking care of emergencies is prohibited by law. There is a widespread belief that the quality of purchasing is often poor, leading to vague contracts and inadequate monitoring. An additional problem of the Swedish health care system is the three party conflict between short-term political interests, professional interests, and the demands of patients.

The proportion of GNP devoted to health care in Sweden varies from 7.4 per cent to 8.8 per cent depending on the basis for calculation. Expenditure was stable during the 1990s. The number of hospital beds has fallen dramatically over recent years and so has the duration of stay in hospital. Expenditure on personnel has decreased, but this has been offset by an increase in pharmaceutical expenditure. Swedish health care has traditionally been hospital-based, but is now under pressure to change towards more primary care. The country has more than 30 000 physicians for a population of 8.8 million (a ratio of about 300 people per physician), but the number of people per primary care physician is about 1 900. The government has set a target of reducing this ratio to 1 500.

The National Board of Health and Welfare (NBHW) is funded through, but independent from the Ministry of Health. It is non-political. The Board has about 500 collaborators of which 100 work in six regional surveillance units. The main objectives of the National Board with respect to the health care sector are: 1) to issue normative material stating the basis for evidence-based medicine and good practice; and 2) to perform surveillance of institutions and authorised personnel providing health care services.

The requirement that health care services shall be of good quality and given on equal terms to all people is enshrined in the 1997 Code of Statutes of the National Board of Health and Welfare as follows: "Continuous and systematic quality assurance and improvement shall be implemented in all medical and dental services." From 1998 a similar regulation concerning the care of the elderly has been in force.

2. National quality registers

There have been many recent initiatives in Sweden to promote performance improvements. The actors have included professional groups and national institutions. Although there has until recently been no systematic attempt to coordinate these activities, one widespread initiative has been the development of national quality registers (Federation of Swedish County Councils and National Board of Health and Welfare, 2000).

The aims of national quality registers are to provide comparative information on outcome and results to participating units, to form a base for evaluation and improvement of medical quality, and to disseminate good medical practice. The intention is that institutions and professionals should be able to compare their performance over time and across providers. Each register is managed by a group that is usually located in one of the Swedish university hospitals. Participating centres send their data to this management group, which assembles the data, undertakes statistical analysis, and disseminates comparative material to participating centres. The participants in each quality register have several meetings per year at which they discuss data from individual centres. The National Board of Health and Welfare and the Federation of County Councils, with the help of the Swedish Society of Medicine, form the reference group and provide financial support for the development of quality registers. The establishment and expansion of national quality registers may be seen as a response to rapid changes in health services, as well as a response to increasing demands for improvements when it comes to patient focus, effectiveness and efficiency, monitoring and evaluation, and quality.

Quality registers contain individual-based data on patient characteristics, diagnoses, treatments, patient experiences and outcomes. Participation in the registers is voluntary on the part of providers. Statistical material is presented at an aggregate level for each participating department and the country as a whole. Registers are initiated by representatives of the medical profession with the primary intention of supporting efforts to improve the quality of clinical work through continuous learning and development. In most cases, the development of registers from a few local hospital departments to a truly national register has taken place gradually.

The first register, the hip arthroplasty register, started in 1979. There are today about 50 registers that have fulfilled the criteria of the National Board of Health and Welfare and the Federation of County Councils, and thus obtain funding. A full list of current quality registers is given in the annex. Box 1 summarizes activity and experience in four. Total funding to support the development of quality registers amounted to SEK 15 million in 2000; it is expected to increase to SEK 20 million per year in the years ahead. The level of funding for each register varies according to the extent of the data collection, the sophistication of the analysis and the degree of interaction between participating centres.

The key to all quality management initiatives is that participants should scrutinize their own results. When a national quality register is established, this is the result of a consensus in the medical speciality regarding fundamental concepts and a related set of quality indicators, and a conviction that the register provides a useful measurement and reporting tool based on these indicators. It is recognised that this tool needs to be developed and refined from year to year.

In addition to facilitating comparisons over time, quality registers also make it possible for an individual department to compare itself with other (anonymized) departments and with national performance. The most well-established registers have abandoned anonymity and present their data publicly. Although there has been strong emphasis on the usefulness of comparisons with other departments, one potential limitation is that departments whose performance is better than the national average may have little incentive to improve quality further.

Quality registers assemble large quantities of data nation-wide every year. This is especially valuable in a geographically large country with a small population, in which many hospitals treat only a few cases of a specific condition each year. The data often promote the dissemination of best medical practice in a faster, simpler and cheaper fashion than the conventional medium of research projects. They also function as a unique "early warning system" for shortcomings in new methods of treatment and new technologies. The hip replacement surgery register offers one good example of such successful use (Box 1).

Box 1. **Four national quality registers in Sweden**

National hip arthroplasty register

Started: 1979

Coverage: 100 per cent of primary hip replacements and re-operations carried out in Sweden.

Content: Patients' age and sex, preoperative diagnosis, type of prosthesis and fixation techniques, number of re-operations.

Primary outcome variable: No need for re-operation.

Major finding/implication: Early detection that "cement-fixation" was accompanied by less need for re-operation, but this operation takes longer and needs more blood transfusions.

National stroke registry

Started: 1995

Coverage: 80 per cent of all departments treating patients with acute stroke.

Content: Patients' age and sex, previous strokes, time from attack to examination in hospital, type of unit (stroke unit or ordinary ward), CT Scan, length of stay (in acute unit and total), diagnosis, medical treatment during period of care and, where applicable, death registration. Aftercare: patients' address three months after the attack, mobility (whether the patient can move without assistance), patients' ADL needs, patients' satisfaction with treatment, and (where applicable) support and assistance after discharge.

Primary outcome variable: Proportion of patients able to live in their home 3 months after stroke.

Major finding/implication: Better outcome for patients treated in stroke units (*i.e.*, teams consisting of physiotherapist, nurse, speech therapist, social worker, and easy access to other specialists).

National cataract register

Started: 1992

Coverage: 95 per cent of all cataract surgery in Sweden.

Content: Patients' age and sex, waiting time, vision at the time of operation, previous eye diseases, type of operation, type of intra-ocular lens, difference between planned and final refraction, induced astigmatism, visual acuity achieved, whether operation has healed after 6 months, perceived eye problems after surgery, and level of activity.

Primary outcome variable: Improvements in vision pre and post surgery.

Major finding/implication: 1) development of a common model to support clinical decisions for surgery throughout the country; 2) measures to shorten waiting lists and waiting times; 3) identification of factors associated with poor visual outcome in spite of successful lens replacement.

National registry for cardiac intensive care

Started: 1992

Coverage: 73 per cent of all patients treated for acute myocardial infarction.

Content: Patients' age and sex, risk factors, previous diseases and drugs used, methods of diagnosis, pharmacological or interventional therapy, complications occurring during hospital stay and, where applicable, death registration.

Primary outcome variable: Mortality rate.

Major finding/implication: No gender bias concerning treatment after adjusting for age. Persistently long delays to thrombolysis. Lower mortality in departments with treatment modalities according to evidence-based medicine.

The data in registers have also been used to support clinical decision-making. For instance, developmental work in eye care makes it possible for individual physicians, in consultation with the patient, to make a better assessment of whether a cataract operation will really improve the quality of life. Some of the quality registers focus on important but neglected areas of treatment (such as hernia surgery), and show how the quality of services provided by different departments can be improved by increasing the use of modern treatments.

Notwithstanding the progress made to date, a great deal remains to be done before national quality registers can realize their full benchmarking potential. The time lag from collecting data to analysis and feedback to providers must be reduced. Local accessibility also needs to be improved, and the information should preferably be provided on-line.

National quality registers have been evaluated twice by an external board. The first evaluation found that one of the positive effects of registers was an increased interest in quality-related issues. However, it also noted that more data could have been provided through these registers and recommended greater openness. The second evaluation came up with similar conclusions, although it acknowledged that progress had been made in terms of data collection and openness.

An initial problem associated with increased openness was the media interest in seeking out and exposing the "bad apples". More recently, there has been however a better understanding of the complexity in interpreting data, and increased attention has been paid to methods of disseminating comparative results on health care quality to both decision-makers and media. This has improved the attitude of managers of quality registers towards openness.

New possibilities also emerge as hospital departments and primary health care centres not only enter data in the registers but also use them for their own planning and quality management efforts. The data are increasingly referred to in annual reports and activity plans, and health authorities can use data from registers as a basis for purchasing decisions.

3. Guidelines

The production of clinical guidelines has become one of the main tasks of the National Board of Health and Welfare, working in collaboration with experts in the field. The work on guidelines runs alongside the work on registers to develop valid and relevant indicators. The intention is that, by introducing indicators of good care in guidelines and demanding an open reporting of results, this will lead to a more transparent and accurate description of health care system achievements.

The overall objective of guidelines is to enhance patients opportunities for receiving equitable, evidence-based care throughout the country. A guideline is intended to contain information on processes to follow when organising care for a certain condition. Where relevant and possible, indicators of such processes should be consistent with indicators used in the national quality register for the condition. Examples of indicators used both in quality registers and guidelines can be found, for instance, in the case of hip and knee replacement surgery (*e.g.*, proportion of re-operations, nosocomial infections). The guidelines are designed to serve as a common document for the various counties and their institutions to produce their own guidelines in which local considerations can be taken into account. They should be evidence-based, and reflect three ethical principles for prioritization: equal value of all human beings, priority given to those in greater need and cost-effectiveness.

Three common criteria have been identified and accepted as potential indicators of cost-effectiveness for use in Swedish guidelines: cost per life year saved, cost per quality-adjusted life year (QALY) and cost per disability-adjusted life expectancy (DALE) gained. There remains however a lack of relevant data in many areas of health care to implement these indicators, especially concerning specific priority groups (*e.g.*, patients with low autonomy, psychiatric patients), but work has started to fill these data gaps.

National guidelines are released in three documents, intended for different target groups: first, a main document for medical personnel developed by a working group in consultation with a reference group which includes representatives from patient organisations; second, a summary document for political and administrative decision-makers developed by the National Board; and third, an

91

information document aimed at patients and their relatives, prepared through a close co-operation between the National Board and patient organisations. National guidelines are widely distributed to all County Councils and all relevant professional and patient organisations, in order to achieve a broad consensus and general acceptance. The intention is that purchasers should request from providers an account of how the guidelines are used, and the results as measured through the quality registers and other indicators. Purchasers may require that such reporting is made public.

4. Assessment

The Swedish experience with quality registers has shown that much painstaking work is needed to develop valid and reliable indicators of health care quality. For example, mortality is a useful outcome measure for some but by no means all conditions. Careful work is needed also to adjust for different case mix.

Although openness has been an ambition of the National Board, success to date has been limited. The arguments against public reporting have centred on potential unintended consequences of publishing performance data (Smith, 1995). However, the legitimacy of a country's health care system depends on citizens believing that the system lives up to their expectations. This perception can be influenced by both political rhetoric and the public's own experiences. The experiences of the politically-strong groups may be different than the experiences of those in greatest need for health care, who may not have the same ability to express effectively their experiences and expectations. Public access to information on outcomes not only on a patient-group level but also on a population level is one way to counteract this potential bias. It is a national responsibility to provide decision-makers with as many facts as possible in order to make more informed political decisions.

Performance indicators are particularly important in areas concerning those in greatest need, such as the elderly, psychiatric patients and patients with low autonomy. However, the experience to date has been that the most valid measures are from highly specialized areas such as cardiology, hip replacement and cataract surgery. These experiences are transferable to other conditions, but success will require considerable commitment.

The public's main complaint regarding Swedish health care concerns waiting lists and waiting times. Although most county councils have made political promises that no patient should have to wait for an elective surgery more than three months, some people still have to wait for up to 12 months for certain procedures. County councils have agreed that any patient could ask for an operation in a different county if the waiting time exceeds 3 months. However, to date patients have tended to stay in their home county and continue to complain, rather than seek help in a different part of the country. Variation is large between regions, and waiting times bear no apparent relationship to resources, as measured by the number of personnel or expenditure. The registers for cataract surgery and hip replacement have waiting times as one variable and, at least in the case of cataract surgery, the register has helped to clarify the discussion by defining who should be on the waiting list and from which point to measure waiting time.

The major responsibility for improving the responsiveness of health care services lies with the county councils, and a special project is ongoing in which waiting times for 24 procedures are published on the homepage of the Federation of the County Councils (*www.lf.se*). Furthermore, various projects are seeking to improve both responsiveness and quality. Registers data have been used as tools in these processes.

Looking ahead, the objective of the planned updating of the Code of Statutes of the National Board of Health and Welfare is to report openly and on an annual basis results on the responsiveness and outcomes of health care. Subject to careful confidentiality requirements, these reports will provide aggregate data on quality of care from several perspectives: the patients, medical and other professions, and health care managers (by looking at issues such as production and resource utilisation). The intention is to put in place a comprehensive system of surveillance which will allow politicians, the public, patients, professionals, managers and the media to compare and scrutinize regularly the performance of any primary care health centre, ward, clinical institution, hospital or county council.

REFERENCES

FEDERATION OF SWEDISH COUNTY COUNCILS AND NATIONAL BOARD OF HEALTH AND WELFARE (2000),
National Health Care Quality Registries in Sweden 1999, Stockholm (available on-line at: *www.sos.se*/FULLTEXT/ 0000-046/0000-046.*pdf*).

SMITH, P. (1995),
"On the unintended consequences of publishing performance data in the public sector", *International Journal of Public Administration*, No. 18, pp. 277-310.

Annex

ACTIVE QUALITY REGISTERS IN SWEDEN (AS OF 2001)

Cancer

National Quality Register for Rectal Cancer Surgery

National Prostate Cancer Register

National Register of Bladder Cancer

Scandinavian Sarcoma Group Register

Swedish Register on Esophageal and Gastric Cardia Cancer

National Quality Register on Cervical Cancer Screening

Register on Stomach Cancer

Prospective Register on Malignant Melanoma of Skin

Endocrine diseases

National Diabetes Register

National Register for Juvenile Diabetes

Mental illness, syndromes and behavioral disorders

National Quality Register on Eating Disorders at Special Psychiatric Units

Psychiatric Register for Multidimensional Evaluation

Diseases of the nervous system

Register on Surgery in Epilepsy Treatment

Swedish Multiple Sclerosis Register

Diseases of the eye

National Cataract Register

Quality Register on Retinal Detachment

Diseases of the circulatory system

Swedish Register on Coronary Angiography and Coronary Angioplasty

Swedish Heart Surgery Register

National Register for Cardiac Intensive Care

National Register on Cardiac Arrest Outside Hospitals

The Swedish Pacemaker Register

National Stroke Register

Swedish Vascular Surgery Register

Register on Quality Assurance in Secondary Prevention of Coronary Artery Disease

Register on Adults With Congenital Heart Disorders

Swedish Register on Endocarditis

Respiratory diseases

Oxygen and Home Respiratory Register

National Quality Register on Otorhinolaryngoly Care

Diseases of the digestive organs

National Quality Register on Hernia Surgery

Musculoskeletal diseases

National Hip-Fracture Registry

National Register on Total Hip Replacement

National Knee Replacement Surgery Register

Swedish Rheumatoid Arthritis Register

Outcome of Lumbar Spine Surgery

Swedish Register on Spinal Cord Injury

National Register on Pain Rehabilitation

Genitourinary diseases

National Register for Quality Improvement in Gynecological Endoscopy

Swedish Register for Active Treatment of Uremia

Pregnancy and obstetrics

National register for Maternal Health Care

Children and adolescence

National Register of Children on Growth Hormone Therapy

National Register for Lip, Jaw, Cleft Palette Treatment

National Peri-/Neonatal Quality Register

Quality Register on Pediatric Heart Surgery

Other areas

National Quality Register on Trauma Patients

Swedish Register on Anesthesiology

Chapter 5

PROVIDING PERFORMANCE INFORMATION FOR CONSUMERS: EXPERIENCE FROM THE UNITED STATES

by

Thomas Reilly, Gregg Meyer, Carla Zema, Christine Crofton, David Larson,
Charles Darby and Katherine Crosson[*]

Abstract

This paper provides a market-based example of using performance measurement to promote health care quality improvement. Underlying this approach is a model of informed consumers making choices among competing health care providers based on cost and quality. Providing information to consumers on quality can create incentives for providers to improve their performance as they attempt to maintain or expand their market share. The paper focuses on efforts in the United States to provide performance information to consumers. It provides an overview of current performance measurement and reporting efforts and summarizes empirical literature on the effects of such efforts on quality improvement. In brief, these efforts are in their early stages and have not yet had a large impact. The paper concludes by offering reflections on steps that can be taken to make the consumer reporting effort more effective. It suggests that there needs to be a sustained education/promotion effort to raise consumer awareness about quality and the availability of information that can be used to help make better choices. The awareness campaign needs to be closely integrated with a multifaceted infrastructure to provide clear cost and performance information and decision support. Work needs to be continued on horizontal and vertical measure development that is standardized and focused on consumers, with appropriate risk adjustment. Incentives from the market, regulation, and purchasing policy need to be aligned to assert consistent pressure for quality improvement. And, consumer reporting initiatives need to be evaluated to promote continuous improvement.

---

[*] The authors are with the Agency for Healthcare Research and Quality, United States. Address correspondence to Thomas Reilly, Ph.D., Agency for Healthcare Research and Quality, 6011 Executive Boulevard, Suite 200, Rockville, Maryland 20852. The opinions expressed are those of the authors and do not necessarily reflect the views or policy positions of the Agency for Healthcare Research and Quality.

1. Background

1.1. Overview of the choice environment

The United States has a complex, decentralized, fluid health care system. To understand consumer choice in this environment, one needs to examine the roles of purchasers, health plans, providers, and consumers.

i) Purchasers

The provision of health insurance coverage in the United States is largely employer-based (about 62 per cent of Americans have coverage through their employer). Employers are given tax incentives to purchase some kind of health care coverage for their employees. Employers typically contract with one or more health plans for this coverage. However, the type of coverage offered by employers is highly variable. Some employers contract with multiple health plans, giving employees a choice of which plan to join. Others contract with a single plan and require employees who want coverage to join that plan. In 2000, 55 per cent of people with employer-based coverage had a choice of health plans, up from 50 per cent in 1996 (Kaiser Family Foundation, 2000).

Public purchasers provide insurance coverage for subgroups of the population. The federal Medicare program provides coverage for 39 million aged (over age 65) and disabled Americans. The joint federal/state Medicaid program provides coverage for 41 million low income and disabled individuals. Other federally funded programs, including those of the Department of Defense, Department of Veterans Affairs, and Federal Employees Health Benefits Program, cover an additional 18 million Americans. In general, these public purchasers offer multiple health plan options from which their enrollees can choose. However, in some geographic areas choice is limited. For example, the Medicare program contracts with managed care organisations to provide services to Medicare beneficiaries living within a defined service area. In some areas it is not sufficiently profitable for these organisations to contract with Medicare. In such areas Medicare consumers have limited choice. About 70 per cent of Medicare beneficiaries live in areas where they have health plan options, while about 30 per cent live in areas where there is only one (fee-for-service) choice available.

About 39 million Americans had no health coverage during 2000. These uninsured individuals must pay providers for their care out-of-pocket, find providers who provide charity care, or find other sources of care.

ii) Health plans

At a very general level, health plan options can be divided into fee-for-service and managed care. Under a fee-for-service arrangement, the purchaser pays a regular premium to an insurance company who reimburses providers for each covered service supplied to a patient. Consumers are generally free to go to any provider they choose. This arrangement allows maximum choice of providers, but includes few incentives for providers to control utilization and costs.

There are a variety of managed care arrangements but they all place some limitations on the choice of providers and create incentives to control costs. Purchasers contract with managed care organisations (MCOs) to provide a comprehensive set of health care services in exchange for a periodic per capita payment set in advance. The MCO bears the risk of any difference between the per capita payment and actual costs. The MCO contracts with a limited set of providers to provide health care services to plan members. With some exceptions, consumers who join the MCO are restricted to providers in the plan's network. Members choose one of the plan's primary care physicians, who is then the point of contact for care and referral to specialists. MCOs employ utilization management techniques and financial incentives to encourage providers in their network to control utilization.

There are several variants on the managed care model. Health maintenance organisations (HMO) and point-of-service plans (POS) employ managed care principles, but differ in the extent to which they allow consumer choice of providers. Preferred provider organisations (PPO) include features of both fee-for-service and managed care.

From the consumers' perspective, the health plan represents one level of health care choice. As noted above, some purchasers offer consumers multiple plans from which to choose, others offer only one plan.

iii) Providers

The choice of provider is another level of choice for American consumers. As noted above, the type of health plan determines the degree of choice among providers. People in fee-for-service plans have more or less unrestricted choice of physicians, hospitals, and other providers. People in managed care plans are generally limited to choice of the providers in the plan's network or pay a fee for going outside of the network. Providers frequently contract with multiple plans, so in many markets there is overlap in networks across plans.

iv) Consumers

In an ideal world, consumers would consider both cost and quality in their choice of health plans and providers. Several consumer characteristics make this challenging. First, at the health plan choice level, there is ample evidence that many consumers do not currently understand the differences between the health plan options very well. For example, Lubalin and Harris-Kojetin (1999) report that 67 per cent of respondents to a national survey said that they did not have a good grasp of the differences between fee-for-service and managed care, and many did not know the most fundamental aspects (*e.g.*, that physician choice is limited, that a referral is often needed for specialist care). Second, many consumers are only beginning to realize that the quality of health care is variable and their choices of health plans and providers can affect the care they receive (Epstein, 2000; Sofaer, 2000).

The variable nature of American health care coverage coupled with current consumer characteristics make for a complex environment in which to provide information to guide consumer choice.

1.2. *Examples of performance reporting efforts for consumers*

To date, most performance reporting efforts in the United States have focused on providing information to support the choice of health plans. Two initiatives have been prominent – the Heath Plan and Employer Data Information Set (HEDIS) and the Consumer Assessment of Health Plans Study (CAHPS). There have also been provider-level reporting initiatives in selected areas. A brief overview of these efforts follows.

i) *Health Plan and Employer Data Information Set (HEDIS)*

HEDIS is a set of standardized performance measures that assess the quality of health care and services provided by managed care plans (Farley *et al.*, 1998). It was developed by the National Committee for Quality Assurance (NCQA) in conjunction with public and private purchasers, health plans, researchers, and consumer advocates. There are eight categories or domains of measures:

- effectiveness of care (*e.g.*, breast cancer screening, childhood immunization status, beta-blocker treatment after a heart attack),
- availability and accessibility of care from providers such as primary and mental health care physicians,
- satisfaction with the experience of care,
- use of services,
- health plan stability (*e.g.*, disenrollment rates, physician turnover rates),
- costs of care,
- informed health care choice (*e.g.*, new member orientation, language translation services),
- health plan descriptive information.

99

Data for the measurements are drawn from three main sources: administrative data, including enrollment and claims/encounter data; medical records; and member surveys conducted by certified vendors. Health plans voluntarily report HEDIS data to NCQA, although increasingly public and private purchasers are requiring plans to collect these data as a condition of participation.

NCQA, which is a private nonprofit accrediting body, uses HEDIS results in their accreditation determinations. They also make the data publicly available through their *Quality Compass* database (note: plans that submit HEDIS data to NCQA for accreditation are not required to have their data reported in *Quality Compass*). HEDIS data can be used by purchasers to help determine which health plans to offer to their constituents and by consumers to choose among the plans available to them.

ii) Consumer Assessment of Health Plans Study (CAHPS)

CAHPS is an initiative to collect and report information on consumers' experiences with their health plans. It includes a rigorously tested survey protocol for collecting information from health plan enrollees on factors such as:

- access to specialists,
- quality of patient-physician interaction,
- customer service,
- reasonableness of paperwork and approvals, and
- ratings of care received.

The developmental work for CAHPS was sponsored by the Agency for Healthcare Research and Quality, with applications for Medicare, Medicaid, and commercial populations. There is a core questionnaire that applies to all settings and supplements that can be added to address the needs and interests of specific populations. For example, the Medicare program added supplements on access to prescription medications and physical, occupational, and speech therapy to address the special needs of elderly and disabled populations.

The CAHPS protocol defines standardized sampling and survey procedures that have been shown to be effective at eliciting scientifically sound responses in these settings in a cost efficient manner (Agency for Healthcare Research and Quality, 1999). A sample of 400-600 enrollees per health plan is randomly selected to take part in the CAHPS survey. The CAHPS questionnaire is completed by mail or telephone by sampled enrollees, who provide information on their experience in getting care through the plan. Results are summarized by health plan and comparative reports on plan performance are made publicly available.

CAHPS has been adopted widely. CAHPS surveys are sponsored by the Medicare program, a number of state Medicaid agencies, and a wide variety of private purchasers. A CAHPS survey is also included in HEDIS as the tool to measure patients' experiences with care. It is estimated that CAHPS data are collected on health plans available to over 90 million Americans. Like HEDIS, data from CAHPS can be used by purchasers to help determine which health plans to offer to their constituents and by consumers to choose among the plans available to them. We will use CAHPS as a case study to highlight lessons learned about performance measurement and reporting.

iii) Provider-level reporting

There are also a limited number of provider-level reporting efforts in the United States. One unsuccessful effort was by the Medicare program to report hospital-level mortality data for the Medicare population. Each year from 1986 to 1993, Medicare released actual and statistically expected mortality rates of hospitals in the United States. The data were intended to aid consumers and physicians in selecting a hospital. Although the mortality information received considerable attention in the press, its release was very controversial among health care policy makers and the hospital industry. Critics argued that the mortality data were not an accurate indicator of hospital quality. In particular, there was intense criticism that the expected mortality rates did not adequately account for the hospitals' case mix. In 1993, the Medicare program discontinued the hospital mortality reporting effort (Mennemeyer *et al.*, 1997).

Another more successful example is an initiative by the state of New York to make risk-adjusted mortality data for patients undergoing coronary-artery bypass grafting (CABG) available by hospital and surgeon (Chassin *et al.*, 1996). The state has developed a registry to collect clinical data on all patients undergoing cardiac surgery. Data on demographic variables, risk factors, and complications are collected by each hospital and forwarded to the registry on a quarterly basis. Hospital data are checked to ensure that all patients are included by comparing the list of patients to a statewide database of hospital discharges. The state ensures the accuracy of submitted data with an independent audit of a sample of data from a sample of hospitals that compares the data in the registry to information in the medical records. With the guidance of a Cardiac Advisory Committee, the state developed a risk-adjustment model that uses data in the registry to compute mortality rates for CABG patients taking into account the severity of each patient's presenting illness and coexisting conditions. The risk-adjusted mortality rates by hospital and surgeon are made available to the public each year. Although there is evidence that consumers do not make extensive use of the reports, the state believes that the public release of the data has played an important part in galvanizing hospitals to seize opportunities to improve. The state of Pennsylvania has a similar reporting effort.

HEDIS, CAHPS, and the provider-level efforts discussed above are prominent examples that illustrate performance measurement and reporting in the United States. There are a number of other related initiatives that are detailed elsewhere (see Lubalin and Harris-Kojetin, 1999).

2. Effects of reporting performance information

This section provides an overview of selected studies assessing the effects of reporting performance data for consumers, purchasers, and health plans and providers.

2.1. *Consumers*

Recent review articles indicate that performance reporting efforts have not had a large impact on consumers to date (Marshall *et al.*, 2000; Mukamel and Mushlin, 2001; Schauffler and Mordavsky, 2001). Estimated effects generally are small and not uniform across markets. At this stage, performance reporting appears to have had a limited impact on consumer decision making.

Research is identifying factors that are limiting the effectiveness of these efforts. A few examples follow. First, while consumers recognize that information on cost and covered benefits is essential when choosing a health plan, they are just beginning to recognize the importance of considering performance information, such as technical quality and consumer ratings (Edgeman-Levitan and Cleary, 1996; Isaacs, 1996; Robinson and Brodie, 1997; Tumlinson *et al.*, 1997).

Second, consumers often find performance information confusing, thereby decreasing its salience (Hibbard and Jewett, 1996, 1997). For example, a number of the report cards that were evaluated presented a large amount of performance data. Consumers are often overwhelmed by such information and simply disregard it in favor of information on cost and coverage, with which they are more familiar (Hibbard and Jewett, 1997). In addition, the salience of existing measurement efforts, which are largely focused at the health plan level, has been questioned by consumers, who most closely identify their care with individual providers and institutions.

Third, we have not isolated the situations in which consumers might find performance information most useful. Recent studies have found that the use of performance reports is greater among disenrollees (Cleary, forthcoming 2001; Schultz *et al.*, 2001). Those who are actively changing their health plan may be more receptive to performance information than those who are already in a health plan with which they are satisfied.

Fourth, consumers seek information from sources they know and trust. For example, 65 per cent of consumers rely on family and friends for information on health plans (Kaiser Family Foundation, 2000).

Many organisations that report performance information are not yet widely established as reliable, trustworthy sources of information among consumers.

Fifth, decision-making in this context is very complicated. Consumer preferences for information are diverse and still not fully understood. For example, Shultz *et al.* (2001) found that consumers prefer aggregate or summary performance measures; however, Gibbs *et al.* (1996) found that detailed information is more useful to consumers than summary measures.

2.2. *Purchasers*

Most purchasers collect performance information. Studies have estimated that approximately 75-90 per cent of purchasers collect health plan-level performance data (Fraser *et al.*, 1999; Hibbard *et al.*, 1997; Maxwell *et al.*, 2001). However, while the majority of purchasers have access to health plan performance information, results are mixed on the extent to which purchasers actually use the information.

Purchasers can use quality information for health plan choice, dissemination to consumers, and a variety of other purposes (National Committee for Quality Assurance, 1995a). Survey estimates of the percentage of private purchasers that use performance information for health plan choice generally range between 48 and 83 per cent (Marquis and Long, 2000, 2001; Maxwell *et al.*, 2001). Marquis and Long (2001) found that the likelihood of employers using health plan performance information increases with firm size. Surveys generally target larger purchasers so the estimates of the use of performance information for health plan choice are probably overestimates.

An increasing number of purchasers disseminate performance information to consumers. Maxwell *et al.* (2001) and Marquis and Long (1999, 2000) report that 22-35 per cent of large private purchasers disseminate quality information to consumers. The Medicare program makes health plan and selected provider-level performance information available to all 39 million Medicare beneficiaries (Goldstein and Fyock, 2001).

Case studies have highlighted other uses of performance measures among purchasers (Hoy and Wicks, 1996; Meyer *et al.*, 1998; Zema and Rogers, 2001). For example, one innovative use by state Medicaid programs is auto-enrollment. In many states, Medicaid beneficiaries who do not choose a health plan within a specified length of time are automatically assigned to a plan. States use health plan performance information as part of the algorithm determining which health plans receive the auto-assignments. However, these case studies usually target "cutting edge" purchasers and are not typically generalizable.

2.3. *Health plans and providers*

At the health plan level, Scanlon *et al.* (2001) and Smith *et al.* (2001) report that performance reports are used by some health plans and providers to target and set goals for specific quality improvement efforts as well as to evaluate and monitor current performance.

At the provider level, much of the evaluation work has focused on several statewide reporting efforts on the outcomes of cardiac care at the hospital and surgeon level. As noted previously, studies of these efforts suggest that although they have not had a significant impact on consumers, facilities have used the reports for quality improvement efforts (Chassin *et al.*, 1996; Marshall *et al.*, 2000; Rainwater *et al.*, 1998; Schauffler and Mordavsky, 2001; Schneider and Epstein, 1998). Based on such evidence, Marshall *et al.* (2000) argue that public reporting of performance data can improve quality because provider organisations are sensitive to their public image, even in the absence of market pressure based on consumer choice.

In sum, there have been a number recent studies evaluating the effect of performance reporting efforts. To date, results on the effects of these efforts are mixed.

3. Reflections on improving the effectiveness of reporting for consumers

A workgroup sponsored by the federal government made up of purchasers, consumer advocates, and consumer information researchers recently identified five areas that would lead to improved effectiveness of reporting performance information for consumers (Workgroup on Consumer Information, 2000): *a*) educating and motivating consumers to use performance information, *b*) improving the supply and delivery of consumer-oriented performance information, *c*) improving the supply and availability of performance measures, *d*) identifying market characteristics that support consumer use of information, and *e*) evaluating the utility and impact of consumer information efforts. We next offer some reflections on how we can improve consumer-reporting efforts through these areas.

3.1. *Educating and motivating consumers to use performance information*

As noted previously, consumers in the United States are only beginning to realize that the quality of health care varies and that their choices of health plans and providers can have important implications for the care they receive. We need to implement a sustained education/promotion effort to significantly increase consumer awareness of these fundamental points. When planning such an initiative several considerations need to be addressed (Sofaer, 2000; Sutton *et al.*, 1995):

- *Purpose*. The purpose of such an effort is to raise consumer awareness that quality varies and their choice of plans and providers will affect the quality of the care they receive. Inevitably, some consumers will be motivated by these messages, others will not. Those consumers who are motivated should be directed to sources of performance information that can support their choice.

- *Audience*. The audience for the initiative is people who are eligible to make health care choices and those who act on behalf of eligible populations (*e.g.*, some elderly consumers rely on their children for guidance in matters of health plan choice). The effort especially should be targeted to audiences who are likely to be most receptive to the message (see "Openings" below).

- *Message*. The message should be as simple as possible. It needs to communicate what we want consumers to know, what we want them to do, and why it is to their benefit to do it. For example, a message could be as simple as, "You have health care options, your choices can affect the quality of care you and your family receive, call this number for information that can help you make a good choice (toll-free number)." How the message is framed will be important. Positive framing suggests the benefit from making a good choice, negative framing suggests the harm that could be caused by a bad choice. Prior research and experience suggests that negative framing is more effective in eliciting behavior, but this must be weighed against the cost of unduly frightening consumers.

- *Openings*. The initiative should target "teachable moments" when consumers are most likely to be receptive to the message. People are unlikely to seek information until they actually need it. The education/promotion effort would want to identify times and places where consumers are most likely to need information about their health care choices (*e.g.*, initial program enrollment, open season for making changes in enrollment, notifications of plan terminations or withdrawals).

- *Channels*. The initiative would want to provide the message over and over again through multiple channels. Research would be needed to identify the important sources through which the target audience gets information. One source certainly would be through community-based information intermediaries (*e.g.*, advocacy groups). To be most successful, the initiative must establish partnerships to help spread the message through groups that consumers know and trust. Working closely with the news media would also clearly be required. The ideal is to provide persistent and inescapable cues and messages through multiple sources. The general content of the message should be delivered as consistently as possible, recognizing that it will need to be tailored to meet the needs of different parts of the audience.

This initiative cannot be a one-time effort. To significantly raise consumer awareness it will be necessary to mount a sustained education/promotion effort using multiple sources and interventions.

Activities that raise the general public awareness of quality issues also can help (Galvin, 1998). For example, the Institute of Medicine (1999) recently released a report that indicated up to 98 000 patients die each year in the United States due to preventable medical errors in hospitals. This report raised significant public concern and interest about patient safety and quality. Beginning in 2003, the US Department of Health and Human Services will begin releasing an annual report to Congress on the status of health care quality in the nation. The National Healthcare Quality Report will track the nation's progress in improving the effectiveness, safety, timeliness, patient centeredness, and equity of care provided to Americans. Such efforts can help focus public attention on health system performance.

3.2. *Improving the supply and delivery of consumer-oriented quality information*

The education/promotion effort is designed to raise consumer awareness about quality issues and that there is information to help them make better choices. This effort needs to be closely integrated with an effective infrastructure to provide performance information to consumers. Three topics are important to consider in developing this infrastructure: the presentation of performance information, dissemination channels, and decision support.

i)   *Presentation of performance information*

Several guidelines are useful for presenting performance information in ways to help consumers make choices (Hibbard *et al.*, 1997; Hibbard, 1998; Lubalin and Harris-Kojetin, 1999; Sofaer, 2000; Sofaer and Fox, 1998).

First, provide context. As noted above, many consumers lack familiarity with basic features of their health care choices (*e.g.*, difference between fee-for-service and managed care). Before we can meaningfully talk about performance, consumers need to understand the basic characteristics of their options. Materials designed to support consumer choice therefore need to provide contextual information about the options under consideration (*e.g.*, characteristics of different types of health plans).

In addition, informational materials need to provide context on how performance measures can support consumers' choice. A basic assumption of utility theory of choice is that preferences are stable (*i.e.*, consumers have well defined preferences and simple provision of information is all that you need to worry about). However, a large body of research shows that preferences may not be well defined, especially in situations where choice is complex and unfamiliar (*e.g.*, health plan choice). In these situations, preferences may be constructed in the process of deciding. Thus, choices may be sensitive to the way information is presented and framed. When faced with complexity, consumers will adopt simplified cognitive strategies. They will give more weight to factors that are well understood and have precise meaning. Many performance measures are hard for consumers to understand. Therefore they are likely to have low salience and may not be used in decision making. Materials need to provide simple, clear contextual information to help consumers understand and interpret the measures. How performance information is described will determine whether consumers understand it, how they evaluate it, and whether they use it. Box 1 presents some lessons learned from CAHPS about providing context in performance materials.

Second, keep it simple. Consumers frequently report that they want more information. However, in practice large amounts of information can be confusing and overwhelming. People can process information from a limited number of variables. Providing more than 5-7 variables actually reduces the efficiency of decision making for many consumers. In health plan choice consumers may be considering cost, coverage, availability of providers, and performance. Materials presenting performance information need to be careful not to overwhelm consumers with too many performance measures. Several strategies have been identified to try to reduce the information-processing burden:

- *Develop composite performance measures.* This approach combines individual performance measures into a smaller number of summary measures. For example, the Foundation for Accountability (FACCT) combines many HEDIS and CAHPS measures into five summary measures organized around consumer needs – the basics, staying healthy, getting better, living with illness, and

---

**Box 1.   CAHPS case study: some lessons learned about providing context
in performance materials**

You can't develop "consumer-oriented" quality information without talking to consumers. In CAHPS, our conversations with consumers took many forms: focus groups, through which we questioned different types of consumers about how they identified high-quality health plans and providers; cognitive testing, through which we asked consumers to react to examples of data displays, background text, graphic enhancements and other format features; and ultimately, outcome evaluations, through which consumers responded our "bottom line' question: Does CAHPS data help you choose a high-quality health plan appropriate for your family and circumstances?

One outstanding lesson CAHPS team members learned through testing our materials with potential users concerned the distinction between *knowing* information and *knowing how to use* information. The National Adult Literacy Survey reports that only 18 per cent of Americans have the cognitive skills to correctly use "matrixed" information, such as amortization schedules, maps – and most health plan quality reports. The distinction between "knowing" and "knowing how to use" was underscored by a comment from one of our early focus group participants. After reviewing (and comprehending) different examples of data displays, he said that he found the information helpful, but he would like to receive it *after* he selected a health plan when he "would really have time to study it". These types of reactions told us very clearly that CAHPS reports for consumers would need to include not just statistics describing consumer assessments of plans and providers, but specific instructions on how to use that information to choose a high quality health plan. These instructions took several different forms:

- A clear statement explaining that the quality of plans and providers varies, and that the plan or provider you choose can affect the quality of the care you receive.
- Graphic symbols and icons (*e.g.*, stars for ratings, a telephone icon to indicate where to go with questions) to direct the reader's attention to critical information.
- Bolded and bulleted text to highlight information relating to interpreting survey results.
- Graphic notation to quickly connect the user to specific types of information, such as assessments of the quality of care given to children.
- In one version of a computer report, an on-line host (with audio capability) talked the user through several steps leading to plan selection.

Through iterative testing, we learned our target audience required these and other types of assistance to enable them to apply survey findings to their selection decision.

---

changing needs. The problem with such approaches is that summary measures can reduce variation between plans and thus undermine the choice model.

- *Remove potential trade-offs.* Some analysts assume that cost will be a dominant factor. They suggest creating cost strata, making the cost decision first, and then looking at performance information within the cost stratum selected. This reduces the burden of cognitive processing. However, it also compromises the policy perspective that posits that cost and quality are equally important.

- *Layer information.* Some consumers want a lot of detail, many are overwhelmed by it. Providing information in layers allows consumers to drill down to the level of detail they want. Providing a clear, simple road map helps them navigate the information. Compared to print products, web-based tools are especially suitable to providing layered information.

- *Global ratings from experts.* Using accreditation or certification as a summary measure of performance suggests that the health plan or provider meets a minimum standard set by a respected state or national accrediting authority. This is intended to signify that the consumer does not need to delve further into the data but can rest assured that they are choosing a plan or provider that meets a set of professional standards. Many physician accreditors are now changing their previous lifetime certification to an ongoing process of continuing maintenance of certification, which will make such information more salient. The task for the consumer is to evaluate the credibility of the expert providing accreditation.

Third, help people understand meaningful differences. Ideas like statistical significance are very difficult for most consumers to understand. Contextual language needs to be provided to help consumers identify meaningful differences. Without guidance consumers will make their own judgments, which often misinterpret small differences. When possible, it is useful to calibrate differences in terms that are meaningful to consumers (Eddy, 1998). For example, if one were comparing plans on rates of annual mammograms, materials might say that a 10 per cent difference in mammography rate on the average corresponds to a xx per cent difference in the likelihood of detecting breast cancer early when it can be treated more effectively.

Fourth, format information in a way that is easy to follow. Information needs to be presented in a simple, clear fashion. NCQA has developed a set of useful guidelines for formatting the presentation of comparative data (NCQA, 1995b).

Fifth, make it clear that the information is trustworthy. Performance information needs to be seen as coming from a credible source (e.g., not from an organisation that stands to benefit from the rating). The problem faced by some organisations presenting performance information is that they are not known by consumers. For example, the Health Care Financing Administration administered the Medicare program but was largely unknown by Medicare beneficiaries. When it began its performance reporting efforts, it needed to establish an identity as a credible, trustworthy source of information.

ii) *Dissemination channels*

The infrastructure for providing performance information to support consumer choice needs to include multiple dissemination channels to accommodate the diversity of consumer needs and preferences (Sofaer and Fox, 1998). These would be made available by public and large private purchasers for their respective populations and might include:

- *Toll-free telephone service.* Such a service could serve at least two functions. The promotion/education effort discussed above aims to increase consumer awareness of quality issues and refer interested consumers to a source for further help. A toll-free telephone service is a good first source of help. Customer service representatives can assess the needs and preferences of the caller and refer them to an appropriate resource (*e.g.*, website, print material, in-person services). If one were willing to invest more in this service, it could also provide information directly to consumers. Callers could be triaged to customer service representatives who are trained to provide information to help consumers make health plan and provider choices.

- *Print materials.* This is the least expensive and most traditional way to make performance information available to large audiences. However, it is the least flexible in terms of presentation of the performance material.

- *Internet.* This is a very versatile resource that allows layering of information, decision support, and linkage to other relevant information and services. It can be used by the growing body of people who are familiar with the Internet and how to access information through it.

- *In-person services.* Many consumers, especially the elderly, want to talk directly with a trusted, expert source about their health care choices. Community-based counseling and consumer advocacy groups can often serve as a partner in filling this role. This channel also offers a main avenue through which decision support can be provided (see below). In-person services fill an important purpose for many consumers, but are expensive and by necessity usually limited in scope.

The ideal is to create an infrastructure that makes performance information available through multiple channels to accommodate differences in how consumers prefer to access information.

iii) *Decision support*

Health care choice can be a very complicated cognitive task. For example, in choosing a health plan consumers must consider information on cost, coverage, access to providers, and performance, and they may need to compare this information across as many as 15 health plans. Many consumers need help (Edgeman-Levitan and Cleary, 1996; Hibbard *et al.*, 1997; Hibbard, 1998; Lubalin and Harris-Kojetin, 1999; Sofaer and Fox, 1998; Sofaer, 2000). Decision support resources are an essential part of the infrastructure for providing information to consumers.

Decision support tools need to be designed to serve several functions (Hibbard, 1998; Sofaer, 2000; Sofaer and Fox, 1998):

- Provide context for thinking about the decision;
- Divide the cognitive task into small steps;
- Elicit consumer values and preferences;
- Address the trade-offs of various decisions (*e.g.*, assure that all relevant factors are considered and properly weighted).

Currently decision support resources fall into three categories:

- *Person-mediated.* As noted previously, many consumers want to work through their decision with someone in person. Information intermediaries who provide this service need to know the important aspects of choice, the characteristics and needs of the population they serve, the meaning of performance measures, and how to help people make trade-offs. This implies that training programs and materials need to be developed for information intermediaries who provide decision support services.

- *Computer-aided.* A number of commercial firms have developed interactive computer-aided decision support tools for health plan choice. The general design of these products is that they elicit information from the user about plan characteristics that are important to them (including different facets of performance), strength of preferences, and trade-offs among characteristics. Based on the data entered by the user, the tool uses an algorithm to calculate a customized score for each health plan. The plans are displayed with the highest scoring plan representing the presumed best choice for the user. Typically the scoring algorithm is proprietary for commercial decision-support tools. A major dilemma for public purchasers is how to deal with the tension between the vendor's proprietary right to guard the content and design of their product and the need for public disclosure of the algorithms the product uses to prioritize health plans.

- *Worksheets.* These are printed materials that attempt to accomplish the functions of decision support. They are inexpensive and can be used by consumers in a wide variety of settings.

3.3. Improving the supply and availability of quality measures

We need to continue to improve the supply and availability of quality measures. Issues that will be important to address include horizontal and vertical measure development, consumer focus, standardization, risk adjustment, and involvement of stakeholders.

i) *Horizontal and vertical measure development*

To date, most performance measurement and reporting efforts in the United States are based on assessments at the health plan level. We need to achieve a greater balance in measurement at this level (horizontal development). The Institute of Medicine recently defined a broad set of aims for quality in health care (*i.e.*, care should be safe, effective, efficient, timely, patient centered, and equitable). Current measurement systems do not fully represent these dimensions of quality. Further work is needed to expand current measurement to more fully capture the entire spectrum of quality.

We also need measurement that takes us "deeper" than assessment at the plan level (vertical development). From the consumer's perspective, the most essential of these measurements is the

107

assessment of health care providers (Cleary and Edgeman-Levitan, 1997). Only a few measurement efforts currently exist at this level. For example, the Medicare program has started reporting performance information for nursing homes and the Agency for Healthcare Research and Quality is working on a version of CAHPS applicable to physician group practices. However, much more development in this area is needed. Progress will likely be slow and difficult in view of the methodological issues associated with assessment of individual providers [e.g., small numbers, risk adjustment, patient confidentiality, political sensitivity (Epstein, 2000)]. However, we need to push the envelope to medical groups, hospitals, nursing homes, home health agencies, kidney dialysis facilities, and other settings.

ii) Consumer focus

Performance measurement focused on guiding consumer choice needs to attend to what consumers want to know. This is not always just the technical quality of care. For example, the quality of hospital care from the consumer perspective includes: respect for patient's values, preferences, and expressed needs; coordination of care; information, communication, and education; physical comfort and pain management; emotional support and alleviation of fear and anxiety; involvement of family and friends; and transition and continuity to home or community (Edgeman-Levitan and Cleary, 1996). It is important to represent these consumer values in our performance measurement systems. This is not to say that clinically oriented quality measures are unimportant. However, such measures often have limited meaning, and thus salience, to consumers. Consumer focus means that when clinical measures are used in consumer choice materials, clear contextual language needs to be provided that explains what the measure is and why it is important. Box 2 provides some lessons learned from CAHPS about a consumer focus in quality measurement.

Box 2.   **CAHPS case study: some lessons learned about consumer focus
in quality measurement**

To motivate consumers to read and use quality information, you need to meet them on their own ground. Only after you successfully respond to the questions that *they* identify as important will you have sufficient credibility to educate them about the issues that *you* define as important. An important part of meeting consumers on their own ground is providing them with information about health care quality as they perceive it. Some comments from focus groups illustrate how consumers perceive quality:

Provider includes me in the decision-making

"You know, the kids get that ear thing...I want to know what's causing this. Well, [the doctor] probably discussed this with five other patients behind us. And [he's] in there peeking in the kid's ear and you can see the little water or whatever it is. And he showed me. If I asked him, he'll show it to me. That's where my trust is."

Doctor speaks in a way I can understand

"[Too often, doctors use] the long words which are medical...They'll talk to you with these long words, these long terms, and you're like, 'I got what?' They could cut it down to where you could more or less tell [what they're talking about]."

Plan educates me about staying well

"Also, the plan I'm in, they educate you a lot about staying well. Not just when I get sick, I call them, but they actually contact me, keep me informed about different training. I can get involved or someone in my family, about staying well. And that's real important to me."

---

iii) Standardization

A decade ago, one of the major impediments to providing comparative data to support consumer choice was the absence of standardized measurement systems. Health plans conducted customer satisfaction surveys and the like for use in marketing, but there was no consistency in measurement between plans to allow reliable comparisons of performance. The development and wide scale adoption of HEDIS and CAHPS represented a crucial breakthrough in our ability to collect comparative data. They both include standardized measurement specification and data collection procedures used for all health plans. It is only through this standardization that we have been able to obtain comparable performance data that can reliably be used for consumer choice. Box 3 presents some lessons learned from CAHPS about standardization.

Standardization needs to be pursued in other potential areas of consumer reporting, particularly at the provider level. Efforts are currently under way in the United States to fill this need. Accrediting bodies such as NCQA and the Joint Commission for Accreditation of Healthcare Organizations (JCAHO) are working to establish core sets of standardized measures to be used by organisations seeking accreditation. The federal government continues to develop and expand existing standardized reporting systems (*e.g.*, CAHPS) and to adapt standardized measurement systems used for regulatory purposes (*e.g.*, the Minimum Data Set for nursing homes). In 1998 the President's Advisory Commission on Consumer Protection and Quality in the Health Care Industry called for the creation of the National Forum for Health Care Quality Measurement and Reporting (the Forum). The Forum is a public/private enterprise designed to promote standardization of quality measures by endorsing common sets of core measures for national use. Rather than developing quality measures, the Forum identifies and evaluates existing measures, choosing for endorsement those that meet national priorities for improving health care quality as well as scientific and technical criteria (Miller and Leatherman, 1999). The on-going success of these standardization efforts is critical to continued improvement in consumer reporting.

Box 3.   **CAHPS case study: some lessons learned about standardization**

One of our main motives in developing CAHPS instruments and reports was to improve the supply and availability – and quality – of quality measures. We learned that:

- At the time we were developing CAHPS, most quality measures applied only to a specific health care delivery system. Developers of instruments, health plans, and health care providers developed consumer assessment tools to meet their specific needs. This meant that there were a number of quality instruments out there but no standardization. No single instrument could be used to compare member responses across different type of plans. In preparing CAHPS instruments, we made sure each item and response option in the core instrument would apply across different delivery systems (*e.g.*, fee-for-service or managed care) and populations (*e.g.*, publicly and privately insured).

- Another problem was that most of the instruments available were proprietary and could be used only with the permission of the developers. The surveys we develop, as well as reporting formats and complete implementation instructions, are made available electronically at no cost to anyone who requests them.

- Many measures had not been tested thoroughly nor were they tested with consumers. It takes both time and a sizable budget to develop and test these questionnaires. Most health plans or purchasers lacked the time, personnel and money to invest in this process. The problem here is that if you don't test, you don't know whether respondents understand survey items or response options in they way you intend, or if they understand numerical summaries of the data or something as basic as your purpose in providing the information.

---

iv) Risk adjustment

Providers (and health plans) differ in the mix of patients they serve. Some have a higher concentration of patients with complications or characteristics that are outside of the provider's control and affect outcomes of care (*e.g.*, presence and severity of comorbid conditions). Reporting efforts that compare health plans or providers need to adjust measurements to account for such differences. Otherwise, a given health plan or provider may have a lower score than another on a performance measure not because they provide a lower quality of care but because they have a more complicated patient mix.

The appropriateness of risk adjustment in public reporting efforts has been a major concern for health plans and providers and at times has been a significant point of contention. Understandably, providers want performance measures to reflect the quality of care they provide, not the characteristics of their patient populations over which they have no control. The methodology of risk adjustment has made significant strides but needs to continue to improve. It will not ever be possible to perfectly adjust performance measures for case mix. However, the effort needs to progress toward the point that providers and consumers can have reasonable confidence that important confounding patient characteristics have been accounted for and differences in measurement reliably reflect differences in performance. Public and private purchasers are beginning to implement risk-adjusted payment mechanisms. As this trend continues, risk adjustment methodologies should continue to be refined.

A concern often expressed around public reporting of performance data is that, without adequate risk adjustment, providers will avoid high-risk patients. Evaluations of public reporting efforts need to carefully monitor whether such unintended consequences are occurring.

v) Involvement of stakeholders

Those who are potentially affected by the measurement should have an opportunity to provide input into measure development and reporting activities. For example representatives of health plans and providers will want to have an opportunity to provide their perspective on measures, data collection protocols, risk adjustment, and the like. The Forum provides one example of how this can be done (National Quality Forum, 2001). The Forum is governed by a 17-member Board of Directors representing health care consumers, purchasers, health plans, providers, and experts in health services research. Supporting the Board is a standing panel of experts in quality improvement and measurement charged with identifying principles and priorities to guide the national measurement and reporting strategy. Four member councils provide organisations the opportunity to take part in the national dialog about how to measure and report health care quality. There is a Consumer Council, Purchaser Council, Provider and Health Plan Council, and Research and Quality Improvement Council.

As another example, it is through the effective involvement of stakeholders that efforts like HEDIS and CAHPS have been successful at developing widely accepted, standardized performance measurement systems that have been broadly adopted.

3.4. Identifying market characteristics that support consumer use of information

Despite some notable idiosyncrasies, the US health care industry functions much like a normal market (Workgroup on Consumer Information, 2000). The structure of this market is defined by many things, including:

- the nature of competition among health care organisations (*e.g.*, the number, variety, and distinctiveness of options);

- the number and size of purchasers and their purchasing strategies;

- the mechanisms employed by regulators to protect consumers, ensure access, monitor quality, and establish minimum standards.

Such factors, along with consumer choice, can shape market behavior. If we want to maximize incentives for quality improvement these factors need to be aligned and work together. This is not

---

Box 4.   **CAHPS case study: market characteristics that support consumer information**

In July of 2001, Blue Cross of California announced plans to end their system of awarding bonuses to doctors for controlling costs and instead began to link bonus payments directly to patient satisfaction. Under this program, physician groups could receive up to a 10 per cent bonus on quarterly capitation payments by meeting criteria related to provision of high quality care. These criteria include data from patient interviews, the speed with which patient grievances are heard and resolved and CAHPS data.

Movement of the market in this direction has at least two positive effects on health care quality: it sends powerful messages to health care providers about the validity and importance of consumer assessment of their experience and to consumers themselves about their ability to directly influence the quality of care they receive.

---

always currently the case in American health care. At times the forces of consumer choice, regulation, and purchasing strategy pull health care organisations in different directions.

One initiative attempting to bring about better alignment of incentives to promote health care quality is the Leapfrog Group. This is a consortium of Fortune 500 companies and other large purchasers who provide health benefits to 26 million Americans. Under Leapfrog, these employers have agreed to base their purchase of health care on principles encouraging higher quality, particularly in the area of patient safety. The principles are (Leapfrog Group, 2001):

- educating and informing enrollees about patient safety and the importance of comparing health care provider performance, with initial emphasis on the Leapfrog safety measures;

- recognizing and rewarding health care providers for major advances in protecting patients from preventable medical errors;

- holding health plans accountable for their role in improving patient safety;

- building the support of benefits consultants and brokers to utilize and advocate for the Leapfrog purchasing principles with all of their clients.

Initially, the Leapfrog effort will make information on whether plans and providers meet the "safety leaps" available to their employees. In the future, this could evolve into a more direct purchasing strategy. When this happens, the initiative would integrate the provision of performance information to consumers, purchasing strategy, and plan accountability. Such alignment of incentives can serve to assert consistent pressure for quality improvement and should be encouraged where possible.

Box 4 presents a CAHPS example of integrating purchasing policy and consumer-based performance information.

3.5. *Evaluating the utility and impact of consumer information efforts*

In order to move the consumer reporting effort forward it will be necessary to continue to evaluate these initiatives and identify ways to improve based on the results of the assessments. This should be standard practice in consumer reporting initiatives.

This said, we need to focus on the right set of outcomes, at the right time, and avoid premature assessment of long-term outcomes. The effort to inform consumers about the quality of food products (*e.g.*, salt and fat content) fundamentally changed the way food products are produced in this country. Products that are lower in salt and saturated fat are being produced in response to incentives generated by consumer demand for higher quality products. It needs to be kept in mind though that it took many years for this process to take hold. There were sustained education/promotion initiatives to raise consumer awareness of the dangers of salt and cholesterol, coupled with clear reporting of quality (*e.g.*, salt and fat content) on the product itself.

Given how unfamiliar consumers are currently with their health plan choices, it is unreasonable to expect that early attempts at providing performance information will fundamentally change the quality of health care. A much larger, sustained effort will be required.

We need to clearly articulate the steps through which consumer reporting interventions are expected to achieve improved health care quality. One can then evaluate the extent to which we are making progress on intermediate outcomes and make adjustments as necessary. As intermediate goals are achieved we will make progress on the long-term goal of quality improvement.

A range of evaluation activities will be helpful in this enterprise and can be used to guide on-going improvement in the effectiveness of performance reporting for consumers (Sofaer, 2000):

- formative research (*e.g.*, focus groups and cognitive testing on comparative materials);
- needs assessments (*e.g.*, for design of training programs for information intermediaries);
- feasibility studies (*e.g.*, to estimate the costs of large scale interventions);
- laboratory studies (*e.g.*, on framing strategies);
- process evaluations (*e.g.*, how was a consumer reporting program actually implemented in the field);
- outcome measurement (*e.g.*, to gauge the effect produced by an awareness or reporting intervention).

Box 5 presents an example of some lessons learned from CAHPS about evaluation.

Box 5. **CAHPS case study: some lessons learned about evaluation**

One of the hallmarks of CAHPS is that the project provided sufficient time and budget to evaluate our products and procedures as we developed them and after they were in use. Both process and outcome evaluations provided valuable information to help refine updated versions of products.

Process evaluation refers both to iterative testing of draft materials with the target audience as well as obtaining user feedback about how final versions of products and procedures work in their intended settings. Both activities are critical elements of a thorough program evaluation and can provide valuable information about why how the products succeeded or failed. For example, in one of our early evaluation sites, our analyses revealed that consumers failed to select the plan that received the highest rating (which happened to be the plan with the lowest membership) and frequently chose a plan with much higher membership but low CAHPS ratings. We were puzzled by this pattern until we learned, through the process evaluation, that the highest rated plan had been eliminated from the roster of alternatives because they had mentioned these ratings in advertisements (a practice which, as they learned too late, violated state rules). We also learned that enrollment counselors had encouraged people to select the lowest rated plan, figuring that the ratings had to be inaccurate since it had been the alternative with the highest membership for several years! In the absence of the process evaluation, we would have concluded that our intervention, the CAHPS report, was ineffective in influencing people to select high quality plans.

In general, outcome evaluation seeks to answer the question, "Did the intervention achieve the expected results?" A challenge here for the CAHPS team was to determine exactly what results we expected. "Voting with your feet", or leaving a health plan whose members have assessed its quality as relatively low, might appear to be the obvious indicator. But there are other indicators as well. For example, in our evaluation in Washington state, we asked plan members whether CAHPS information was easy or hard to understand (only 11.7 per cent rated it "hard" or "very hard") and how helpful the information was for the decision to stay with that plan or not (70 per cent described it as "somewhat" or "very helpful"). We also asked these consumers to identify the source that provided the most important information about the health plan. Of eight alternatives (CAHPS report, print material from employer, benefit fair, internet, print material from plans, talking with co-workers, newspapers/magazines), the CAHPS report was identified most often (by 28.1 per cent of respondents) as the most important source of information. Obtaining information to multiple outcome questions like these provides a richer, fuller picture of the effects of providing CAHPS information to potential users.

Assessment of the extent to which we are making progress in the areas identified by the Workgroup on Consumer Information (see discussion above) would be an important component of an overall evaluation scheme.

4. Summary and conclusions

Measuring quality is fundamental to improving it. When there is no public disclosure of performance information, competition is based on cost. Providing health care performance information is an important part of checks and balances in health care. When consumers have information on cost and quality they can make choices based on their best overall value (Epstein, 1995; Hibbard *et al.*, 1997; McGlynn, 1997).

Performance information can support decision making at several levels. Information on health plans can help purchasers select plans with which they want to contract and can help consumers choose among the plans available to them. Performance information on providers can help health plans identify providers to include in their networks and can help consumers select the providers from whom they want to receive care. The provision of performance information therefore has the potential to support choice mechanisms that can create incentives to improve performance throughout the health care delivery system.

It is also important to reiterate that the public reporting of performance data can improve quality even in the absence of market pressure based on consumer choice because provider organisations are sensitive to their public image and want to perform well. A combination of such internal motivation coupled with market pressure from consumer choice has the potential to be a potent force for quality improvement.

The effort to inform consumers about quality is in its childhood. To be a significant contributor to quality improvement the effort needs to move beyond its current state. In this paper we have offered reflections on how the effort can continue to move forward. There needs to be a sustained education/ promotion effort to raise consumer awareness about quality and the availability of information that can help them make better choices. The awareness campaign needs to be closely integrated with a multifaceted infrastructure to provide clear cost and performance information and decision support. Work needs to be continued on horizontal and vertical measure development that is standardized and focused on consumers, with appropriate risk adjustment. Incentives from the market, regulation, and purchasing policy need to be aligned to assert consistent pressure for quality improvement. And, consumer reporting initiatives need to be evaluated to promote continuous improvement.

REFERENCES

AGENCY FOR HEALTHCARE RESEARCH AND QUALITY (1999),
  CAHPS 2.0 *Survey and Reporting Kit*, Washington, DC.

CHASIN, M., HANNAN, E. and DEBUONO, B. (1996),
  "Benefits and hazards of reporting medical outcomes publicly", *New England Journal of Medicine*, Vol. 334, No. 6, pp. 394-398.

CLEARY, P. (2001),
  Personnel communication on 9/10/01 regarding forthcoming study of health plan choice among employees of the Washington Health Care Authority.

CLEARY, P. and EDGEMAN-LEVITAN, S. (1997),
  "Health care quality: incorporating consumer perspectives", *Journal of the American Medical Association*, Vol. 278, No. 19, pp. 1608-1612.

EDDY, D. (1998),
  "Performance measurement: problems and solutions", *Health Affairs*, Vol. 17, No. 4, pp. 7-25.

EDGEMAN-LEVITAN, S. and CLEARY, P. (1996),
  " What information do consumers want and need?", *Health Affairs*, No. 15, pp. 42-56.

EPSTEIN, A. (1995),
  "Performance reports on quality – Prototypes, problems, and prospects", *New England Journal of Medicine*, No. 333, pp. 57-61.

EPSTEIN, A. (1998),
  "Rolling down the runway: the challenges ahead for quality report cards", *Journal of the American Medical Association*, Vol. 279, No. 21, pp. 1691-1696.

EPSTEIN, A. (2000),
  "Public release of performance data: a progress report from the front", *Journal of the American Medical Association*, Vol. 283, No. 14, pp. 1884-1886.

FARLEY, D., McGLYNN, E. and KLEIN, D. (1998),
  Health Plan Reporting Patterns for HEDIS Performance Measures, The RAND Corporation, Santa Monica, CA.

FRASER, I., McNAMARA, P. and LEHMAN, G.O., ISAACSON, S. and MOLER, K. (1999),
  "The pursuit of quality by business coalitions: a national survey", *Health Affairs*, No. 18, pp. 158-165.

GALVIN, R. (1998),
  "Are performance measures relevant?", *Health Affairs*, Vol. 17, No. 4, pp. 29-31.

GIBBS, D.A., SANGL, J.A. and BURRIS, B. (1996),
  "Consumer perspectives on information needs for health plan choice", *Health Care Financing Review*, No. 18, pp. 55-73.

GOLDSTEIN, E. and FYOCK, J. (2001),
  "Reporting CAHPS quality information to Medicare beneficiaries", *Health Services Research*, Vol. 36, No. 3, pp. 477-488.

HIBBARD, J.H. (1998),
  "Use of outcome data by purchasers and consumers: new strategies and new dilemmas", *International Journal for Quality in Health Care*, Vol. 10, No. 6, pp. 503-508.

HIBBARD, J.H. and JEWETT, J.J. (1996),
  "What type of quality information do consumers want in a health care report card?", *Medical Care Research and Review*, No. 53, pp. 28-47.

HIBBARD, J.H. and JEWETT J.J. (1997),
  "Will quality report cards help consumers?", *Health Affairs*, No. 16, pp. 218-228.

HIBBARD, J.H., SLOVIC, P. and JEWETT, J.J. (1997),
  "Informing consumer decisions in health care: implications from decision-making research", *The Milbank Quarterly*, No. 75, pp. 395-414.

HIBBARD, J.H., JEWETT, J.J., LEGNINI, M.W. and TUSLER, M. (1997),
"Choosing a health plan: do large employers use the data?", *Health Affairs*, No. 16, pp. 172-180.

HOY, E.W. and WICKS, E.K. (1996),
"Forland RA. A guide to facilitating consumer choice", *Health Affairs*, No. 15, pp. 9-30.

INSTITUTE OF MEDICINE (1999),
To Err Is Human: Building a Safer Health System, National Academy Press, Washington, DC.

ISAACS, S.L.. (1996),
"Consumers' information needs: results of a national survey", *Health Affairs*, No. 15, pp. 31-41.

KAISER FAMILY FOUNDATION AND THE AGENCY FOR HEALTH CARE POLICY AND RESEARCH (2000), *Americans as Health Care Consumers: An Update on the Role of Quality Information*, Menlo Park, CA.

LEAPFROG GROUP (2001),
Fact Sheet, Washington, DC.

LUBALIN, J. and HARRIS-KOJETIN, L. (1999),
"What do consumers want and need to know in making health care choices?", *Medical Care Research and Review*, No. 56, pp. 67-102.

MARQUIS, M.S. and LONG S.H. (1999),
"Trends in managed care and managed competition, 1993-1997", *Health Affairs*, No. 18, pp.75-88.

MARQUIS, M.S. and LONG, S.H. (2000),
"Who helps employers design their health insurance benefits?", *Health Affairs*, No. 19, pp. 133-138.

MARQUIS, M.S. and LONG, S.H. (2001),
"Prevalence of selected employer health insurance purchasing strategies in 1997", *Health Affairs*, Vol. 20, No. 4, pp. 220-230.

MARSHALL, M.N., SHEKELLE, P.G., LEATHERMAN, S. and BROOK, R.H. (2000),
"The public release of performance data: what do we expect to gain? A review of the literature", *Journal of the American Medical Association*, No. 283, pp. 1866-1874.

MAXWELL, J., TEMIN, P. and WATTS, C. (2001),
"Corporate health care purchasing among fortune 500 firms", *Health Affairs*, No. 20, pp. 181-188.

McGLYNN, E. (1997),
"Six challenges in measuring the quality of health care", *Health Affairs*, Vol. 16, No. 3, pp. 7-21.

MENNEMEYER, S., MORRISEY, M. and HOWARD, L. (1997),
"Death and reputation: how consumers acted upon HCFA mortality information", *Inquiry*, Vol. 34, No. 2, pp. 117-128.

MEYER, J.A., WICKS, E.K., RYBOWSKI, L.S. and PERRY, M.J. (1998),
Report on Report Cards, Vol. I and II, Economic and Social Research Institute, Washington, DC.

MILLER, T. and LEATHERMAN, S. (1999),
"The national quality forum: a 'me-too' or a breakthrough in quality measurement and reporting?", *Health Affairs*, pp. 233-237.

MUKAMEL, D. and MUSHLIN, A. (2001),
"The impact of quality report cards on choice of physicians, hospitals, and HMOS: a midcourse evaluation", *The Joint Commission Journal on Quality Improvement*, No. 27, pp. 20-27.

NATIONAL COMMITTEE FOR QUALITY ASSURANCE (1995a),
Health Plan Performance Data: Are Purchasers Providing Results to Consumers?, Washington, DC.

NATIONAL COMMITTEE FOR QUALITY ASSURANCE (1995b),
NCQA Consumer Information Project, Focus Group Report, Washington, DC.

NATIONAL QUALITY FORUM (2001),
The National Forum for Health Care Quality Measurement and Reporting, Washington, DC.

RAINWATER, J.A., ROMANO, P.S. and ANTONIUS, D.M. (1998),
"The California hospital outcomes project: how useful is California's report card for quality improvement?", *Joint Commission Journal for Quality Improvement*, No. 24, pp. 31-39.

ROBINSON, S. and BRODIE, M. (1997),
"Understanding the quality challenge for health consumers: the Kaiser/AHCPR Survey ", *Joint Commission Journal on Quality Improvement*, No. 23, pp. 239-244.

SCANLON, D.P., DARBY, C., ROLPH, E. and DOTY, H.E. (2001),
"The role of performance measures for improving quality in managed care organizations", *Health Services Research*, No. 36, pp. 619-641.

SCHAUFFLER, H.H. and MORDAVSKY, J.K. (2001),
"Consumer reports in health care: do they make a difference?", *Annual Review of Public Health*, No. 22, pp. 69-89.

SCHNEIDER, E.C. and EPSTEIN, A.M. (1998),
"Use of public performance reports", *Journal of the American Medical Association*, No. 279, pp. 1638-1642.

SCHULTZ, J., CALL, K.T., FELDMAN, R. and CHRISTIANSON, J. (2001),
"Do employees use report cards to assess health care provider systems?", *Health Services Research*, No. 36, pp. 509-530.

SMITH, F., GERTEIS, M., DOWNEY, N., LEWY, J. and EDGMAN-LEVITAN, S. (2001),
"The effects of disseminating performance data to health plans: results of qualitative research with the medicare managed care plans", *Health Services Research*, No. 36, pp. 443-463.

SOFAER, S. (2000),
"Informing older consumers about health care quality: issues in implementing a research and action agenda", Paper prepared for conference on Informing Consumers about Health Care Quality, December.

SOFAER, S. and FOX, K. (1998),
"Providing Medicare beneficiaries with useful quality information to compare HMOs", Report for the Medicare Quality Information Project, The Commonwealth Foundation.

SUTTON, S., BALCH, G. and LEFEBVRE, R. (1995),
"Strategic questions for consumer-based health communications", *Public Health Reports*, No. 110, pp. 725-733.

TUMLINSON, A., BOTTIGHEIMER, H., MAHONEY, P., STONE, E.M. and HENDRICKS, A. (1997),
"Choosing a health plan: what information will consumers use?", *Health Affairs*, No. 16, pp. 229-238.

WORKGROUP ON CONSUMER INFORMATION (2000),
"Informing consumers about health care quality: a proposed agenda for research and action", Paper prepared for conference on Informing Consumers about Health Care Quality, December.

ZEMA, C.L. and ROGERS, L. (2001),
"Evidence of innovative uses of performance measures among purchasers", Health Care Financing Review, No. 22, pp. 35-47.

Chapter 6

CAN A TULIP BECOME A ROSE? THE DUTCH ROUTE OF GUIDED SELF-REGULATION TOWARDS A COMMUNITY-BASED INTEGRATED HEALTH CARE SYSTEM

by

Niek Klazinga, Diana Delnoij and Isik Kulu-Glasgow[*]

Abstract

The Dutch health care system has both in financing and health care provision a hybrid nature. Financing is realized through a mixture of public and private insurance executed by care insurers with a (semi) private status. Health care is provided through professions and institutions that function to a large extent as not-for-profit private entities within a highly regulated context, reimbursed through a mixture of budgetary, pro-capita and fee-for-service schemes. The role of the state has changed over the years. Roughly one can claim that in the fifties and sixties the welfare state was created, in the seventies and eighties government tried to control the growing costs through managing the structure of health care by planning regulation and in the nineties the processes within the system (regulated market) were the main policy paradigm. At the turn of the century the steering paradigm is shifting towards the input (needs assessment) and outcome (performance measurement) of the system. Not only production and costs, but also performance in terms of health outcomes and consumer satisfaction are deemed relevant management factors. This shift is facilitated by the present perceived performance crisis (waiting times are a pressing political issue) and a public call for more transparency. One of the challenges in creating this new steering paradigm lies in linking the various quality management activities set up since 1989 with a stronger public health orientation and community participation. Performance indicators can only be of use if they are part of existing management cycles either set up for internal process control and improvement or for external accountability. This paper will explore the following:

- First the nature of the Dutch health care system and the rationale of the existing policy and management mechanisms will be explained in more detail. Self regulation plays an important part in the Dutch health care system. This is partly due to the historical (not for profit) private nature of the main part of the system and a consensus culture for policy making.

- Secondly the results of a national policy on quality of care will be discussed. This policy, based on the premise that care providers should develop quality systems for internal process control and external accountability towards consumers and insurers, has been in place since 1989. Various components of the national quality policy will be discussed both for health care institutes (*i.e.* quality systems and certification/accreditation) and professions (relicensing, external peer-review, practice guidelines, clinical indicators and audit). The functioning of these various components will be discussed and linked to the debate on performance indicators.

- Thirdly an analysis will be provided of the strengths and weaknesses of the Dutch approach in optimizing the overall performance of the health care system. To do this, data on the public

---

[*] Department of Social Medicine, Academic Medical Centre, University of Amsterdam, Meibergdreef 9, 1105 AZ Amsterdam, The Netherlands, phone +31 20 566 4892, fax +31 20 697 2316, email *n.s.klazinga@amc.uva.nl*.

---

health situation will be presented that are collected regularly for the Public Health Forecasting Scenario's (RIVM 1997). By focussing on the performance of individual health care institutes and organized groups of professionals, the overall performance of the system is not an integrated part of the existing management cycles. Although government initiates specific public health policies in areas of concern, the preventative function, the cure and care function and the social care function are to a large extent separate entities. The analyses will show how the development of community-based integrated care takes place in a health care system dominated by self-regulation.

1.   What are we talking about: conceptualization and operationalization

In the title of the conference "Measuring Up: Improving Health System Performance in OECD Countries" at least four different concepts are introduced. These are the concepts "health system", "performance", "improvement" and "measurement". The assumption is that the four concepts can be operationalized and linked to one another in a meaningful way. In this paper we will explore to what extent this can be done for one country, The Netherlands. This paper therefore presents a case study that illustrates the complexity of linking the four concepts but it may also contain some lessons for other countries going through similar processes. In a recent paper on the applicability of complex adaptive system theory on health care systems, Plsek argued that it is helpful to speak about health care systems in organic rather than mechanical metaphors (Plsek, 2000). It is for this reason that we decided to present the Dutch health care system as a tulip. The tulip is a national symbol. Its leaves are rather well organised around the stem and, when fresh, it has no smell. Some people like the symmetry of the tulip, others see it as a rather dull flower. The ambition is to turn it into a rose. Flowers with a more compassionate symbolism, a larger amount of loosely but compact integrated leaves and a nice smell. In this paper we will try to describe the route the Dutch health care system takes in turning from a tulip into a rose.

In essence we conceptualize the health care system as the compilation of organized efforts of society (public as well as private) to help its population to produce health. We conceptualize performance as the realization of the common felt goals of the health care system on medical effectiveness, responsiveness, efficiency and equity. We conceptualize improvement as the policies and activities related to quality of care and we conceptualize measurement as the attempts to transform information on the health of the Dutch population and production of its health services into indicators that can be used in the existing management- and policy frameworks. Emphasis in this paper will be on the dimensions of medical effectiveness and responsiveness as this is our own field of expertise but discussions on efficiency and equity of the Dutch health care system, which are usually led by health economists (Van Doorslaer et al., 2000; Elsinga and Rutten, 1997; Scheerder and Schrijvers, 1998), will not be ignored. As with every case-study in international comparative research, the more understanding the reader has of the specific internal dynamics of the system the more prudent he or she will be in drawing generalizable conclusions (Øvretveit, 1998). Therefore we start our paper with a short description of some important characteristics of the Dutch health care system. Then we will present an overview of the results of a national policy on quality of care that has been in place since 1989 and is based on the principles of guided self-regulation. It has resulted in many initiatives in the field of quality system development emphasising the presence of functioning quality systems rather than focusing on indicators. Thirdly the strength and weaknesses of the Dutch approach will be discussed. In the fourth paragraph the Dutch situation will be compared with developments in other OECD countries.

2.   The Dutch health care system: becoming a tulip

Like many Western health care systems, the modern Dutch health care system has its roots in the second half of the nineteenth century. Industrialization and the development of the nation state created conditions under which public health issues were addressed collectively and later on regulation of academically trained medical professions and hospitals took place. It should be noted, however, that until the seventies of the twentieth century the role of the national government with

---

Box 1. **Characteristics of and problems in the Dutch health care system**

- Health care is financed through a mix of private and public insurance schemes. The public insurance schemes are regulated through the Sick Fund Law (ZWF), covering most of the curative sector (*e.g.* hospitals, physicians) and prescription drugs, and the Catastrophic Illness Act (AWBZ), covering most of the care (*e.g.* nursing homes, homes for the elderly, home care).
- Private insurers and Sick Funds have merged in the past decade into a limited number of care insurers of which the majority works on a regional level.
- The Netherlands has a well-developed primary health care system in which GPs play a gatekeeper role.
- Municipal Public Health Offices who fall under the jurisdiction of (a collection of) municipalities execute preventive care on population level.
- At present there is a labour shortage in many health care professions
- Because of waiting lists, incidents and quality problems health care is high on the political agenda

---

respect to health care was limited. Major initiatives were taken by the emerging medical profession itself and the transformation of hospitals from care institutes for the poor into science-based cure institutes was mainly the achievement of local communities and the church. During the first half of the twentieth century, government was not able to introduce a common insurance scheme for health care costs. The German occupier introduced the Sick-Fund law, which still forms the basis of the present social health insurance, in 1941. Historically it makes sense that the provision of health care is mainly privately organised on a not-for profit basis. Self-regulation has always been the dominant management philosophy of the Dutch government and a limited set of laws and an inspectorate of health were since 1865 the main ways the government controlled and assessed the performance of the health care system. The annual reports of the inspectorate of health can be read as a compilation of health system performance indicators *avant la lettre*. Box 1 presents the basic features of the Dutch health care system, and the dominant problems it currently experiences.

Government became more interested in health care in the seventies. In addition to the social health insurance act (ZFW, "Ziekenfondswet"), which covered acute care costs for around 61 per cent of the population earning less than two times the average income (the other 39 per cent had private insurance), a national insurance scheme for catastrophic illness (covering the costs of chronic care and mental health care) was introduced in 1967. This law, the AWBZ ("Algemene Wet Bijzondere Ziektekosten"), proved to be an incentive for the development of nursing homes and home for the elderly. Although the AWBZ was based on the changing care needs of an ageing population, the main driving force for the government to become involved in health care policy making was the economic recession and the need for cost containment. Like in other countries in the seventies the quickly rising costs of health care were regarded as an undesirable collective burden and between 1974 and 1987 the Dutch government tried to influence the costs of the system through planning regulation. Various attempts were made to limit the expansion of health care, notably through health manpower planning (*i.e.* the number of yearly medical students dropped from 2000 to 1485), reduction of bed-capacity (4 per cent norms) and a budgetary regime. The enforcement of planning regulation in a health care system in which the majority of services are of a private- not for profit nature and the formal instruments for government control are limited, created a lot of tension. In 1987 it was concluded that the prevailing policies were stifling the health care system. The change was made towards a steering philosophy based on the principles of a regulated market. This philosophy seemed to fit best with the history of self-regulation and the ambitions of providers and patients, as well as those of Sick Funds and private health insurers.

Although policy plans, like the Dekker plan in 1987, embraced the principles of a regulated market, budget systems as the one for hospitals introduced in 1983 remained in place. The performance of the

---

health care system was increasingly monitored on costs. The annual financial overviews of costs in the health sector were gradually transformed into expenditure targets and caps. The government was changing its monitoring role into a management role. Cost data and production data of the various health sectors alongside data on waiting lists in the nineties became performance indicators that actually seemed to be used for policy making.

Performance indicators on the *effectiveness* of the health care system were developed in the aftermath of the WHO health for all policy but have during the past 20 years never really been taken up as instruments for navigating the health care system (Van Herten, 2001). *Efficiency* of the health care system was not expressed in indicators but the prevailing philosophy was that the internal market would enhance efficiency. Performance data on *equity* were used as part of the discussions on necessary reforms in the insurance system. When attempts to combine the social health insurance for acute care (ZFW) and chronic care (AWBZ) in the late eighties and early nineties were made, the aim to limit the differences between social and private insurance schemes and thus improve equity was one of the driving forces. When these attempts failed politically, it had to wait until 2001 before a Dutch cabinet came with proposals to combine the two insurance schemes in one basic insurance scheme for the whole population executed by care insurers who are a merger of the former social and private insurers (Ministry of Health, Welfare and Sports, 2001). The *responsiveness* of the system is measured *ad hoc* through satisfaction surveys but is operationalized mainly through policies that enforce the role of the consumer. Patient organisations have become a more important player in the health policy field and legislation on patient rights has enforced the position of the individual patient.

So far, however, there is not an overall performance framework that measures the performance of the health care system as a whole on each of the four dimensions; effectiveness, responsiveness, efficiency and equity. There are many policies and mechanisms in place that focus on improvement of the system and within these mechanisms various services (like hospitals, GP's, home-care organisations, nursing homes) are building indicators into their quality systems for either internal or external use.

However, data on health care are mainly collected per sector. Data on health on population level are collected by the Municipal Public Health Offices and by the RIVM (State Institute for Environment and health) the Central Bureau for Statistics (CBS) and the Social and Cultural Planning Bureau (SCP). In addition medical performance data are collected through various national and regional registries set up by the medical profession (*i.e.* oncology, obstetrics, surgery). Table I provides an overview of information sources on the Dutch health care system.

Thus, the health care system resembles a tulip. All leaves are neatly arranged alongside and each by itself monitors its performance. Real integration of all leaves is not taking place. So far government liked tulips, but over the past two decades they became aware that the public (demand), the soil (economic circumstances and epidemiological need) and even the leaves themselves want roses. Emphasis has so far been on fertilising the soil and facilitating integration of the leaves. The art of smelling by performance indicators is developing slowly.

3. Quality policies and quality systems: the promise of a rose garden

The introduction of government policies based on the principle of a regulated market in the eighties caused mixed reactions. On the one hand the corporate bodies in the Dutch health care system such as the Royal Dutch Medical Association, the Hospital Association, the Sick Funds and the emerging patients organisations welcomed the extension of the possibilities for self-regulation. On the other hand they feared too strong commercial interests in health care that would not be in accordance with the predominantly social and equitable culture of Dutch society. With the negative side effects of the planning policies still in the back of their minds, the general opinion was that the introduction of a regulated market should go alongside a nation wide policy on quality of care. Thus the quality of care of professionals and health care services were to be monitored and improved under the new legislative and financial regime. In 1989 the first national conference on quality of care was held, hosted by the medical association with around 40 corporate organisations of providers, patients and financiers present and government and the inspectorate of health attending in an observer role. During this

Table 1. **Examples of information sources in the Dutch health system**

Parameter	Types of indicators	Frequency of data collection, type of data	Registration name, collecting institute
Demography	• Age-sex distribution of the population • Birth rate, death rate • Life expectancy etc.	Continuously, census data	"Bevolkingsstatistiek" (population statistics), CBS (Central Bureau of Statistics)
Population health	• Incidence and prevalence of diseases in the population • Incidence and prevalence of diseases in general practice • Socio-economic difference in health status etc.	Every 4 years, registrations in nationally representative samples	"Volksgezondheid Toekomst Verkenning", (public health forecasting scenarios) RIVM
Utilisation of health services	• Number of visits to GPs, specialists, physiotherapists per non-institutionalised inhabitant per year	Every year, survey of a nationally representative sample	"Gezondheidsenquête" (health questionnaire), CBS (Central Bureau of Statistics)
Production of health services	• Number of GP contacts • Number of referrals by GPs to specialists per diagnosis per 1 000 enlisted patients • Number of prescriptions per 1 000 enlisted patients	Continuously, registration in a nationally representative sample	"Landelijk Informatie Netwerk Huisartsenzorg" (national GP information network) (LINH), Nivel/NHG/LHV/WOK
	• Number of hospital admissions per diagnosis • Length of stay in hospital per diagnosis • Number of procedures conducted in hospital etc.	Continuously, registration in hospitals	"Landelijke Medische Registratie" (national medical registration) (LMR), Prismant
	• Number of visits to hospital outpatient department by speciality	Yearly, survey of all hospitals	"Landelijke Ambulante Zorg Registratie" (national ambulatory care registration) (LAZR), Prismant
	• Number of admissions to nursing homes per diagnosis • Length of stay in nursing homes per diagnosis etc.	Continuously, registration in all nursing homes	"SIG Verpleeghuis Informatiesysteem" (nursing home registration) (SIVIS), Prismant
	• Number of clients receiving home care • Number of hours home care provided	Yearly (in principle; though absent in recent years), surveys of non-profit home care organisations	"Databank Thuiszorg" (home care registration), Prismant
Supply of health services	• Numbers of doctors, nurses, physiotherapists, speech therapists, occupational therapists, midwives etc.	Yearly, combination of registration and survey data	"Rapportage Arbeidsmarkt Zorg" (health manpower report) (RAZ), Nivel/Prismant/OSA, commissioned by the MoH
	• Number of hospitals, nursing homes, homes for the elderly, home care organisations etc. • Number of hospital beds, nursing home beds etc.	Yearly, different surveys	Various statistics collected by the Central Bureau of Statistics (CBS)
Health care costs	• Costs per sector specified by category (e.g. personnel vs material) and by source of financing (public/private)	Yearly, surveys and accounts	"Exploitatiekosten en opbrengsten" (financial statistics, CBS (Central Bureau of Statistics)

Source: Author.

Table 2.   **Number of licensed professionals ultimo 1999**

Profession	Number
General practitioners	7 704
Medical specialists	12 300
Public health doctors	3 000
Nursing home doctors	1 007
Dentists	7 336
Pharmacists	2 616
Midwives	1 578
Physiotherapists	17 150
Occupational therapists	2 015
Speech therapists	3 910
Dieticians	2 201
Nurses	255 850
Home helpers	125 102

Source: Rapportage Arbeidsmarkt zorg en welzijn 2000, NIVEL/Prismant/OSA.

conference the key points for a national policy were formulated that where officially endorsed during a follow-up conference in 1990.

The main points of the national policy were:

• health care professions and institutions will develop quality systems;

• these quality systems are used for reasons of internal quality improvement as well as external accountability;

• patient organisations and financiers (municipalities, public and private insurers) will be involved in the quality system development process to guarantee mutual trust;

• government will enforce these policies and role of the inspectorate of health will be to control the existence of quality systems.

In 1991 the ministry of health formally underscored these policies and initiated legislation that resulted in a series of new laws, namely on the quality of practice of individual practitioners ("BIG"), a new law on the functioning of quality systems in health care institutes and a law that regulated the formal position of health care providers towards patients/clients ("WGBO"). During the nineties many initiatives were taken to enforce already existing quality assurance mechanisms or to introduce new ones.

When we focus on the initiative taken by professions (Table 2) and institutions (Table 3) the following can be mentioned.

Table 3.   **Number and capacity of clinical institutions in Dutch health care in 1998**

Type of institution	Number
Acute care hospitals	143
Number of beds per 1 000 inhabitants	3.7
Mental hospitals	79
Number of beds per 1 000 inhabitants	1.7
Institutions for mentally handicapped	148
Number of beds per 1 000 inhabitants	2.2
Nursing homes	336
Number of beds per 1 000 inhabitants	3.7

Source: Central Bureau of Statistics (*www.cbs.nl/nl/kerncijfers/kgwo628a.htm*, March 15, 2001).

3.1. Quality system development amongst professionals

- further formalisation of training programmes;
- further formalisation of practice profiles of various professions;
- further formalisation of continuous education (*i.e.* accreditation of courses);
- introduction of obligatory re-licensing for the medical professions (1989);
- introduction of national practice guideline programmes for medical specialists (1982), general practitioners (1987), allied health professions and nursing professions;
- introduction of visitation programmes (site visits by peers) by scientific societies of the various medical specialities (1985, covering all specialities by 1998);
- peer review and audit programmes for specialists, general practitioners, nursing home physicians, specialists in social medicine, allied health professions and nursing professions (1976);
- development of clinical registries by scientific societies;
- development of clinical indicators (1998).

All these methods have there own dynamics and rationale and several studies have described their development and impact (Casparie *et al.*, 1997; Klazinga, 1996; Van Herk, 1997; Grol, 2001; Klazinga *et al.*, 1998). It is fair to state that the development of these programmes has always been a combination of driving forces within the profession (*i.e.* the need for evidence-based medicine, the need to study effectiveness and the need to explain practice variation) and external pressure (accountability towards patients, financiers and the government). Overall, the professional groups have developed a plethora of quality assurance mechanisms. These mechanisms are partly embedded in the institutions in which the professionals work and have also been used to strengthen the organisational formats in which the professions have organized their work (*i.e.* practice groups for GP's and speciality partnerships and hospital staff cooperatives for medical specialists).

3.2. Quality system developments amongst health care institutes

Health care institutes have been more active in applying industrial quality system models on their work than professionals. Off 1987 various attempts have been made to apply theories such as Total Quality Management and Continuous Quality Improvement to health care services. The most favourite models at the moment are the EFQM model, the ISO model and the North American Accreditation[*] model (Klazinga, 2000). Dutch health care institutes have since the eighties seen many quality policy plans and an influx of quality co-ordinators.

In 1995 and 2000 follow-up conferences on the national quality policy took place. For this purpose a series of evaluation studies was undertaken that tried to capture the trends in quality system development in the Dutch health care system. Some of the findings are summarised in Tables 4 and 5 that provide an impression of the use of indicators by Dutch health care institutes in 2000. In the year 2000, two-thirds of the institutional health care providers were involved in project-based quality improvement. One third was preparing for the implementation of a comprehensive, coherent quality system. Five per cent of all the institutions already had such a coherent quality system (Sluijs and Wagner, 2000).

Compared to the situation in 1995, progress has been measured mainly in the field of quality of care documents (*e.g.* the use of handbooks), with regard to the development of protocols, and with regard to the development of quality subsystems (that should eventually become a part of a comprehensive total quality system) (Klazinga, 2000).

---

[*] The EFQM (European Foundation for Quality Management) model operationalises structure and outcome elements of organisations, in contrast with the ISO (International Organisation for Standardisation) model, which mainly conceptualises an organisation in terms of processes. Both models are rooted in industry, as opposed to the North American Accreditation model, which has been developed specifically in health care.

Table 4. **Percentage of institutions in different sectors using indicators in order to monitor quality of care**

Sector	Percentage of institutions
Municipal public health departments	80
Primary health care centres	75
Hospitals	91
Home care non-profit organisations	93
Home care for-profit organisations	95
Homes for the elderly	86
Nursing homes	85
Social services	86
Social-paediatric services	82
Mental health care	76
Care for the handicapped	84

Source: Sluijs and Wagner (2000).

Table 5. **The top-3 of indicators used by health care institutions in different sectors and the percentage of institutions using them**

Sector	Top-3 of indicators	Percentage of institutions
Municipal public health departments	Production data	72
	Formal complaints	65
	Sickness absence/% of personnel quitting jobs	52
Primary health care centres	Formal complaints	61
	Production data	58
	Sickness absence/% of personnel quitting jobs	46
Hospitals	Production data	91
	Formal complaints	91
	Sickness absence/% of personnel quitting jobs	90
Home care non-profit organisations	Formal complaints	90
	Sickness absence/% of personnel quitting jobs	82
	Waiting lists/waiting times	70
Home care for-profit organisations	Formal complaints	75
	Evaluations of care plans	75
	Incidents	65
Homes for the elderly	Data on case mix	74
	Sickness absence/% of personnel quitting jobs	74
	Registration of incidents	62
Nursing homes	Sickness absence/% of personnel quitting jobs	76
	Formal complaints	75
	Incidents	72
Social services	Production data	85
	Waiting lists/waiting times	64
	Sickness absence/% of personnel quitting jobs	59
Social-paediatric services	Waiting lists/waiting times	79
	Sickness absence/% of personnel quitting jobs	61
	Formal complaints	61
Mental health care	Waiting times	55
	Case mix	50
	Formal complaints	47
Care for the handicapped	Formal complaints	79
	Sickness absence/% of personnel quitting jobs	74
	FONA	74

Source: Sluijs and Wagner (2000).

Many activities have been set in motion but a distinction can be made between quality system development focusing on the strengthening of the internal management functions of individual institutes and initiatives focused on creating accountability mechanisms. Of the latter the following developments can be noted:

- In 1996 a council for the harmonisation of external quality assurance mechanisms (HKZ) was set up on the initiative of the insurers, patients and providers associations. This council helps the various sectors in health care to develop certification schemes. These certification schemes are all fully compatible with ISO but are developed by the various health care branches themselves to assure applicability. Once the council approves certification schemes, the national certification body for industry forces certification bodies to use these schemes. Thus the ISO-itis that terrorises some other countries health care systems was contained and integrated in more health care specific accountability models. In 2001 around 20 different schemes are already approved and used for a wide array of services varying from home care, dentistry, centres for dialyses to child care centres.

- Since the early nineties the hospital sector has taken initiatives to develop an accreditation system modelled after the accreditation programmes for hospitals in North America (Joint Commission for the Accreditation of Health Care Organizations in Chicago and the Canadian Council for Accreditation in health Care in Ottawa). In 1999 the Netherlands Institute for the Accreditation of Hospitals was founded and since then a still limited group of hospitals has experienced full accreditation.

Quality system development has so far mainly been attempts to translate models to the reality of health are processes. Indicators are seen as part and parcel of the steering mechanisms implied by quality systems and therefore not as a goal in themselves. By putting the emphasis on getting quality systems in place first it might be that many Dutch health care institutes are lagging behind in indicator development compared to some other countries.

The overall conclusion of the 1995 follow-up conference on national quality policy was that quality systems were developing, but were focusing mainly on internal quality assurance of professions and institutes. The conference concluded that a broader orientation towards the interests of insurers and patients was needed. In 2000 the conference concluded that the principle of self-regulation was still endorsed but that quality system development went slow and was running the danger of freezing the existing positions of professions and institutes instead of being a vehicle for the development of more integrated care arrangements. Both the need for integrated care and more specified mechanisms for accountability were expressed during the 2000 conference. Although the link with performance measurement of the health system as a whole was not made explicitly, it is clear that this is implied by the recommendations of the last national quality conference.

4.   The art of cultivation: strength and weakness of a system based on self-regulation

The quality policies of the past decade have enforced the already existing model of self-regulation. Overall the model works fine and The Netherlands seem to have been able to keep the subtle balance between trust and criticism in health care. Although comparative research is scarce, it seems that the amount of quality assurance activities taken up by the medical and nursing profession themselves, the level of quality system development within health care institutes and the active involvement of patients in their care processes stands out favourably internationally. The corporate character of Dutch health care creates a situation of mutual dependencies that favour decision making in health care based on consensus (Van der Grinten and Kasdorp, 1999).

However, the model of self-regulation is also challenged. The Dutch health care system is a typical mix of public and private initiatives. A lot of organisations have a semi-public (independent advisory councils) or semi-private (health insurers executing social insurance schemes) nature. In the policy paradigm of the European Union this is somewhat problematic, as the EU seems to make a rather sharp distinction between public and private activities. As a result the Netherlands Competition Authority (NMA, "Nederlandse Mededingings Autoriteit") is at present questioning the legitimacy of some of the public/private arrangements made in the Dutch health care system.

Another weakness of the Dutch model is its relative inability to work towards integrated care or organised delivery systems. The present self-regulation enforces existing professions and institutes and incentives for mergers and substitution amongst professions and services are weak. The present legislation and financing structure treats prevention, cure, care and social care as separate entities (*cf.* Box 1). As a consequence necessary shared care arrangements and the integration of preventive activities in the regular activities of cure and care are hard to realise. However, the need for integrated care is recognised and recent cabinet plans propose a merger of the AWBZ and ZFW in one basic insurance package for cure and care. This would most probably enhance the further development of integrated care arrangements.

Another consequence of the focus on separate professions or types of services is that data collected for managerial purposes focus on these professions and services separately (*cf.* Table 1). The past years have seen the rise of branch reports issued by the hospital sector, the nursing home sector and the home-care sector. In addition, as a consequence of the Law on Quality of Care, every health care institute (including every group of professionals such as GP practices) is obliged to issue an annual quality report. Although these reports are a big step forward, they do not provide a coherent picture of the quality of care delivered by a regional mix of services and professionals. In this respect there is a wide gap between the performance data issued by the individual services and professionals and the public health data collected by the municipal health services. One of the major challenges ahead will be to link public health data with the performance data of individual services in a meaningful way (Klazinga *et al.*, 2001). A prerequisite is that the health care system is redesigned in such a way that on a local and regional level, the collective of health services and professionals develops a stronger focus on their overall contribution to the production of health. This community orientation is difficult to realise under a self-regulation model when financial and legislative incentives work in the opposite direction. Although the self-regulation model is functioning well in the Dutch health care system with respect to creating mutual trust and stimulating quality improvement activities, government should provide guidance towards the overall goals of health care, take initiatives to safeguard sufficient coherence in the system on a local and regional level, and assure that the system is population based instead of service based.

5. The Netherlands compared to other OECD countries

The WHO and the OECD have over the past two years taken several initiatives to compare the performance of health care systems. Figures 1, 2 and 3 illustrate the performance of The Netherlands on effectiveness (in disability-adjusted life expectancy), efficiency (in health expenditure as a percentage of GDP) and equity (in out-of-pocket expenditure as a percentage of total expenditure), according to WHO estimates.

In addition to these external benchmarks, several reports comparing the Dutch situation with other countries were produced in The Netherlands itself; a report of the ministry of social affairs, the two-annual report of the Social and Cultural Planning Bureau and an extensive research report on socio-economic differences in health. Table 6 provides a summary of the performance of the Dutch health care system based on these reports (Kramers *et al.*, 2001).

The WHO report put The Netherlands on the 17th place. This caused a lot of debate in the Dutch press but the scoring as such is not highly informative due to the calculation methodology applied and the wide confidence intervals (Klazinga *et al.*, 2001; Groenewegen and van der Wal, 2001; Mulligan *et al.*, 2000). It has however, helped to put the phenomenon of performance indicators of health systems on the political agenda. The other report, including the one from the OECD, contained more concrete handles for action. One issue arising is that the increase in life expectancy in The Netherlands is lagging behind the European Union average. This is particularly the case for women and a major cause of this is smoking. Developments in Dutch perinatal mortality are also unfavourable and are associated with a strong increase in the age at which women bear children and the growing importance of a multicultural society.

Figure 1. **Performance of the Dutch health care system on effectiveness (Disability Adjusted Life Expectancy)**

DALE (total population, at birth)

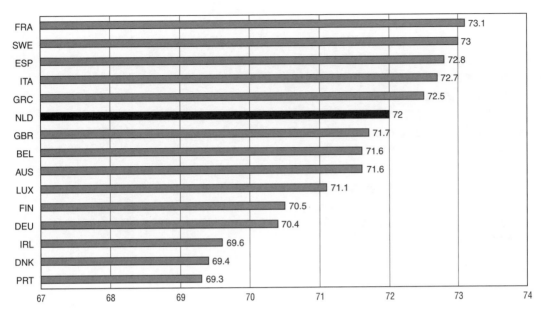

Source: WHO (2000).

Figure 2. **Performance of the Dutch health care system on efficiency (% of GDP spent on health)**

Health expenditure as % of GDP

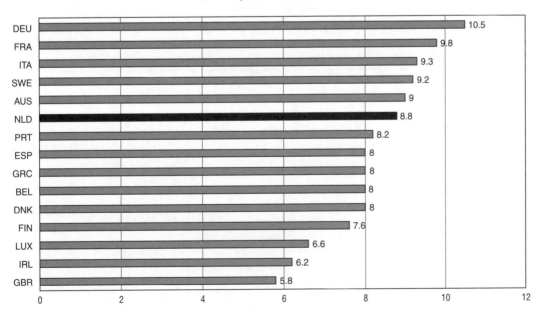

Source: WHO (2000).

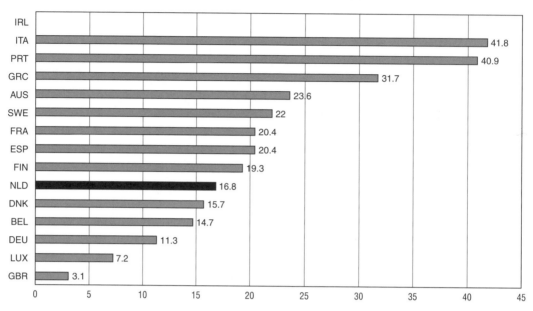

Figure 3. **Performance of the Dutch health care system equity**
(% of care financed by out-of-pocket expenditures)

Out-of-pocket expenditure as % of total expenditure

Source: WHO (2000).

These comparisons enforce public health actions rather than health system reform. The performance indicators used in these reports do not really address the acutely felled problems in the Dutch health care system such as waiting times and labour shortage. Therefore more energy should be put in conceptualising performance measures that measure the performance of the collective of services and professions with regard to their contribution to health. This asks for indicators that are far more specific than the presently used overall public health indicators on effectiveness and the generic

Table 6. **Performance of the Dutch health care system on various indicators compared to other countries in the EU and the OECD, as described by the WHO (2000), the OECD (2000), the Ministry of Social Affairs and Labour (SZW, 2000), and the Social Cultural Planning Bureau (SCP, 2000)**

Netherlands perform worse than average on the indicators:	Netherlands perform more or less average on the indicators:	Netherlands perform better than average on the indicators:
• Development of life expectancy (SCP)	• Level of life expectancy (all reports)	• Premature death in men (SCP)
• Development of infant mortality (SCP)	• Level of infant mortality (all reports)	• Subjective health status (OECD)
• Development of) smoking behaviour (SCP)	• Healthy life expectancy (SCP)	• Patient satisfaction (OECD, SZW, SCP)
• Physician density, number of medical students (OECD)	• Disability adjusted life expectancy (WHO)	• Medical consumption (SCP)
• Waiting lists (OECD)	• Premature death in women (SCP)	
• Percentage of health personnel in direct patient care (SZW)	• Level of responsiveness (WHO)	
• Development of drug expenditures	• Fairness of financial contribution (WHO)	
	• Number of consultations of ambulatory care physicians per capita (OECD)	
	• Development of) health expenditures (all reports)	
	• Level of drug expenditures (OECD)	

Source: Translation of table in Kramers *et al.* (2001).

indicators for responsiveness, equity and efficiency. Apart from looking at outcome indicators one could consider evidence-based process indicators to get a fair picture of the performance of the services in health systems and/or percentages of institutes/professions that are certified, accredited or re-licensed. Above all it must be clear in what type of policy or management cycles the indicators are integrated and unintended consequences of their publication should be avoided. The balance in the use of indicators for internal management purposes versus external accountability is a subtle one.

6. Conclusion: can we smell the rose ?

A health care system is organic and constitutes the result of many social processes. In the Dutch health care system self-regulation has always been one of the founding paradigms. Although government has since the seventies of the twentieth century tried to influence the nature and growth of the Dutch health care system, it has influenced its phenotype rather than its genotype. As a result many policy changes go slowly and depend on mutual consensus. Also, the public/private dichotomy so prevalent in the economic thinking of the EU does not apply smoothly to the Dutch situation. Looking at the ownership of services and insurers the Dutch system is one of the most liberal in Europe. Looking at the extent of not-for profit activities and social character of financing of cure as well as care and prevention activities, it contrasts sharply with the United States. To improve the health system the following conclusions can be drawn looking at national as well as international reports:

The goals of the system are both changing and made more explicit. The five goals in the WHO 2000 report help to reorient the focus of the Dutch health care system. Especially the mix of equity, efficiency, effectiveness, equality and responsiveness is discussed in a more articulate way. Plans are beginning to emerge to develop a national performance framework as in other OECD countries.

The Dutch health care system is still weak in linking public health data on regional and national level with performance data on health services and professions. Data collection and indicator development in public health and health services like hospitals are still separated. Integrating these types of data in one comprehensive framework is vital if we want to monitor both whether we do the right thing (e.g. do we provide the optimal mix of services to our population?) and whether we do things right (e.g. are these services provided efficiently, in a client-oriented manner, according to evidence-based protocols etc.?). The coming years, therefore, additional efforts are needed to develop performance indicators for health care institutes and professions that are population based i.e. focused on the contribution of that service/profession to the health of the community. In the Dutch health care system, sickness funds are the most obvious actors to stimulate the self-regulatory uptake of initiatives in this field by health care providers. However, sickness funds currently have few incentives to focus on regions or local communities. The challenge probably lies in triggering sickness funds to compete with each other on the issue of the quality and continuity of care that they contract for their enrolees, rather than having them compete on the issue of costs. To guard and to ensure quality and continuity of the care that is provided by the contracted providers is much easier for sickness funds that are rooted in regional and local communities, than for those operating nation wide with small market shares in many local delivery networks.

A strong division between prevention, cure, care and social care characterises the present health care system. For the near future a more integrated health care system is warranted. Recent policy plans on changes in the insurance and legislative system may help to promote integration and substitution within the system. Performance indicators should be developed to monitor the various integration processes. In the Netherlands, several studies (Persoon et al., 1996; van der Linden, 2001) have provided overviews of interventions and projects aimed at providing integrated care. Also, the developments in the field of physician-hospital integration have received quite some attention (Plochg et al., 1998; Groenewegen and van Lindert, 2001). However, no systematic inventory has yet been made of integrative processes on the level of delivery networks (e.g. of the mergers, contracting, and strategic alliances between health care institutions). Consequently, the integration process itself is not monitored systematically on the health system level.

All indicators should be part and parcel of quality systems. It is through quality systems that health care services and professions can assure the quality of their performance. Indicators are an important but surely not the only measurement tool that produces information for quality improvement actions. In the Dutch health care system the development and implementation of quality systems is seen as a prerequisite for indicator development. Although organised delivery systems are not a reality as yet, it seems no more than logical that the quality system thinking will be applied on these new organisational arrangements and on the health care system as a whole. The development of performance indicators should therefore be considered as part of the quality system thinking on health system level. A national performance framework should therefore not only be consistent with the dimensions identified in recent international WHO and OECD reports but should also be consistent with the conceptual frameworks provided by for example EFQM and ISO.

There is a large potential benefit in international benchmarking. We should be careful however in choosing a limited set of indicators too easily. First, the indicators should really reflect the performance of the system but second they should not be isolated from their context. A quality system approach on health system level may help us to develop a performance framework that helps steering the health care sector in a balanced way alongside other sectors in society.

Whether the Dutch health care system will finish its transformation from a tulip to a rose in the near future will partly depend on the weather. The cultivation process is well under way. The scent of performance indicators stimulates many noses, the art will be to keep them in the same direction.

REFERENCES

CASPARIE, A.F., SLUIJS, E.M., WAGNER, C. and de BAKKER, D.H. (1997),
"Quality systems in Dutch health care institutions", *Health Policy*, Vol. 42, No. 3, pp. 255-226, Dec.

ELSINGA, E. and RUTTEN, F.F. (1997),
"Economic evaluation in support of national health policy: the case of The Netherlands", *Soc Sci Med*, Vol. 45, No. 4, pp. 605-620, Aug.

GROENEWEGEN, P.P. and VAN DER WAL, G. (2001),
"De toestand van de Nederlandse gezondheidszorg: behoefte aan genuanceerde en concrete maatstaven", *NederlandsTijdschrift voor Geneeskunde*, Vol. 145, No. 36, pp. 1722-1725.

GROENEWEGEN, P.P. and VAN LINDERT, H. (2001),
"Vrije beroep in afhankelijkheid: de veranderende positie van medisch specialisten in de Nederlandse algemene ziekenhuizen", in Arts, W., Batenburg, R. and Groenewegen, P., *Een kwestie van vertrouwen. Over de veranderingen op de markt voor professionele diensten en in de organisatie van vrije beroepen*, Amsterdam University Press, Amsterdam.

GROL, R. (2001),
"Successes and failures in the implementation of evidence-based guidelines for clinical practice", *Medical Care*, Vol. 39, No. 8, Suppl. 2, pp. II46-II54.

KLAZINGA, N.S. (1996),
"Quality management of medical specialist care in the Netherlands. An explorative study of the nature and development", Thesis, Belvedere, Overveen.

KLAZINGA, N. (2000),
"Re-engineering trust: the adoption and adaption of four models for external quality assurance of health care services in western European health care systems", *International Journal for Quality in Health Care*, Vol. 12, No. 3, pp. 183-189.

KLAZINGA, N., LOMBARTS, K. and VAN EVERDINGEN, J. (1998),
"Quality management in medical specialties: the use of channels and dikes in improving health care in The Netherlands", *Jt Comm J Qual Improv*, Vol. 24, No. 5, pp. 240-250, May.

KLAZINGA, N., STRONKS, K., DELNOIJ, D. and VERHOEFF, A. (2001),
"Indicators without a cause. Reflections on the development and use of indicators in health care from a public health perspective", *International Journal for Quality in Health Care*, Vol. 13, No. 6, pp. 433-438.

KRAMERS, P.G.N., ACHTERBERG, P.W. and VAN DER WILK, E.A. (2001),
"De prestaties van de Nederlandse Gezondheidszorg in internationaal perspectief: achtergronden en implicaties voor beleid", *NederlandsTijdschrift voor Geneeskunde*, Vol. 145, No. 36, pp. 1752-1755.

MINISTERIE VAN SOCIALE ZAKEN EN WERKGELEGENHEID (2000),
De Nederlandse verzorgingsstaat. Sociaal beleid en economische prestaties in internationaal perspectief, Hoofdstuk 7 "De gezondheidszorg", Ministerie van SZW, Den Haag.

MINISTRY OF HEALTH, WELFARE AND SPORTS (2001),
Vraag aan bod (Towards a demand driven health care system), The Hague, June.

MULLIGAN, J., APPLEBY, J. and HARRISON, A. (2000),
"Measuring the performance of health systems: indicators still fail to take socioeconomic factors into account", *British Medical Journal*, Vol. 321, pp. 191-192.

OECD (2000),
OECD *Economic Surveys. The Netherlands*, Chapter IV "The health care system", Paris, March.

PERSOON, A., FRANCKE, A., TEMMINK, D. and KERKSTRA, A. (1996),
Transmurale zorg in Nederland: een inventarisatie op basis van bestaande gegevensbestanden, Nivel, Utrecht.

PLOCHG, TH., KLAZINGA, N.S. and CASPARIE, A.F. (1998),
Het medisch-specialistisch mozaïek. Een dubbele' integratie tussen de medische beroepsgroep en de ziekenhuisorganisatie, BMG/VVAA, Rotterdam.

PLSEK, P. (2000),
"Redesigning health care with insights from the science of complex adaptive systems", in *Crossing the Quality Chasm: A New Health System for the 21st Century*, The National Academy of Sciences, Washington, pp. 309-322.

SCHEERDER, R.L.J.M. and SCHRIJVERS, A.J.P. (1998),
"Health care policy making against an OECD background, With some recommendations for non-OECD countries", in Øvretveit, J. (ed.), *Comparative and Cross-cultural Health Research. A Practical Guide*, Radcliffe Medical Press, Oxon.

SLUIJS, E.M. and WAGNER, C. (2000),
Kwaliteitssystemen in zorginstellingen. Stand van zaken in 2000, Nivel, Utrecht.

SOCIAAL EN CULTUREEL PLANBUREAU (2000),
Sociaal en Cultureel Rapport 2000. Nederland in Europa, Hoofdstuk 8 "Gezondheid en zorg", SCP, Den Haag.

VAN DER GRINTEN, T.E. and KASDORP, J.P. (1999),
"Choices in Dutch health care: mixing strategies and responsibilities", *Health Policy*, Vol. 50, No. 1-2, pp. 105-122, Dec.

VAN DER LINDEN, B. (2001),
"The birth of integration. Explorative studies on the development and implementation of transmural care in the Netherlands", Thesis, University of Utrecht.

VAN DOORSLAER, E., WAGSTAFF, A., VAN DER BURG, H., CHRISTIANSEN, T., DE GRAEVE, D., DUCHESNE, I., GERDTHAM, U.G., GERFIN, M., GEURTS, J., GROSS, L., HAKKINEN, U., JOHN, J., KLAVUS, J., LEU, R.E., NOLAN, B., O'DONNELL, O., PROPPER, C., PUFFER, F., SCHELLHORN, M., Sundberg, G. and Winkelhake, O. (2000),
"Equity in the delivery of health care in Europe and the US", J *Health Econ*, Vol. 19, No. 5, pp. 553-583, Sept.

VAN HERK, R. (1997),
"Artsen onder druk. Over het kwaliteitsbeleid van medische beroepen", Thesis, Elsevier/De Tijdstroom, Utrecht.

VAN HERTEN, L.M. (2001),
"Health targets. Navigating in health policy", Thesis University of Amsterdam, TNO Prevention and Health, Leiden.

WHO (2000),
World Health Report. Health Systems: Improving Performance, Geneva.

Chapter 7

TOWARDS INTEGRATED AND COHERENT HEALTH INFORMATION SYSTEMS FOR PERFORMANCE MONITORING: THE CANADIAN EXPERIENCE

by

Michael Wolfson[*] and Richard Alvarez[**]

Abstract

Canada has a great deal of excellent health data; but we are still striving for integrated and coherent information systems in the health domain. There is growing appreciation that the proper kinds of health information systems can:

- significantly improve patient care,

- support much more effective management of the delivery of health services, and

- provide the foundations for major new insights into the determinants of population health.

In addition, these same health information systems, if properly conceived, designed and implemented, can provide the foundations for effective performance monitoring. This paper briefly traces the evolution of these ideas over the past decade, describes the leading current health information initiatives, and links them together into the vision of Canada's "health infostructure".[1]

Introduction

As in most OECD countries, Canada's health information landscape is very complex. One reason is the myriad players in Canada's health system – including solo general practitioners, various group practices, hospitals which are essentially all non-profit public institutions, labs which are often private, nursing home and continuing care programs which are a mixture of public, private and voluntary, and so on. As well, health care in Canada is constitutionally a provincial jurisdiction, so that in a very real way, Canada has over 10 health care systems.[2] As a result, this discussion will generally take a national perspective, and of necessity be highly selective.

The general plan of the paper is to begin with background and context – key elements of the past that have brought us to our current situation. We then give a few empirical examples from our current health information system by way of both illustration, and to motivate the final part of the paper, our vision for the future evolution of Canada's health information system, where a central theme is the need for coherence and integration.

* Assistant Chief Statistician, Statistics Canada.
** President and CEO, Canadian Institute for Health Information.

1. Background and context

1.1. Definition of "health system"

The phrase "health system performance" begs the question of just what is meant by "health system". Conventionally in Canada, this has been hospitals and doctors. However, especially over the decade of the 1990s, which witnessed substantial reductions in the numbers of hospital beds, and increasing media coverage of the aging of the "baby boom" birth cohort, conventional thinking has broadened to include both home and institutional care for the ill while outside hospital. In addition, the technological explosions in diagnostic imaging and lab testing have brought these facilities into the widely appreciated "health system". And the dramatic growth in pharmaceutical costs in overall health spending has clearly highlighted the role of drugs in the system.

The publication of the *World Health Report* in 2000 (WHO, 2000) gave a new interpretation to countries' health system. WHO defined it somewhat more broadly than is conventional in Canadian discourse, by including anything whose primary intent relates to health. This definition brings public health and health promotion programs, for example, squarely into the "health system".

However, there is a widely accepted framework, at least among many senior health officials, many health ministers, and the health research community in Canada, that is considerably wider than the WHO definition. This has arisen in our discourse on the "broader determinants" of health. As we will show later, it is clear that there is more to health than health care, and more than is implied by conventional risk factors like smoking and cholesterol. Broader determinants of health include not only a range of individual behaviours like physical activity, but also individual socio-economic circumstances, and the character of the communities within which we live. From a policy perspective, the health system includes not only programs and policies whose primary intent relates to health, the WHO definition, but also programs and policies whose secondary intent, or even inadvertent effects, are important for population health. These include areas like transportation, education, and social protection.

1.2. Driving forces in the Canadian health information context

Canada is probably similar to many OECD countries in terms of the driving forces at work in the health sector, the broader political and public context within which this sector is playing out. There are at least four main factors playing a major role in Canada:

1. Many leaders in the sector are experiencing the painful realisation that just throwing more money into the system simply is not working. There seems to be an endless demand for more services of various kinds, and most on the face of it appear reasonable. Yet, ministers of health and the public are not able to see clearly the benefits of these expenditures.

2. Health care, if it ever was, is now certainly much more than hospitals and doctors. Chronic care and home care, alternative providers, drugs, new kinds of community interventions are all part of the system, and need to be coordinated so that from the patient's perspective, there is a "continuum of care".

3. There is increasing popular concern that the aging of the baby boomer generation will bankrupt the health care system. In Canada, there are studies going back well over 25 years with such projections (Economic Council, 1979). At the same time, a number of other studies have suggested that these "demo doom" scenarios are overstated (Fellegi, 1988; Wolfson and Murphy, 1997; Evans *et al.*, 2001). These latter analyses have shown that changes in population age structure have not been, and need not be, the main factor driving health care costs. Rather, the key factors include the relative rates of pay of health care professionals compared to the workforce in general, and the management of the diffusion of new technologies in areas such as pharmaceuticals, imaging, and (still mainly in the future) bio-technology.

4. Finally, something our grandmothers likely always knew, we have been accumulating an increasing stock of careful empirical studies on the myriad factors outside the health care system that have profound effects on the health of citizens of OECD countries. These factors

obviously include genetics, and well-recognised "risk factors" like smoking and physical inactivity. But they also include a more pervasive set of social factors including social isolation, income and education, and stress related to social position in work roles. (Evans *et al.*, 1994) As a result, understanding the performance of the (conventional) health care system cannot be divorced from an understanding of health determinants more broadly.

1.3. Major tensions in the Canadian health information context

In addition to sharing a number of driving forces with other OECD member countries – forces that are shaping both our health care systems, and the evolution of our heath infostructure, Canada faces a number of significant tensions. One is relatively unique to Canada, our jurisdictional complexity. General responsibility for health, and the management and delivery of health services, constitutionally, are primarily the responsibility of the ten provinces and three territories. However, based on a history of fiscal transfers from the federal to the provincial governments, Canada's public health care systems generally adhere to a set of core principles established in federal legislation. Hospital inpatient and outpatient services, physician services, and some pharmaceutical products and public health services are covered by interlocking general revenue-financed health insurance plans. In addition, the federal government plays a leading role in health research, and is increasingly playing a leading role in health information.

The health sector has a diversity of stakeholders. Real advances in health information require not only the cooperation of physicians, hospitals, heath regions, nurses, ministries of health, public health, health promotion, and community care officials and managers, but also their sharing in and consensus approval of a vision of Canada's health infostructure.

This diversity of players leads to a degree of tension regarding the most important and salient kinds of health information. Physicians, for example, do not want to be saddled with mundane data entry while in the midst of caring for a patient. Yet when aggregated, such information is critical for a range of applications, not only to improve patient care, but also to manage the system.

At the other end of the spectrum of generality, there is a fascination with broad national-level summary indicators of population health and health system performance. This has reached a pinnacle with the *World Health Report* (WHO, 2000). Relatedly, Smee (Part II, Chapter 3 in this volume) has argued that in the UK, it is proving most useful to focus on a very parsimonious set of key indicators. However, in WHO consultations, for example, as well as in Canadian discussions, concerns have been raised about the practical usefulness of such broad summary indicators. In particular, there is a tension between an indicator that is (at least superficially) easy to grasp, and the kinds of measurements that are relevant to decision-makers, and provide the basis for practical decision making. In essence, there is a call for additional information to "connect the dots" – to bridge the broad impressions given by summary indicators, and the more specific policy levers and choices available to governments and other decision-makers.

Health information costs significant amounts of money, much more than is currently being spent in Canada. At the same time, health ministers are facing demands on all sides to improve patient care. There is, as a result, a major tension between the proverbial urgent and the important. It is politically difficult to invest in information when "patients are going without".

Finally, and as we shall argue below, one of the fundamental requirements for a health information system that is able to "connect the dots" is person-oriented information. This is an information system that integrates individuals' myriad health care encounters so they can be viewed not only piecemeal, but also on a person basis, so individuals' trajectories through the health care system, as well as in terms of broader health-related factors, can be examined holistically. Naturally, such information raises major concerns for individual privacy. As a result, it is absolutely fundamental that there is broad public understanding about the way their health information can and is being used, and that the legislative and policy frameworks for health information strike a reasonable balance between individual privacy and health system needs ranging from individual patient care to overall system monitoring. This tension is well recognised in Canada, but is still some distance from being reasonably resolved.

135

1.4. Past character of performance measurement in Canada

Over past decades, performance measures in the Canadian health care system were rather narrowly defined, motivated by questions of cost control and affordability, and the need for accreditation. The information used was typically single measures, usually focused on efficiency like length of stay in hospital, and based mostly on inputs, like numbers of bed-days, and throughputs like numbers of surgical procedures of various types performed. They drew on snapshots of services at a point in time, rather than more integrated data like person-oriented information. In sum, we generally had "stovepipe" or "silo" health information systems which reflected the separate and unintegrated character of our health care delivery systems.

Moreover, there was also almost a complete split between information on the health care system, and information on the health of the population. What population health measures we had were convenience-based, given the data systems readily available. They focused on mortality or disease-as-reported-in-hospital indicators drawn from administrative data sources, augmented with some survey data on disability and selected lifestyle factors. The motivations for these measures were straightforward – tracking trends, and supporting targeted programs like those related to tobacco smoking. The broader social and economic milieu was ignored.

The audiences for these kinds of information were mainly technical, not practitioners, and certainly not the general public.

There were, however, a few early glimmers of the kinds of health information systems we now envision. These include the Manitoba Centre for Health Policy (*www.umanitoba.ca/centres/mchp*) which, for over two decades, has been a world leader in assembling person-oriented health information, and in partnership with the Manitoba Ministry of Health, producing targeted studies of immediate relevance to the policy issues of the day. Another early leader is Ontario's Institute for Clinical Evaluative Sciences (ICES). They have led, for example, in the production of small geographic area data, with their influential "practice atlases" (Goel *et al.*, 1996).

1.5. Canadian health information context – Intellectual milieu

An essential part of the context for the development of Canada's health information system is the intellectual milieu over recent decades. Canada was internationally recognised for broadening thinking with respect to health with the publication over 25 years ago of the Lalonde Report (1974). This report was very influential in adding the concept of "lifestyle" to the lexicon of population health – enlarging the post-war focus of health ministries on the establishment and public funding of health care insurance.

Another key feature, unique to Canada, has been the Canadian Institute for Advanced Research (CIAR) program in Population Health (*www.ciar.ca*). This multi-disciplinary group of individuals pioneered a broad synthesis of research evidence into a comprehensive theoretical framework of the broad determinants of health, most succinctly summarised in Evans and Stoddart (1990). Figure 1 shows in a very summary form some of the key ideas. In addition to emphasizing the broad range of health determinants shown in the diagram, the Population Health program also emphasized the need to understand individuals' health within a life course framework (Hertzman *et al.*, 1994).

1.6. Canadian health information context – Statistical system

Just as there are many players in Canada's health care system, there are almost as many players in our health information system. Statistics Canada has been central for over a century, with the population census and vital statistics. More recently, Statistics Canada's health statistics program, with the strong support of Health Canada and our many partners, has blossomed in the areas of health surveys and data integration, and has become increasingly responsible for reporting on Canadians' health status and its determinants, broadly conceived.

Figure 1. **A comprehensive framework of broad determinants of health**

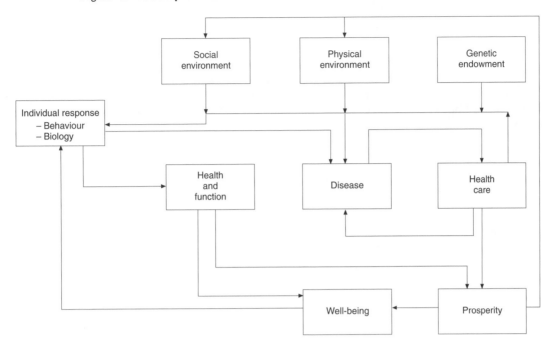

The Canadian Institute for Health Information was created in 1994, following a major review of Canada's health information (Wilk, 1991). One of the main rationales for its founding, given the myriad players in the health sector, was the need for coordination. This is the basis for one of CIHI's core foci, information standards development. CIHI is also the developer and holder of national health care data sets, especially on various kinds of health care encounters, and has recently become principally responsible for regular reporting to the public on the health care system.

Provincial health ministries are the source of, or responsible for, the vast majority of administrative data on health care service encounters (*e.g.* hospital and doctor visits, lab tests, insured drug prescriptions). Provincial governments' registrars are the source of vital event (birth, death, marriage) records. In addition, some provinces have successfully fostered leading academic groups specialising in the statistical analysis of their administrative data, such as the Manitoba Centre and ICES noted above.

Finally, national health research funding agencies have been moving increasingly to provide substantial support for the creation and maintenance of large health data bases. Health research funders in Canada have come to recognise the parallels with other areas of "big science". Just as astronomers could not function without billions of dollars worth of telescopes and related observational tools, population health and health services research cannot function without major investments in richly multivariate cohort databases, and in the skills and institutional settings needed for their analysis.

1.7. *Health information context – Reports and studies*

In the 1980s, fiscal pressures and a growing awareness of the range of factors outside the health care system that affect our health – influenced by shift in intellectual milieu noted above – led to a number of reviews of the health care system. One by one, a series of Royal Commission and Task Force reports ushered in a series of health care system reforms across the country.[3] As part of these reforms, many provincial and territorial governments created health regions (sometimes the size of large school boards), and assigned them responsibility for the day-to-day operation of the health care system. Goals varied, but most jurisdictions aimed to streamline health care services and to bring their planning and delivery closer to local residents. Regionalisation of health systems was recognised as a fundamental requirement for providing more direct accountability to the public. Better management as opposed to more funding became a key focus for many. Other common goals included increasing the focus on health promotion and committing more resources to community based services. (Nevertheless, in practice, many health region authorities remain preoccupied with the conventional issues of running hospitals and closely related health care services.)

Furthermore, these commissions recommended that broader, non-medical factors like income, housing and other social, environmental and demographic factors be considered as part of the health equation. For perhaps the first time, there was a clear institutional recognition that there is more to health than health care.

And there were calls for better health information. This was a common theme emanating from the commission reports, the recognition that good information systems were key to informing health reform. Conversely, the lack of quality information was recognised as a significant barrier to bringing about effective reform. The call for better information was echoed in the (now perhaps commonplace) sentiment that "you can't manage what you can't measure" (Advisory Council, 1999).

More recently, pan-Canadian consultations on health information needs in 1998, jointly undertaken by CIHI, Statistics Canada and Health Canada (CIHI, 1998) identified common themes for action across the country. These consultations found that "a new ethos of performance permeates the entire debate and results in priorities for data to support evidence-based decision-making and comparability of outcomes at all levels". Participants envisaged an evidence-based, results-oriented, client-centred health care system, driven by information built on common standards consistently applied, with key linkages between all actors and to data repositories. The thrust of information would be to optimise access, quality of service, and affordability, to allow meaningful comparisons across jurisdictions, and to support important health reform-driven shifts and patient accountability for knowledge, choice, and health status.

Specifically, this includes:

- the capacity to integrate health and health care data at different levels (*e.g.* province/territory, region, community);

- financial and cost data (for both the public and private sectors in health) for assessing cost-effectiveness of alternative interventions and technologies;

- better information on health outcomes, including comparative data and benchmark indicators across the continuum of care;

- validated information for the general public about personal health assessment, choices of treatment, as well as other health-related information;

- developing the core standards that would allow for linkage of information on population health to determinants of health and to service utilisation;

- better comparative information, including health indicators and trend data; and

- appropriate information on health human resources.

Participants in these consultations also emphasized the importance of urgently ensuring that a framework and guidelines for privacy and confidentiality of health information is in place.

1.8. International factors

Canadians are keenly interested in international comparisons. There is a longstanding interest in health care costs, where (until recently) Canada has had the second highest per capita health care costs in the world, second only to the US. There is also a long history of comparisons using mortality-based indicators like life expectancy and infant mortality.

However, these kinds of indicators are increasingly seen as too limited. There is a growing interest in comparative measures of health status and disability, the roles of social context, details of the operation of health systems, and generally a desire to learn from international experience "what works".

The use of international health information is closely tied to the level of international data standards. Life expectancy and mortality-based indicators are widely used because of the long history of investments in common concepts and methods for population censuses, vital event registration, and disease classification (WHO's ICD; WHO, 1992). The OECD annual compendia (OECD, 2001a, 2001b) have played a major role in facilitating these kinds of analysis.

On the other hand, international comparisons of population health status and disability prevalences, disease incidence, and health care treatment patterns have been almost completely stymied by the absence of commonly agreed concepts and definitions for measurement and data collection. At the same time, there is among OECD member countries an increasing sense of shared challenges, for example in containing health care costs, learning which interventions are cost-effective, and learning which organisational / financing structures work best.

Canada certainly feels the need for laying the foundations for a broader range of international health information and data standards, and then collecting comparable data based upon these standards.

2. Current initiatives

One of the national initiatives for which both Statistics Canada and CIHI were responsible has been the Health Information Roadmap. This initiative responded to many of the needs expressed in a cross-country consultation in 1998, followed by a Strategic Plan endorsed by both the provinces and the Federal Government. The initiative was given start-up funding by the Federal Government in 1999.

The Roadmap has funded a range of new data collection activities, especially the massive Canadian Community Health Survey (CCHS), with a sample size of 130 000. This survey was the response to one of the main messages in the cross-country consultations – that there was a paucity of health information available at the "local" level, particularly on health status, functioning, and risk factors. The CCHS has been designed to provide this kind of information.

At the same time, there was a clear message about the need to provide this information in a clear, coherent, and accessible form. As a result, CIHI in collaboration with Statistics Canada undertook the development of an indicators framework. This framework was born at a consensus meeting in May 1999, and the current version is shown in Figure 2 (CIHI, 1999).

Figure 2. **Canadian framework for health and health system performance indicators**

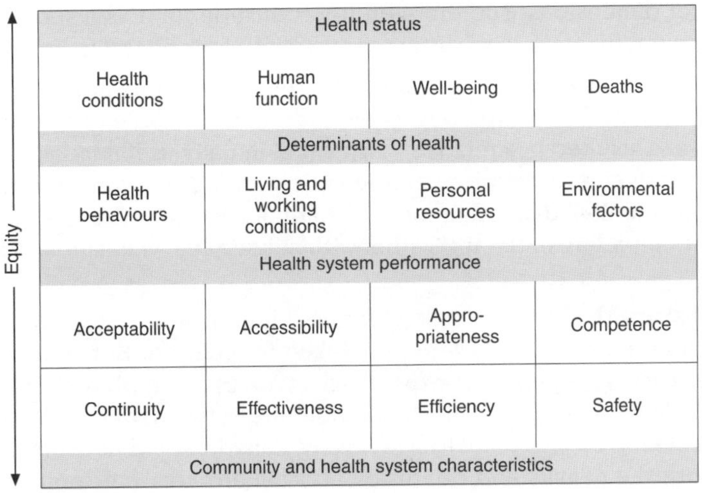

Health status			
Health conditions	Human function	Well-being	Deaths
Determinants of health			
Health behaviours	Living and working conditions	Personal resources	Environmental factors
Health system performance			
Acceptability	Accessibility	Appropriateness	Competence
Continuity	Effectiveness	Efficiency	Safety
Community and health system characteristics			

Equity

The basic intent is to provide not only provinces and territories, but also sub-provincial health regions, indicators of the overall health of the population served, how it compares to other regions of the country, and how it is changing over time. These indicators also span the major non-medical determinants of health in the region, the quality of health services received by the region's residents, and various characteristics of the community or health system that provide useful contextual information. In some indicator areas, good data currently exist. In others, such as indicators of environmental factors and acceptability, serious gaps remain.

Of course, this indicators framework is no more than the tip of the iceberg of a properly functioning health infostructure. Each indicator must be supported by the appropriate data infrastructure, *i.e.* a range of underlying data systems. In the multi-jurisdictional environment of Canada, and with the myriad players in the health sector, there is also a fundamental need for standards, in order that all the bits of data being collected in each jurisdiction and by each kind of health care provider can fit together. There is also a range of increasingly sophisticated methodologies that have become essential in the construction of many indicators, as shown below.

This framework is designed to inform the selection and interpretation of useful and informative health indicators. In order for them to be informative, the indicators must reflect accurately the fundamental elements of the system that we are attempting to measure. As a result, the framework is both comprehensive, and rooted in the determinants of health perspective, discussed above. The implication is that the evaluation of either health system performance or the health of the population must take account of a broad set of factors including, but not limited to, the provision of health services.

Not surprisingly, then, health system performance is directly reflected in only one of the four major dimensions pictured in this model. This dimension includes eight categories[4] designed to capture various aspects of health system performance, including responsiveness (accessibility and acceptability), those related to processes of care (*e.g.* continuity of care or safety), and outcomes directly related to a medical or health intervention (*e.g.* effectiveness).

Three other dimensions figure prominently in this framework, health status, the non-medical determinants of health, and community and health system characteristics. The *health status* dimension includes a broad range of indicators spanning deaths to disability to well-being. In order to better understand variations in health status and health system performance, *non-medical determinants of health* are also highlighted. Non-medical determinants of health are those that fall outside of the sphere of health care, generally speaking, but that have been shown to affect a variety of health outcomes or processes. The last dimension labeled *community and health system characteristics* provides useful contextual information. These indicators should broadly reflect resources (financial or human), the population (*e.g.* population density) and the characteristics of the health system (*e.g.* level of specialisation, utilisation).

Finally, the notion of equity spans all dimensions of the framework, and can be applied to almost any of the constructs or dimensions. Therefore equity is included not as a separate dimension or cell within the framework, but rather as a crosscutting aspect that spans all the four dimensions.

Practically, a twofold strategy has been followed to implement this indicator framework. First, the framework has been populated as completely as possible with available information, even though it is not always ideal. This has resulted in a relatively rich set of initially useful indicators. Second, a number of priority initiatives designed to develop a more coherent and integrated data infrastructure have been launched, such as the Canadian Community Health Survey, with the intent of further populating the framework, and of upgrading initial indicators with subsequent measures that better capture the intended concepts.

It is worth emphasizing the iceberg analogy for health indicators. Life expectancy is perhaps the most commonplace of indicators, and is generally taken for granted. But consider what is below the "water line". To be measured properly, life expectancy involves a complete death registration system, and a complete periodic population census. In Canada, these two data collections have costs on the order of one hundred million dollars annually. Obviously, Canada would not spend this much money for just one indicator. Both the census and death registration are very much multi-use data collection systems, only one of whose outputs is the measurement of life expectancy. The basic implication is that health indicators must be designed and developed in a way that is very closely tied to the development of information systems more generally. Information systems and indicators must be mutually reinforcing.

3. Illustrations

CIHI and Statistics Canada have chosen to guide their strategies for health information development by two straightforward questions: How healthy are Canadians? and How healthy is the health care system? The answers to these questions are now being provided in a series of annual reports (CIHI, 2000 and 2001; Statistics Canada, 2000 and 2001). In this section, a few examples drawn from these reports and other studies, will be shown. In each case, there are two objectives: One is to highlight a result of intrinsic importance. The other is to peer beneath the results, and draw out implications for the health information system.

3.1. *Health care expenditures*

To begin, the most widely used health indicators are based on deaths and dollars. The first is life expectancy; the other is health care spending, often expressed as a proportion of the size of the economy. Figure 3 shows time series data on the three largest components of health care spending for Canada. After rather rapid growth up to the early 1990s, spending leveled off, but recently has begun rising again. Perhaps even more notable is that drug costs have overtaken physician fees to be in number two spot, after hospital spending.

Beyond the basic trends, a key question is not only how the provinces compare to one another, but also how Canada compares to other OECD countries. The OECD has played a key role in providing internationally comparable data (OECD 2001a, 2001b), and the recent development of their manual on health care costs (OECD, 2000) is a significant advance for the quality of these data.

Of course, the obvious question in relation to health care costs is what we are buying for the money; what are the improvements in population health that all this spending on health care services is yielding, and which services are most cost-effective. Here, we are fundamentally at sea. The reason,

Figure 3. **Selected health expenditures, Canada, 1975 to 2001**

Current dollars

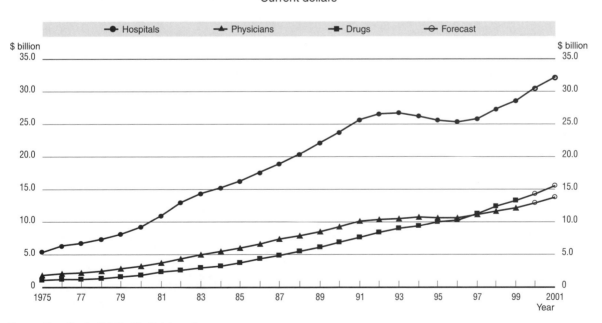

Source: Canadian Institute for Health Information.

simply, is that we have absolutely no connections in our health information systems, at the patient level, between costs and outcomes.

In policy terms, this is an extraordinary lacuna. Given tremendous spending pressures, the health information system offers no guidance on where funds could be cut with least harm, or reallocated to maximum benefit in terms of population health.

3.2. Heart attacks

The next example jumps down into the core of the health care system, and focuses on one of the most prevalent health problems – heart disease. A key indicator in the framework is the one year heart attack (acute myocardial infarction or AMI) survival rate. CIHI's detailed hospital morbidity data, based on standard computerised discharge abstracts, linked on a person-oriented basis to each other, and to Statistics Canada's Canadian Mortality Database, supports measurement of this indicator not only overall, but also by health region.

Figure 4 provides data on AMI survival rates. For statistical reasons, these data cover only large health regions (with a population of 100 000 or more). These inter-regional comparisons, to be as fair as possible, are based on region-specific mortality rates adjusted for differences in the age, sex, and co-morbidity distributions of the patients. (Johansen et al., 2002)

The 1-year AMI mortality rates (horizontal axis) are shown in a scatter plot juxtaposed with the major kind of intervention, revascularisation, which is either or both PCTA (percutaneous transluminal coronary angioplasty) or CABG (coronary artery bypass graft surgery) (rates shown along the vertical axis).

The sloping straight line is a least squares regression fit which, reassuringly, shows that there is some positive association between revascularisation within 14 days and AMI survival. However, there is a very substantial variation across this set of health regions, both in mortality rates (between 10 and 27 per cent) and in revascularisation rates (almost nil to 25 per cent) within 14 days of the attack.[5] This

Figure 4. **One-year mortality rate in relation to percentage of AMI patients revascularised within 14 days**

Health regions with populations over 100 000, 4 provinces, Canada, 1995-96

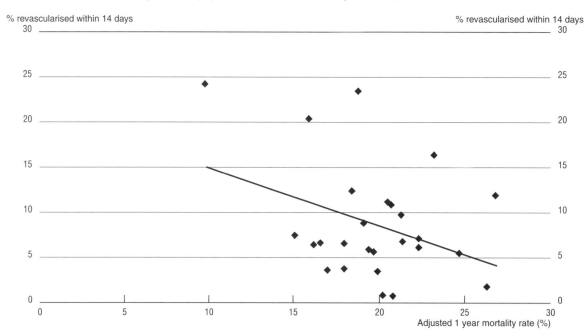

Source: Johansen *et al.* (2002).

set of results is in the same spirit as the small area variations analyses pioneered in Canada by the ICES in Toronto, with its health atlases for Ontario (*e.g.* Goel *et al.*, 1996).

However, this analysis makes an important advance by showing not only the high variability in these procedure rates, angioplasty and coronary bypass surgery for heart attack cases, but also the high variability in a key outcome, one year survival. Moreover, there is not a terribly strong link between these major interventions and the key health outcome, survival after a heart attack. These are rather provocative results. If there are good reasons for these regional variations, our current data systems are unable to show them. If there are not good reasons, this is an alarm bell regarding the quality of patient care, and the quality of health system management.

Of course, there are a number of caveats that must be borne in mind regarding these results. These caveats all turn on data that are still missing. There is no information, for example, on the extent and timing of thrombolysis, the clot-busting drugs that are often administered within hours of presenting with an AMI, nor on the kinds of drugs patients are prescribed upon discharge from the hospital, and their compliance with these prescriptions. Similarly, there are no data on health-related behaviours and risk factors like smoking, hypertension, physical activity and cholesterol – either before the AMI or after discharge. Such data, if available, would have been added to the available clinical data as part of the risk adjustment methodology used to render the survival rates more comparable across health regions.

Nevertheless, measures like these are an absolutely essential building block for the kinds of health information system needed to support assessments of health system performance. Figure 4 in fact represents a very recent and major improvement in Canada's health info system, one of the Health Information Roadmap initiatives, since it depends on the linkage of hospital records to each other and to death certificates to form a "person-eye view", or person-oriented information (POI).

3.3. *Low volume surgery*

One factor that could be at play in the variations in heart attack survival just shown is the skill and capability of the teams undertaking the heart surgery. There is considerable published evidence that low volumes of specialised procedures may lead to poor patient outcomes.

In the case of coronary artery bypass graft surgery, a recent review found 11 published studies on volume/outcome relationships. All showed better outcomes in hospitals that did more operations. The study estimated that patients cared for in hospitals that did fewer than 500 surgeries a year were 39 per cent more likely to die than others (Dudley *et al.*, 2000).

As a result, surgical procedure volume is one of the measures CIHI produces from the hospital morbidity data system. In Canada, 33 hospitals performed almost 22 500 bypass surgeries in 1998/99. There was a ten-fold difference in the number of patients across hospitals – from just over 200 to more than 2000. These services are not concentrated equally across the country. Only 4 per cent of Ontario patients were operated on in hospitals doing less than 500 procedures a year. This compares with 16 per cent in B.C., 33 per cent in the Prairies, 47 per cent in Quebec, and 23 per cent in the Atlantic provinces (Figure 5).

These patterns of hospital volumes could be one of the explanations for the variations seen for 1-year AMI survival in Figure 4. The POI database under development at Statistics Canada will allow an analysis of the relationship between procedure volumes and health outcomes.

3.4. *Health care utilisation and social background*

The examples so far have focused on clinical questions – heart disease, surgical procedures, and variations across small geographic regions. But there is far more to health system performance than caring for heart attacks, and far more than is available from solely a clinical perspective.

Figure 6 (Knighton *et al.*, 1998) displays the health care utilisation of infants, in their first year of life. The infants have been classified by their mother's education, divided into quartiles along the horizontal axis. The first set of bars show the proportions of these babies who were born early – gestations less than 37 weeks. There is a clear gradient, with less well educated mothers having higher rates of early births, and the rate of

Figure 5. **When volume counts, percentage of surgery by hospital volume, Canada, 1998-99**

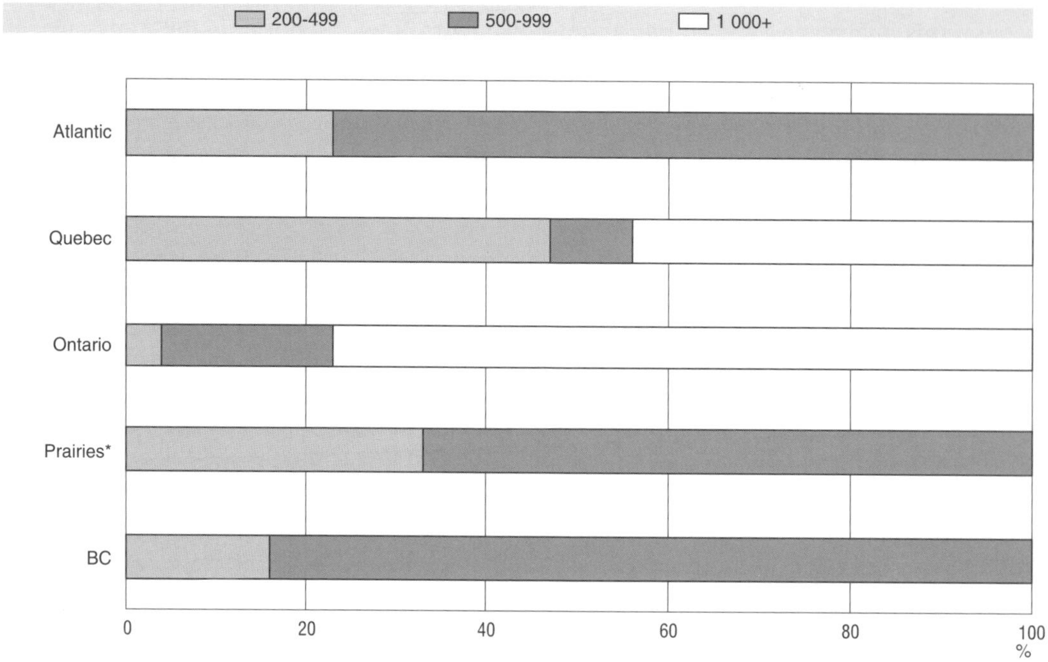

200-499
500-999
1 000+
Atlantic
Quebec
Ontario
Prairies*
BC
0
20
40
60
80
100
%

Source: CIHI (2001).

Figure 6. **Health of Manitoba infants by maternal education**

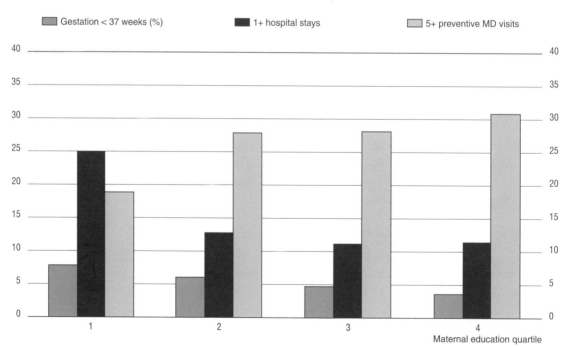

Gestation < 37 weeks (%)
1+ hospital stays
5+ preventive MD visits
40
35
30
25
20
15
10
5
0
1
2
3
4
Maternal education quartile

Source: Knighton *et al.* (1998).

this adverse birth outcome declining with every step up the socio-economic status (SES) ladder.[6] As a result, we would expect these infants from lower SES homes to use more health care services.

This relationship is borne out by the second set of bars, showing the percentages of infants with at least one hospital stay during the first year of life. However, the third set of bars shows the extent to which the infants were exposed to preventive health care services, such things as well-baby visits and immunisations. In this case, the rates increase with the mother's education quartile.

In Canada, these services are all free of charge, from the first dollar. As a result, there are no financial barriers for mothers in any social class to using any of these services. Yet their use is differential, and preventive services like vaccination are skewed to the more educated. This result has been one of the key findings establishing the existence of important *non-financial* barriers to health care access – clearly important from the viewpoint of health system performance.

This result builds on the pioneering work of the Manitoba Ministry of Health and Manitoba Centre for Health Policy mentioned earlier. It also builds on a unique pilot project in which population census data were linked to Manitoba health care records (Houle *et al.*, 1997). This was a precedent-setting project because of the sensitivity of the data sets involved. As a result, prior to the linkage, there was extensive consultation, including the Privacy Commissioner of Canada (1989-1990), and approval from the Minister responsible for Statistics Canada. Based on Statistics Canada's rigorous formal policy on record linkage (Statistics Canada, 2001), the benefits in terms of health information that could be generated from the linked files were carefully weighed against the equally serious concerns regarding individual privacy. On balance, results such as these demonstrate that it is possible to generate fundamentally important findings that would otherwise be very difficult or impossible using other approaches. At the same time, the record linkage involved, conducted as it was under the statutory authority of the federal Statistics Act, has successfully protected all individual information.

Unfortunately, these linkage projects remain very difficult. They have encountered years of delay due to the complexities and incoherence of federal and provincial acts and policies that govern the flows of individual data. It remains for Canada and its constituent jurisdictions to strike the right balance between legitimate concerns for individual privacy and the immense potential benefits from improved health information. This has been widely recognised in many studies and reports, and in current federal/provincial/territorial initiatives on health information. One of the most fundamental prerequisites for a proper health information system is a harmonised and appropriate set of privacy legislation and policies.

3.5. *Life expectancy and variants*

So far, the indicators and examples all involve the health care system. But a proper assessment of health system performance requires much broader indicators than these. An obvious and indeed ubiquitous indicator is life expectancy. But the populations of OECD countries are substantially beyond the "epidemiological transition". There are relatively few deaths at early ages from infectious diseases. Most of us can expect to live long lives, but lives that will often be burdened over many years by chronic disease and debilitating conditions. As a result, indicators are needed that bring together how many years of life we can expect, life expectancy (LE), and how healthy we can expect to be during those years of life.

One such indicator is disability-free life expectancy (DFLE). Figure 7, based on a study by Belanger *et al.* (2002), shows estimated LE and DFLE for women based on two different disability severity levels. Moreover, we have divided these LE and DFLE measures first between the 24 per cent of women who are smokers over their lifetimes, and non-smokers; and then between the 33 per cent of women with active leisure time pursuits (> 1 500 kcal/kg/day), and those who are not active. (The patterns are very similar for males, the main difference being that the bars are shorter.)

Not surprisingly, smoking and physical inactivity are both bad for longevity. While being physically active and not smoking does not allow us to avoid significant periods of disability over our lifetimes, they still give us an expectation of substantially longer periods of disability-free life. From a policy perspective, it is also interesting to note that physical activity (compared to inactivity) is associated

145

Figure 7. **Female life expectancy at age 45 by "lifestyle" and disability**

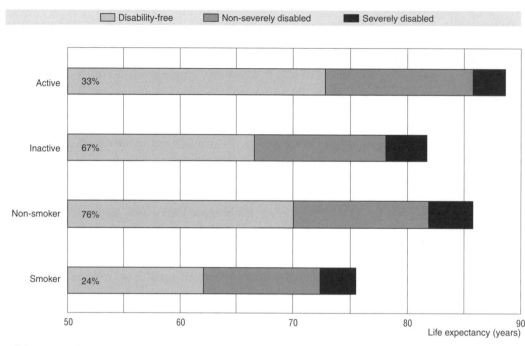

Source: Bélanger *et al.* (2002).

with an increase in life expectancy and DFLE that is almost as large as that associated with being a non-smoker (compared to being a smoker). Even casual observation, however, suggests that the health system devotes far more time and resources to smoking issues than to physical inactivity. Indicators such as these, therefore, can play a valuable role in setting broad health priorities.

It is also important to appreciate the information systems underlying this rather simple-looking graph. Assembling these measures required not only the usual population census and death registration data that underlie life expectancy. The measures also drew on longitudinal data on disability status for a sample of individuals, combined with their risk factors – in this case smoking and physical activity, and their chances of dying. These latter data came from Statistics Canada's National Population Health Survey, which almost uniquely among OECD countries is longitudinal. Moreover, with the permission of the vast majority of respondents, their survey records have been linked to mortality records, allowing mortality rates to be differentiated not only by clinical diseases, but also by disability status and risk factor. Thus again from a health information system perspective, the assembly of person-oriented information (POI) has been essential to the production of an obviously useful family of indicators.

3.6. *"Complex interventions"*

The next example draws on the results from a major clinical drug trial. Randomised clinical trials form the gold standard basis of "evidence-based medicine". The kinds of variation shown above in the treatment of AMI is an example of small area variations which, for over a decade, have been casting doubt on the rigor and scientific basis for many health care interventions. As a consequence, there has been a broad adoption of the principle that health care interventions ought to be "evidence-based", and a correspondingly substantial growth in the number and scale of clinical trials, a major source of such evidence.

One example is using the drug tamoxifen in a new way. Tamoxifen is already established as effective in preventing contra-lateral breast cancer in women who already have the disease. The

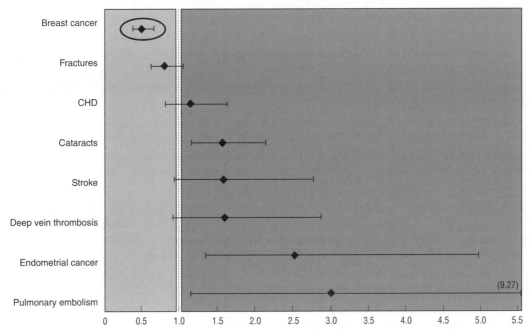

Figure 8. **Relative risks of "preventive" tamoxifen**

Source: Fisher *et al.* (1998).

question is whether tamoxifen would also be beneficial in preventing breast cancer in women who are otherwise healthy, but according to specified criteria, at higher risk. For example, one reason for elevated risk is having a close relative with breast cancer.

Figure 8 (Fisher *et al.*, 1998) displays the main results of the largest clinical trial designed to answer this question. The horizontal axis shows relative risks based on almost five years of follow-up – 1 is neutral; less than 1 means the chances of the event happening were reduced. The horizontal bars show the 95 per cent confidence intervals for the effects of this drug used in this preventive manner.

Breast cancer incidence, shown at the top of the figure, was cut in half, and the confidence interval is quite tight. The drug clearly has a beneficial impact on breast cancer incidence for the population targeted in the clinical trial. However, for other clinical endpoints examined in the trial, like the incidence of coronary heart disease (CHD), stroke, deep vein thrombosis (DVT), endometrial cancer and pulmonary embolism, there are highly uncertain, but often substantially adverse effects.

Given these results, the potential use of the drug tamoxifen as a preventive agent for breast cancer in otherwise healthy women is an example of what can be called a "complex intervention", since it may well have both positive and negative effects. Since most of the trial was not in Canada, and to some extent people self-select to participate, the population enrolled in the clinical trial may not be fully representative of the target population in Canada. And as clearly evident in Figure 8, even these best available clinical trial results have a substantial degree of uncertainty, represented by the wide statistical confidence intervals for some endpoints.

Such complex interventions pose a number of challenges in making a reasoned judgment as to whether, or how, the intervention should be adopted. If a large proportion of the population is potentially affected, costs to governments, insurance plans or individuals, depending on how these are financed, will likely be important. Since these interventions may have both positive and negative effects, an informed judgment should be based on a careful assessment of the likely joint or overall impacts of all these effects on the population that would be the intended beneficiaries. Unfortunately, the Fisher *et al.* tamoxifen trial did not find any statistically significant differences in overall mortality rates between the tamoxifen and the control groups, so the trial itself offers no guidance on this most basic question. When there are mixed results, as in the example just given, and population heterogeneities matter, differences between the trial population and the intended population of beneficiaries can be important.

The circumstances of this trial exemplify the analytical challenges for assessing complex interventions. Even though there has been a substantial increase over recent decades in clinical trials, there has been nowhere near as great an increase in the capacity to estimate, prospectively, the likely population impacts of such interventions. Doing so requires much more sophisticated health information systems than generally appreciated.

Fortunately in Canada, these needs have been considered, and are implicit in a number of health information initiatives. Person-oriented information (POI) in particular, both administrative and survey, and in some cases linked together, already highlighted in previous examples, provides the foundation for constructing statistical descriptions of the natural histories of diseases – their onset, progression, and case fatality.[7]

These same kinds of data also proved the foundations for estimating the effects of various risk factors on the incidence of disease – risk factors that include both the more conventional "lifestyle" sort like smoking, and clinical risk factors like hypertension, but also more distal and likely much more profoundly important risk factors like education, income, employment status, social support and other socio-economic factors. POI data sets are also needed to trace the effects of a disease, over the course of an individual's life, on their health care service use.

But all these data alone are insufficient for the prospective analysis of complex health interventions. The key additional piece is a simulation model – software plus data that weave together all the derived "nuggets of empirical regularity" (e.g. statistical descriptions of relative risks, disease onset and progression patterns, treatments, case fatality) estimated from diverse, often essentially POI sources, and allows the rigorous posing of "what if" questions. Such a capacity has long been taken for granted in Ministries of Finance, for both macro-economic and taxation policy. But the idea is still very new for health ministries.

This kind of simulation capacity sits near the top of the information system hierarchy, so that a country's health information system must be designed with this use in mind. Statistics Canada has taken the lead in this area with the development of POHEM, our POpulation HEalth Model. Its application in the case of preventive tamoxifen is illustrated in Will *et al.* (2001). And the results of this analysis are sobering: depending on assumptions, it could well be that preventive tamoxifen, notwithstanding its beneficial effects on breast cancer incidence, could have a net negative effect on the longevity of Canadian women.

3.7. Mortality and income inequality

As a final example (Ross *et al.*, 2000), we examine the juxtaposition of two very broad indicators, in Figure 9. This graph may at first appear similar to Figure 4 on AMI survival and revascularisation. As before, one axis shows a health outcome, in this case the vertical axis shows the age-standardised working age male mortality rate. But the horizontal axis shows something relatively new in health research – the degree of income inequality in the metropolitan area where individuals live.

The white circles represent US metropolitan areas, with their diameters proportional to their populations. The black circles are Canadian metropolitan areas, while the triangles are for Australian metropolitan areas. The scatter of white circles shows a clear association in the US – greater income inequality (measured by the share of total income going to the bottom half of the population in each city, the "median share") is associated with higher mortality. Canada and Australia, in comparison to the US, have lower mortality rates, less income inequality, and most interestingly, no significant association between the two.

These kinds of results have provoked a spate of new research. One strand is challenging the very existence of the relationship among US cities (*e.g.* Deaton and Lubotsky, 2001; Mellor and Milyo, 2001). The concern being raised is that the relationship shown is solely "ecological", *i.e.* among metropolitan areas, taking no account of individual-level relationships. It is well accepted that for individuals, higher

Figure 9. **Working age (25-64) mortality rate by median share of income**
Metropolitan areas in the United States, Canada and Australia

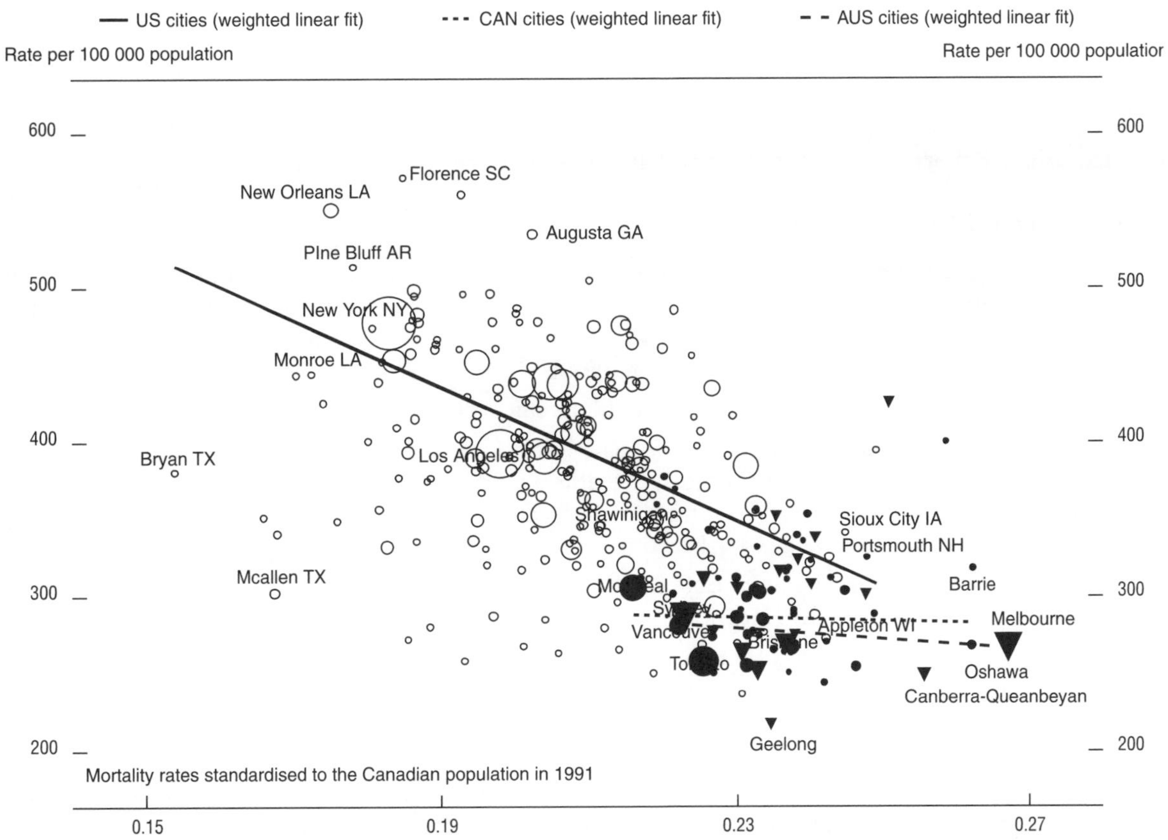

income is associated with greater longevity. It is also logically possible that this fact alone can account for the observed relationship (Gravelle, 1999), though this is most unlikely for the US (Wolfson *et al.*, 1999). Moreover, preliminary multi-level analysis using the National Longitudinal Mortality Study in the US, which has 10 year mortality follow-up data for 750 000 men, is strongly suggestive that even after explicitly accounting for individual-level factors, particularly income, the inequality-mortality association in the US is still statistically significant (Backlund and Rowe, personal communication).

Another strand of research spawned by these results is trying to understand why the association between income inequality and mortality is clearly evident in the US, but not in Canada – what makes Canadian cities different? For example, could it be the influence of Canada's publicly funded health care system which insures everyone, or the more egalitarian distribution of income in Canada? Another conjecture focuses on cities themselves – the general absence of gated communities and ghettos in Canada relative to the spatial concentrations of affluence and poverty seen in the US.

In any case, from the viewpoint of health system performance, and the information systems needed to monitor, manage and develop policy for the health system, this is perhaps the most challenging of empirical examples. It moves well beyond the conventionally defined health care system, and raises very broad questions about the determinants of health.

To assess and understand the relationships indicated in Figure 9, individual-level data, as well as data on the communities within which we live, are necessary. Moreover, these data must be used in multi-level analyses. Such multi-level analysis, which combines, for example, census small area data on neighbourhood

149

characteristics with individual level health system survey data, is becoming more prevalent. For example, health ministry analysts have been using such data to assess regional differences in health needs.

This is an area where Statistics Canada has been playing a key role by providing data for smaller geographic areas. In turn, diverse users can couple these small area characteristics with their own data or various health surveys. Indeed, Canada is likely in the early years of a flowering of this kind of information development and analysis.

4. Towards a coherent and integrated statistical system

4.1. A *summary vision*

The examples above illustrate the basic importance of a very broad range of health information. The challenge and basic goal is a health information system where all these kinds of data co-exist in a coherent and integrated manner. Such a system can be described in many ways; the diagram in Figure 10 gives only one view, but a very important one.

The pyramid here is intended to convey the hierarchical character of such an information system.

- The foundation is a combination – one part is basic administrative data on the full ranges of individuals' health system encounters; the other is a sample of responses from a systematic set of health surveys that go well beyond clinical disease to gather information on health and socio-economic status, and a range of risk factors.

- The foundational administrative data must be relevant to the myriad providers at ground level, otherwise there will be little incentive for them to generate high quality data.

- The system must have a bottom up aspect – so data can be rolled up to local/regional/provincial/ and then national levels.

- At the apex (flattened slightly to indicate that there is no one overall summary indicator), the information system must offer a valid and salient but parsimonious set of top level summary indicators for the health system as a whole, particularly a basic measure of population health, and its distribution, and the costs and resources used in the health system.

- And the information system must have a top down aspect: overall or summary indicators cannot exist in splendid isolation; they cannot risk a disconnect to practical policy choices. There must be a built in "drill down" capability. And there must be a capacity, somewhere in the middle of the pyramid, to join the resources devoted to interventions with their outcomes. The information

Figure 10. **Vision of a coherent and integrated statistical system**

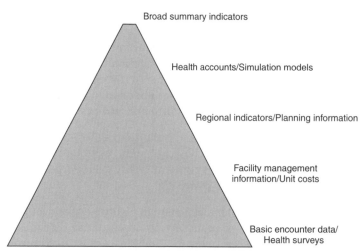

Broad summary indicators

Health accounts/Simulation models

Regional indicators/Planning information

Facility management information/Unit costs

Basic encounter data/ Health surveys

system has to support continuous monitoring and feedback on results achieved, as well as research and analysis to determine how well various activities are "working".

4.2. Main strategies

In order to achieve this vision, there are several key strategies which need to form the core of health information developments in Canada:

- a consensus on a parsimonious set of indicators, generally accessible via periodic reports, as part of the health sector's accountability to its publics;

- a standardised electronic health or patient record, accessible on a need-to-know basis, both for immediate patient care, and in anonymised (but not aggregated) form for management information and research;

- statistical frameworks which not only provide the data that roll up into summary indicators, but also an underlying richness of detail to allow interested parties to "drill down" to understand the "why" of various trends or patterns;

- an appreciation of the institutional diversity of health care and governance within Canada, which requires emphases on common standards and inter-operability, with much data and information focused on local needs, but at the same time being centrally accessible; and

- a sensitivity to international developments, for example in indicators of health system performance, and the benefits of sufficient comparability of health information, so Canada can learn from the experiences of other countries.

In sum, this requires building up our administrative data systems, and in turn, establishing common concepts and definitions for capturing the basic administrative data on health system encounters. It also requires the adoption and implementation of these standards. The federal government has recently created a new non-profit corporation with an endowment of $500 million to be spent primarily with the objective of creating electronic health records for Canadians – not only within each jurisdiction, but with a sufficient base of commonality that Canadians' health records will ultimately be accessible, on a strict need to know basis, across the country. The primary objective is improved patient care. But very close is the objective of building a "health infostructure" that supports performance assessment, improved system management, and public accountability.

Of course, these developments must be framed and supported by harmonised privacy policies and legislation. At the same time, this policy and legislation should not impede the kinds of data flows needed not only for more effective patient care, but also for the statistical analysis that is essential for the system management and performance measures sketched above.

The person-oriented data, embodied in electronic health records, in combination with improved and sustained population health surveys, are also key to public accountability. And these major extensions to Canada's endowment of health information will never reach their full potential without a major increase and re-focusing in our health analysis and research infrastructure. The newly formed Canadian Institutes for Health Research has greatly strengthened the priorities for population health and health services research and training, in addition to basic biological and clinical research, and is seeking to build bridges amongst researchers in all these areas.

Canada is therefore well positioned to make significant advances toward an integrated and coherent health information system.

NOTES

1. "Health infostructure" has become a widely used phrase in Canada to describe an interconnected and inter-operable health information infrastructure.

2. In addition to the 10 provinces' systems, there are also systems for the Northern Territories, for on-reserve First Nations, and for other populations under federal jurisdictions such as the military and those in federal prisons.

3. These include: Advisory Committee (1989, Alberta), British Columbia Royal Commission (1991), Collins and Twomey (1984), Commission (1998, New Brunswick), La Commission (1988, Québec), Manitoba Health (1992), Nova Scotia Royal Commission (1989), Ontario Panel (1987), and Saskatchewan (1990).

4. These eight dimensions of quality in health care were developed by the Canadian Council on Health Services Accreditation (1996).

5. Note that the general conclusion are not substantially affected if revascularization within 7 days or 30 days is used instead of 14 days.

6. Note that this variation in birth outcomes is not just apparent at the bottom of the social scale; it is also a "middle class" phenomenon – hence the much broader salience of including socio-economic factors centrally in health information systems.

7. Still, there are obvious and major gaps. For example, rigorous evaluation of pharmaceuticals, especially given their growing costs, the increasing subtleties of the distinctions between new and existing drugs, and the likelihood of more specific targeting of drug approvals for selected indications, will require some form of systematic post-marketing surveillance. Appropriate person-oriented administrative data systems, built on electronic health records, could achieve this at relatively low marginal cost.

REFERENCES

ADVISORY COMMITTEE ON THE UTILIZATION OF MEDICAL SERVICES (1989),
    An Agenda for Action, Government of Alberta, Edmonton

ADVISORY COUNCIL ON HEALTH INFOSTRUCTURE (1999),
    Canada Health Infoway. Paths to Better Health, Final Report, February, www.hc-sc.gc.ca/ohih-bsi.

BÉLANGER, A., MARTEL, L., BERTHELOT, J-M. and WILKINS, R. (2002),
    "Gender differences in disability-free life expectancies for selected risk factors and chronic conditions in
    Canada", Special issue on International Perspectives on Health Expectancies for Older Women, Journal of Women
    and Aging, Vol. 14, No. 1/2.

BRITISH COLUMBIA ROYAL COMMISSION ON HEALTH CARE AND COSTS (1991),
    Closer to Home, Crown Publications, Victoria.

CANADIAN COUNCIL ON HEALTH SERVICES ACCREDITATION (1996),
    A Guide to the Development and Use of Performance Indicators, Ottawa.

CIHI (1998),
    Health Information Needs in Canada, Ottawa. www.cihi.ca/wedo/infonds.shtml.

CIHI (1999),
    National Consensus Conference on Population Health Indicators: Final Report, Ottawa. www.cihi.ca/wedo/phidoc.shtml.

CIHI (2000),
    Health Care in Canada: A First Annual Report, Ottawa. www.cihi.ca/Roadmap/Health_Rep/healthreport2000/pdf/
    Healthreport2000.pdf.

CIHI (2001),
    Health Care in Canada, Ottawa. www.cihi.ca/HealthReport2001/toc.shtml.

COLLINS and TWOMEY (1984),
    A Green Paper on Our Health Care System Expenditures and Funding, Government of Newfoundland and Labrador,
    St. John's.

COMMISSION D'ENQUÊTE SUR LES SERVICES DE SANTÉ ET LES SERVICES SOCIAUX (1988),
    Rapport de la Commission d'enquête sur les services de santé et les services sociaux, Gouvernement de Québec, Québec.

COMMISSION ON SELECTED HEALTH CARE PROGRAMS (1988),
    Report of the Commission on Selected Health Care Programs, Government of New Brunswick, Fredericton.

DEATON, A. and LUBOTSKY, D. (2001),
    "Mortality, inequality and race in American cities and states", NBER Working Papers 8370, National Bureau of
    Economic Research, Inc.

DUDLEY, R.A., JOHANSEN, K.L., BRAND, R., RENNIE, D.J. and MILSTEIN, A. (2000),
    "Selective referral to high-volume hospitals: Estimating potentially aviodable deaths", JAMA, Vol. 283, No. 9,
    pp. 1159-1166.

ECONOMIC COUNCIL OF CANADA (1979),
    One in Three: Pensions for Canadians to 2030, Government of Canada, Ottawa.

EVANS, R.G. and STODDART, G.L. (1990),
    "Producing health, consuming health care", Social Science and Medicine, Vol. 31, No. 12, pp. 1347-1363, also
    reprinted in Chapter 2 in R.G.Evans, M.L.Barer and T.R.Marmor (eds.), Why Are Some People Healthy and Others
    Not? The Determinants of the Health of Populations (1994), Aldine de Gruyter, New York.

EVANS, R.G., BARER, M.L. and MARMOR, T.R. (1994),
    Why Are Some People Healthy and Others Not? The Determinants of the Health of Populations, Aldine de Gruyter, New York.

EVANS, R.G., McGRAIL, K.M., MORGAN, S.G., BARER, M.L. and HERTZMAN, C. (2001),
    "Apocalypse no: Population aging and the future of health care systems", Canadian Journal on Aging, Vol. 20,
    Supplement 1, pp.160-191, Summer.

FELLEGI, I.P. (1988), "Can we afford an aging society", Current Economic Observer, Statistics Canada, October, Ottawa.

153

FISHER, B., COSTANTINO, J.P., WICKERHAM, D.L., REDMOND, C.K., KAVANAH, M., CRONIN, W.M., VOGEL, V., ROBIDOUX, A., DIMITROV, N., ATKINS, J., DALY, M., WIEAND, S., TAN-CHIU, E., FORD, L. and WOLMARK, N. (1998),
"Tamoxifen for prevention of breast cancer: report of the National Surgical Adjuvant Breast and Bowel Project P-1 Study ", *Journal of the National Cancer Institute*, Vol. 90, No. 18, pp. 1371-1388.

GOEL, V., WILLIAMS, J., ANDERSON, G., BLACKSTIEN-HIRSCH, P., FOOKS, C. and NAYLOR, C.D. (eds.)(1996),
Patterns of Health Care in Ontario: The ICES Practice Atlas, 2nd Edition, Canadian Medical Association, Ottawa. *www.ices.on.ca*.

GRAVELLE, H. (1999),
"Diminishing returns to aggregate level studies", *British Medical Journal*, Vol. 319, No. 7215, pp. 955-956.

HERTZMAN, C., FRANK, J. and EVANS, R.G. (1994),
"Heterogeneities in Health Status and the Determinants of Health", in R.G. Evans, M.L. Barer and T.R. Marmor (eds.), *Why Are Some People Healthy and Others Not? The Determinants of the Health of Populations*, Aldine de Gruyter, New York.

HOULE, C., BERTHELOT, J-M, DAVID, P., WOLFSON, M.C., MUSTARD, C. and ROOS, L. (1997),
"Matching census database and Manitoba health care files", in W. Alvey and B. Jamerson (eds.), *Proceedings of an International Workshop and Exposition*, pp. 305 to 319, Federal Committee on Statistical Methodology, Office of Management and Budget, Washington, D.C. *www.fcsm.gov/working-papers/choule.pdf*.

JOHANSEN, H., NAIR, C., MAO, L. and WOLFSON, M. (2002),
"Revascularization and heart attack outcomes", *Health Reports*, Vol. 13, No. 2, pp. 35-46.

KNIGHTON, T., HOULE, C., BERTHELOT, J-M. and MUSTARD, C. (1998),
"Health care utilization during the first year of life: The impact of social and economic background", in Miles Corak (ed.), *Labour Markets, Social Institutions, and the Future of Canada's Children*, pp. 145-155, Statistics Canada, Ottawa.

LALONDE, M.(1974),
A New Perspective on the Health of Canadians: A Working Document, Department of Health and Welfare, Ottawa.

MANITOBA HEALTH (1992),
Quality Health for Manitobans: The Action Plan, Manitoba Health, Winnipeg.

MELLOR, J.M. and MILYO, J. (2001),
"Reexamining the evidence of an ecological association between income inequality and health", *Journal of Health Politics Policy and Law*, Vol. 26, No. 3, pp. 487-522.

NOVA SCOTIA ROYAL COMMISSION ON HEALTH CARE (1989),
Towards a New Strategy, Government of Nova Scotia, Halifax.

OECD (2000),
A System of Health Accounts, Version 1.0, Paris.

OECD (2001*a*),
OECD Health Data 2001, CD-ROM and User Guide, Paris.

OECD (2001*b*),
Health at a Glance, Paris.

ONTARIO HEALTH REVIEW PANEL (1987),
Toward a Shared Direction for Health in Ontario, Ministry of Health, Toronto.

PRIVACY COMMISSIONER OF CANADA,
Annual Report, 1989-1990, p. 30. *www.privcom.gc.ca*.

ROSS, N.A., WOLFSON, M.C., DUNN, J.R., BERTHELOT, J-M., KAPLAN, G. and LYNCH, J. (2000),
"Relation between income inequality and mortality in Canada and the United States: Cross-sectional assessment using census data and vital statistics ", *British Medical Journal*, Vol. 320, pp. 898-902.

SASKATCHEWAN COMMISSION ON DIRECTIONS IN HEALTH CARE (1990),
Future Directions for Health Care in Saskatchewan, Queen's Printer, Regina.

STATISTICS CANADA (2000),
"How healthy are Canadians? A special issue", *Health Reports*, Vol. 11, No. 3, Minister of Industry, Ottawa.

STATISTICS CANADA (2001),
"How healthy are Canadians? 2001 annual report", *Health Reports*, Vol. 12, No. 3, Minister of Industry, Ottawa. *www.statcan.ca/english/ads/82-003-XPB/toc.htm* (summary of paper).

STATISTICS CANADA (2001),
Policy on Record Linkage. www.statcan.ca/english/recrdlink.

TASK FORCE ON HEALTH (1992),
Health Reform: A Vision for Change, Government of Prince Edward Island, Charlottetown.

WHO (1992),
The Tenth Revision of the International Statistical Classification of Diseases and Related Health Problems, Vol. 1, Geneva, Switzerland.

WHO (2000),
World Health Report, Geneva. www.who.int/whr/2000/en/report.htm.

WILK, M. (1991),
Health Information for Canada, Report of the National Task Force on Health Information, Statistics Canada, Ottawa.

WILL, B.P., NOBREGA, K.M., BERTHELOT, J-M., FLANAGAN, W., WOLFSON, M.C., LOGAN, D.M. and EVANS, W.K. (2001),
"First do no harm: Extending the debate on the provision of preventive tamoxifen", British Journal of Cancer, Vol. 85, No. 9, pp. 1280-1288.

WOLFSON, M.C. and MURPHY, B. (1997),
"Aging and Canada's Public Sector: Retrospect and Prospect", in K.G. Banting and R. Boadway (eds.), Reform of Retirement Income Policy, International and Canadian Perspectives, Queens University School of Policy Studies, Kingston, Ontario.

WOLFSON, M., KAPLAN, G., LYNCH, J., ROSS, N. and BACKLUND, E. (1999),
"Relation between income inequality and mortality: empirical demonstration", British Medical Journal, Vol. 319, No. 7215, pp. 953-955.

155

Part III

PERFORMANCE MEASUREMENT ACTIVITIES AT THE INTERNATIONAL LEVEL: HOW CAN INTERNATIONAL COMPARISONS ASSIST NATIONAL POLICY-MAKING?

Chapter 8

OPENING THE BLACK BOX: WHAT CAN BE LEARNED FROM A DISEASE-BASED APPROACH?[1]

by

Stephane Jacobzone, Pierre Moise and Lynelle Moon[*]

Abstract

What are the appropriate levels and methods of funding, and the optimal mix of services for improving health care system performance? Policy-makers confronted with this question often look to other countries for answers. What they find is much variation across countries, with little understanding of how this relates to performance. The purpose of our paper is to demonstrate how a disease-based approach for comparing health care systems can help us better understand what drives health care system performance.

The OECD Ageing-Related Diseases (ARD) study has examined how institutional structures and economic incentives influence variations in diagnoses and treatments of certain diseases. The consequences in terms of costs and health outcomes were also explored. The study focused on ischaemic heart disease, breast cancer and stroke.

The first part of our paper places the ARD study within a framework for monitoring health care system performance. In the second part, we present some of the results of the ARD study relevant to health care system performance. They reveal striking differences in the utilisation of various health care technologies. Economic factors play a role, but exert more influence on the supply of these technologies than their demand. As a result, the levels of resources employed in health care systems vary more according to supply incentives than "demand" patterns that reflect disease prevalence.

However, disease rates are not "exogenous" to health care systems; epidemiological trends are themselves shaped by factors endogenous to health care systems. They can be influenced by preventive and diagnostic policies that are themselves subject to health policy and economic factors. Some countries may achieve lower mortality and improved outcomes mainly by using upstream population-based approaches, whereas others experience an intensive use of high technologies and curative care.

We examined outcome measures in terms of case fatality and survival rates. Our results show that outcomes of medical interventions can be sensitive to treatment patterns, which themselves are influenced by medical and non-medical factors. We found it more difficult to measure costs which limited our ability to assess the value of health expenditures, but we did find that countries with higher prices for inputs were generally those with the highest expenditure levels.

The policy implications of this study need to be assessed in the light of the various social preferences upon which health care systems are built. To better understand the implications of this

---

[*]   OECD Secretariat.

---

information, significant investments in integrated information systems, including registries and linked datasets will be required.

Introduction

Health care systems face complex demands from more empowered and better-informed patients. The production of health care involves several "product lines" and several types of interventions. The general aggregate indicators which have been used for international comparisons may no longer be adequate to summarise this complexity. These were essentially developed with an aggregate health and macroeconomic perspective. In order to obtain a fuller understanding of health systems in developed countries, more detailed data are needed. These include detailed performance indicators, with a microeconomic analysis of individual health records. In particular, disease-specific indicators of utilisation rates, treatments and outcomes are required. There is also a need for health policy studies and health policy work to be relevant in a clinical perspective.

A study, called the OECD Ageing-Related Diseases (ARD) study, was developed in response to the limitations in available information. It aims to offer more precise comparisons of activity and outcomes across countries with particular regard to the increasing needs of ageing populations. This is relevant for OECD health systems, as recent evidence shows health expenditure for people aged 65 and over is three to five times higher than for people aged 0-64 and accounts for an estimated 35 to 50 per cent of health expenditure as a whole (Jacobzone, forthcoming).

In spite of this progressive shift, modern health care systems in many OECD countries are still built upon the Pasteurian paradigm of protection against infectious diseases and sudden catastrophic expenditure. However, "modern" diseases in OECD countries are highly likely to be associated with old age, and are, for the most part, non-communicable. They often require ongoing treatment and significant expenditures until the end of life. For most OECD countries, this epidemiological transition has had profound implications for health systems, which are not always fully taken into account in policy frameworks. These systems are now increasingly buying extensions of and increases in the quality of life at older ages, rather than preventing mortality in younger age. The latter function is still performed, but it is no longer the main function in terms of the relative share of current and likely future expenditures in OECD countries.

This takes us to technology, the key factor in understanding differences in resource use and in performance across countries. The supply aspects of medical research and development, and the fact that it is generally geared towards finding more effective medical treatments – and not always the least costly ones – are the key challenges faced by policy makers. This is why this study has a clear emphasis on the use of several technologies. The study represents an assessment *ex post* of the impact of technology use on performance. This assessment *ex post* should be seen as a necessary supplement of the assessment *ex ante*, which occurs under the health technology assessment procedures implemented in a number of countries. Therefore, this study completes the performance measurement and improvement cycle introduce by Jeremy Hurst (Hurst, Part I, Chapter 2 in this volume). This paper first discusses the value of a comprehensive disease-based perspective in answering the key health policy questions in the field of performance monitoring. The paper follows with a discussion of the potential drivers of performance for the diseases studied, and how this can lead to improvements in performance. It concludes by discussing the various perspectives of various stakeholders in the field of performance monitoring and how they are illustrated through the current study.

I.   Reporting on performance: the value of a comprehensive disease-based perspective

1.1. A framework for performance monitoring

Policy makers in the field of health and social policy are increasingly asking questions about the value and quality of care obtained from health care expenditure at a cross national level (Anderson,

1997). The needs for this information are twofold. First, policy makers need clear answers in terms of cost, access and outcomes for health care systems. Second, these answers are needed to address some of the unresolved questions of previous macroeconomic analyses. For example, many macroeconomic analyses of trends in health costs, and of differences in expenditure and outcomes across countries, have come to the conclusion that differences in the diffusion of modern technologies could explain some of the unexplained differences across developed countries.

There is significant potential for disease focussed studies in international comparisons of the effectiveness of health expenditure. Clinical studies may not necessarily fit with policy-makers' needs, in terms of their focus and data coverage. In order to be able to examine causality, clinical studies tend to be very specific, using often narrowly defined populations receiving treatments under highly controlled conditions. However, because of these constraints, the results may not be representative of actual practice. This is where studies based on large datasets from routine care can be valuable. Examples of such comparisons come from the US/Canada, but remain of limited scope at the international level (Tu *et al.*, 1997a, *b*). The OECD's role in this process has been to provide a strong economic and health policy component.

Understanding which types of medical technologies diffuse efficiently and what policies influence diffusion is crucial for answering policy makers needs in developed countries. There is a need to explore whether there are links between the diffusion of technology, prices and the incentives faced both by providers and patients. The ARD project represents an attempt at examining these links through combining microdata from large individual patient discharge datasets, and a detailed analysis of health systems regulation and technological capacities. This leads to a concrete implementation of the framework introduced in Hurst (Part I, Chapter 2 in this volume). Although economic evaluation of technologies are often just performed before the decision to authorise entry, the actual diffusion of technologies in health care systems should be a primary concern of policy makers, since they result in actual expenditures and should be assessed against their true contribution to performance.

Two key elements were needed for this framework:

– *a disease approach*. This ensured that the analysis can be performed from a relevant angle.

– *large patient-based health records datasets*. These allowed for the analysis of the "average" treatment received by a given type of patients.

These two elements are discussed in the following subsections.

1.2. A *disease approach and its relationship to performance monitoring*

To assist in our discussion on the contribution that can be made by a "disease-based approach" to performance monitoring, it is first helpful to illustrate the health care system in relation to a particular disease as illustrated in the model presented in Figure 1. This disease-based model contains the main components of the health care system, and the relationships between these components and the disease.

The three main components of the disease-based model depicted in Figure 1 are:

1. the potential epidemiological phases (determinants, disease phase, and functional limitations),

2. interventions/treatments, and

3. resources/inputs.

For the first group, the determinants or risk factors are the precursors for the disease. These include both environmental and individual determinants, such as social, economic, lifestyle and biomedical factors, with some of these acting more directly than others (proximal and distal determinants). The second phase, the disease phase, represents the initial and/or more acute stages of the diseases, where signs and symptoms of the disease are apparent. The third and final phase occurs when any functional limitations may be apparent, including both physical and mental limitations.

161

Figure 1. **Disease-based model of health care system**

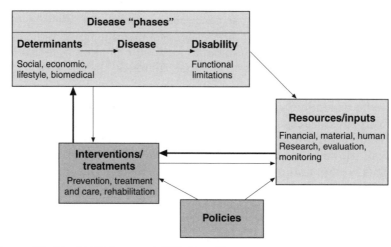

Source: Adapted from Evans and Stoddart (1990), Figure 5 and AIHW (2000), Figure 1.1.

The interventions box includes all aspects within the continuum of care such as disease prevention, treatment and care related to the disease, rehabilitation, and long-term care. The resources box represents two types of inputs into the health care system:

- the more visible inputs such as financial, human and material resources;
- the less observable inputs from research, evaluation and monitoring.

The bold arrows in Figure 1 represent the main activity between these boxes. As represented in the lower section of the diagram, the resources for the health care system are primarily directed to providing the interventions and treatments. The interventions in turn are directed at treating or managing the disease determinants, the more direct consequences of a disease, and any functional limitations related to the disease.

Other influences occur between these boxes, indicated by the arrows with light lines. First, aspects related to the level and severity of a particular disease, its determinants or resulting functional limitations (disease-phase group), influence both the type and mix of interventions (interventions box), and the level of inputs dedicated to the disease (resources box). Second, depending on the existence of constraints within a health care system, the type and mix of interventions may influence the level of inputs consumed. In summary, although the main influences are in the direction of the bold arrows, there are also influences that occur in other directions.

Policies and incentives within a health care system are an important influence on the relationship between the components of the health care system. The remaining box in Figure 1 represents this aspect. The influence of policies and incentives on both treatment variations and variations in the level of inputs to the health care system is also one of the primary focuses of this study.

An example of the type of information that can be collected using this model is given in Box 1. This illustrates the relevant data collected for the various diseases included in the study.

By examining variations in the components of the disease model shown in Figure 1, the ARD study is also aiming to further understand the effects of these influences on two performance-related issues – health outcomes and costs. The relationship of these to the disease model is represented in Figure 2, with the performance issues shown in the ovals on the left of and below the disease model.

The first performance-related issue identified in Figure 2 is "health outcomes". Health outcomes can be defined as changes in health status caused by health system activities. Health outcomes measures are directly related to health status measures reflecting the different phases of a disease, so

---

Box 1. **The disease model in the Ageing Related Diseases study**

The disease specifications are focussed on acute myocardial infarction, angina, breast cancer and ischaemic stroke. Information is collected for males and females separately, and for 3 broad age groups: 40-64, 65-74 and 75+ years.

Epidemiology

Information was collected on:

- *Determinants*: concentrating on tobacco smoking, cholesterol and hypertension for the relevant diseases. This is supplemented with some information on socioeconomic and other determinants of health from published sources.

- *Incidence*: collected from community-based registers, or from large patient health records. For stroke and cancer, registers are needed to capture cases both admitted to hospitals and those cared for in the community or other institutions, and to ensure the necessary follow up.

- *Mortality*.

- Supplemented with some info on *disability*, largely from published sources.

Treatments

- Based around the continuum of care (prevention, acute care, rehabilitation; and supplemented with information on long-term care). However, this is often limited by data availability.

- Information was collected on a number of treatment components, including key procedures, drug treatment, and the organisation of care (for example angioplasty (PTCA) and bypass (CABG) for heart attacks, mammography, radiotherapy for breast cancer, Magnetic Resonance Imaging, CT scans and stroke units for stroke).

Resources

- Information was collected on technology supply (for example CT scanners, MRI, catheterisation laboratories, cardiac surgery centres, mammography machines, radiotherapy machines), physician supply with the relevant specialty, although definitions of specialties were difficult to track across countries, and direct expenditures.

Policies

- Qualitative information was collected using a standard table listing policy administrative and incentive issues. Examples include the financing mix, the role of copayments and cost sharing for demand side incentives, the existence of queuing/waiting times, the regulation and planning regarding the introduction of new technologies, and the reimbursement mechanisms for providers.

---

the relevant component is located alongside the corresponding section of the disease-based model of the health care system. For a particular disease, health outcome measures should ideally relate to all three identified "phases" of the disease.

The second performance-related issue identified in Figure 2 is costs. The costs related to a particular disease can be divided into the direct and indirect costs, located in Figure 2: the relevant component of the disease model. The direct costs are associated with the resources and inputs for the disease model of the health care system and include both public and private expenditure. Indirect costs can be thought of as the costs related to the mortality and morbidity from a particular disease (for example, the costs due to the associated lost productivity), and are therefore located under the disease phase component of the model. Box 2 introduces examples of indicators collected under the various diseases of the study in relation to the performance aspects.

Figure 2.   **Relationship of performance aspects to disease model**

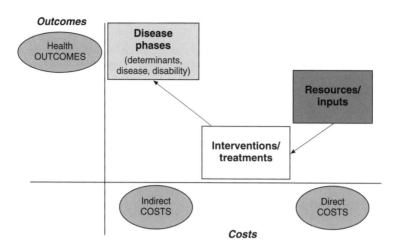

The performance-related issues shown in the ovals in Figure 2 are those included in the study – health outcomes and costs. These two aspects *together* have important connections to the broad aims of health policies – to improve health outcomes whilst minimising costs. Inevitably there are some trade-offs to be made when balancing these two aspects. However, it is important to remember that it is both of these in relation to the other that is generally important from a policy perspective.

These two aspects relate to the model presented as a proposed OECD Performance Framework (Hurst and Jee-Hughes, 2001). The three components of that framework are:

- health improvements/outcomes,
- financial contribution/health expenditure
- responsiveness and access.

Box 2.   **Links with performance monitoring**

The following information relevant to performance monitoring has been included where relevant and possible in the study in the breast cancer, ischaemic heart disease and stroke components:

Health outcomes

- Hospital fatality rates
- Case fatality rates
- Supplemented with information on disability-related outcomes from published sources.
- Survival 5 year after diagnosis for cancer
- Trends in mortality by age and gender group

Costs

- Direct costs (aggregate public and private expenditure)
- Per unit expenditures for a number of "bundles of goods"
- Supplemented with information on indirect costs from a small number of countries.

The first two of these align closely with the two performance issues presented in Figure 2 ("health outcomes" and "costs"). Although the third component of the framework was not explicitly included in the model based on the scope of the project, one important dimension has been explored throughout the study: its relation to age and the access of older persons to appropriate care.

In addition, other performance aspects could be added to the disease-based performance model presented in Figure 2. Many other aspects commonly included in performance frameworks (Hurst and Jee-Hughes, 2001; Or, 2001), such as appropriateness, responsiveness, access, safety and respect/caring relate to the interventions/treatments component of the model. These are all connected with the provision of the health services. Several of the measures that were collected under the study could be considered as part of future national performance frameworks in OECD countries.

1.3. The value of a disease-based approach in performance monitoring

The value to be gained in using a disease approach is in its ability to provide information on a complete subset of the health care system. This provides analysis using more specific measures than is the case with a more aggregate level approach. Also, it provides the basis for examining relationships between components of the health care system, in a way that is clinically relevant and understandable by patients and providers.

A disease approach closely follows the organisation of health care. Health professionals often specialise in a particular area that is associated with a specific disease group, which is notably the case for medical specialists. Similarly, specific health policies and programs are often centred on a particular disease.

A disease approach also increases the homogeneity of a particular patient group. For example, the health outcomes for a well-defined diagnosis are easier to interpret than for a broader group of patients. This is due to less variation being attributable to patient differences rather than due to differences in health service provision. Thus, by using a well-defined diagnosis group, we overcome the problem of heterogeneity to some extent by controlling for a portion of the unobserved heterogeneity both within and between jurisdictions. This is particularly important for cross-national studies, where the relevance of statistical tools for controlling unobserved heterogeneity remains limited.

However, one drawback of the disease approach is the risk of being too specific compared with the broader questions asked by policy makers. In order to minimise this risk, the current study concentrates on several "key" diseases for modern health care systems, with a view to providing a more general perspective on health care systems by combining the results from all the disease analyses.

There is also substantial value to be gained from the international comparisons of health systems that this type of approach permits. It is at the international level that comparisons of health care systems and policies can be made. In addition, international comparisons also make it possible to compare different approaches to care that may contribute to our knowledge of best practice. However, it is also important to be cautious when interpreting or applying results from international comparisons, as what may be advantageous in one country is not necessarily appropriate for another country due to differences both in the political situations and in the social values.

1.4. Building the knowledge: making use of existing patient-based health records

A disease approach needs to be supported by a solid information infrastructure in order to properly measure performance. The strategy chosen in the current study was to make extensive use of existing patient-based health records, obtained through contacts between the Secretariat and national administrations in OECD countries. This wealth of health records currently collected by national administrations make it a relatively cheap source of information, given its size, in the health field, and one which deserves further analysis. The alternative would have involved developing specific clinical based surveys, which are usually costly to administer and their size and general relevance for policy remains inevitably limited.

i)   Availability

The ever increasing availability of patient-based health records has greatly facilitated the ability to monitor health care system performance on an individual disease basis. Advances in information technology have both greatly increased the amount of information that is easily accessible and provided the greater computing power necessary for estimating complicated statistical equations. Thus, hospital administrative databases have evolved beyond their original design to monitor hospital activity for planning purposes to include a host of patient-based clinical, policy and economics-related variables that can be used for research. Some of these databases are listed in Moise (2001).

Based on Figure 2, there are two dimensions of performance that can be measured, outcomes and costs. The same variables from hospital administrative databases used for health care services administration and research can also be used for monitoring health care system performance. In theory, the cost aspect of performance can be monitored with Diagnosis Related Groups (DRG)-based hospital administrative databases since these can be linked to resource use. However, in practice, using DRG-based hospital administrative databases to measure costs can be difficult. On the other hand, it is much easier to measure some aspects of the outcome component of performance. All hospital administrative databases record inhospital deaths. Linked hospital administrative databases (see below) are also able to keep track of deaths following discharge, providing a more complete measure of case fatality. Furthermore, linked databases can keep track of readmissions, another outcome measure.

The value of hospital administrative databases as tools for measuring health care system performance increases with the breadth of coverage. The most comprehensive databases, in each case covering the entire nation, are found in Australia, Canada, Denmark, Finland, Sweden and the United States (Medicare – only persons aged 65 and over) and many have been in existence for years. More recently, other countries have started developing their own nationally representative hospital administrative databases. In many cases these have evolved from sub-national databases. In Italy for example, the *Scheda di Dimissione Ospedaliera* has evolved from databases representing a few regions in the early 1990s to a nationally representative database.

Hospital administrative databases can only be used to monitor performance aspects of the acute care part of the health care system. A disease-based approach to measuring performance requires supplemental sources of information to cover the nonacute parts of the health care system. In the current study information from hospital administrative databases was supplemented with data taken from surveys, disease registers (especially for breast cancer and stroke) and *ad hoc* studies. For example, for the ischaemic heart disease part of the project we used data from the MONICA study to provide a link between health outcomes and the utilisation of health care interventions. The MONICA information provided us with information on drug therapies not available with hospital discharge databases. A list of some of the supplemental sources of information we used for the project is found in the various reports.

ii)   Linking

Hospital administrative databases are designed to record only inhospital activities, which presents a problem for measuring health outcomes of discharged patients (although the act of being discharged, whether dead or alive, is itself a measure of outcome). Thus, there is a need to monitor the results of medical interventions both during the hospital stay and *after* patients are discharged from hospital, that is, health outcomes should be measured during an "episode of care", defined as: the period in which a patient is admitted to hospital for treatment until the resolution of the health problem. Of course, there are the problems of defining exactly when the health problem has been resolved, unless the result is death, and the logistics of following many patients over a considerable period of time. To minimise these problems episodes of care are usually defined for a specific period of time, usually no longer than a year, although in the case of long-lasting diseases such as cancer, outcomes are typically measured for periods greater than one year up to 5 or 10 years.

The most effective method for measuring the health outcomes of patients following discharge is to assign a patient identifier to each admission record. The process of assigning an identifier to a patient record in hospital administrative databases is known as "linking", because for each patient, all records corresponding to a hospital admission can be linked together through the patient identifier. Data derived from linked databases may be referred to as "patient-based", as opposed to "event-based" data in which each are specific to a given patient but only for one hospital stay. In addition, there is also interdatabase linking such as between hospital data systems and death registers, disease registers, ambulatory care administrative databases and various surveys.

The capability to link to other databases increases the ability to monitor health care system performance by allowing for better measuring health outcomes. This is particularly important for older patients. This is because the aged are more likely to have multiple encounters with the health care system. Therefore, it is important to be able to create a proper episode of care for the elderly otherwise a significant amount of health care activity could be lost or inaccurately measured.

In addition, the potential exists for linking hospital administrative databases to surveys regarding issues of particular concern to the elderly. Long-term care and home care are two issues where there have been an increasing number of surveys in recent years. The launch and further development of large longitudinal surveys such as the National Long-Term Care Survey and the Health and Retirement Survey in the United States, and the progressive development of similar surveys in Europe are positive signs for the future. However, in many countries, the potential for a full assessment of performance remains currently limited, as information systems remain fragmented along the continuum of care, and as legal constraints challenge the possibility of linking data for the purpose of performance monitoring.

The crucial importance of patient privacy should not hide the important research and evaluation benefits, which can be derived from linked datasources. It is crucial to ensure the public's confidence in the security of data gathering systems while allowing for better access to information for research purposes. This relative balance differs across countries. In at least part of Australia, Canada, Denmark, Finland, Sweden and the United States the importance of linking information has been recognised, both over time and over care settings, and corresponding information infrastructure has been implemented. These countries have made significant strides in linking their hospital administrative databases to other information sources, although this is done at the state and provincial level in Australia and Canada respectively, and only for the population 65 and over in the US. However, efforts are also being developed in other countries, such as in the UK Oxford area, and in France, with "non identifiable" patient identifiers, which allow tracking rehospitalisations over time, without making it possible to link hospital discharge data with any other administrative files.

iii) *Measuring outcomes*

The primary identifiable health outcome common to all hospital discharge databases is inhospital case fatality.[2] Unlike the broader measure of mortality, case fatality has the added advantage of a more direct link between intervention and result. Thus, inhospital case fatality provides a more precise outcome measure of the acute-care part of the health care system. Furthermore, by using linked databases, an even more precise picture of case fatality can be measured for a specified episode of care: for example from 30 days to one year, or even beyond.

The importance of linking hospital discharge databases also comes in to play with another measure of health outcomes: readmissions. At the aggregate level, the use of mortality measures only one aspect of health outcomes, death. In the same vein, case fatality figures only cover the death portion of the health outcomes. Readmissions are a relatively easy way to measure non-fatality related health outcomes; they include the diagnosis most responsible for a readmission following an earlier admission, and can thus be used to measure the morbidity outcome of the initial admission.

Beyond these objective measures, the ability of hospital records to fully measure outcomes could be greatly enhanced by introducing short modules, including patient satisfaction and patient's perception for key indicators such as responsiveness, suffering/pain and satisfaction about the interaction with health professionals. Such indicators exist in a few countries, for example in the Voluntary Hospitals in Japan (VHJ) system in Japan, or in specific research modules in the United States.

Their extension in the future could greatly enhance the capacity and relevance of research in this field, making use of patient health records.

2. Understanding the drivers of performance

Earlier investigations of the drivers of performance have focused on explaining differences in health care expenditure across countries. These descriptive studies have often tried to transpose at the international level factors identified in national studies which contribute to growth in medical spending. Potential growth factors identified include increased coverage, ageing populations and variations in prices. Using an economic growth accounting framework, Newhouse (1992) maintains these factors account for only 50% of the growth in medical care spending; the remaining 50 per cent "residual" should be attributed to technological change.

2.1. Technology, economic incentives and the use of medical interventions

In the policy debate, many analysts tend to attribute the rapid growth in health expenditures to ageing, whereas, in fact, this growth mainly results from the diffusion of new technologies. The entry of medical technologies in health care systems of developed countries is highly dependent upon prevailing institutional and economic incentives (Weisbrod, 1991). Weisbrod posits that the United States, as the only significant "actor" in both the health care R&D (production) and consumption sectors, exerts the largest influence on technological change. Invention of new technologies is affected by policies which foster relationships between academia, government financed-research, and property right legislation, with the US health care system giving very generous incentives. However, the types of incentives prevalent in the US. system tend to favour cost-increasing technologies rather than cost-saving ones.

Once technologies are established, the patterns of diffusion within countries are subject to economic incentives inherent in their health care systems. These are related to the relative propensity of government and health care systems to pay for those technologies. This is illustrated in a number of theoretical studies, but with very few empirical cross-national studies. Recent US work (Cutler and McClellan, 1996) has shown that, for heart attack patients, a key factor behind increasing health expenditures has been the rate of the diffusion of technologies. At an international level, the TECH network (McClellan and Kessler, 1999; TECH, 2000) provides an example of an analysis of such factors, building on the earlier results of the McKinsey report (McKinsey Global Institute et al., 1996).

The diffusion of technologies is of particular concern to health policy makers, since many developed countries are facing decreasing marginal returns from medical technologies. Technologies are often assessed under well-defined circumstances in medical trials, with limited population samples. Afterwards, their use might be extended well beyond the intended target group to patients whose characteristics are disimilar to those of the initial patient group tested in the trial. This is why the issue arises, "Whether certain technologies have 'gone bad'" (Phelps, 1997). The marginal cost-effectiveness of medical interventions varies in different groups of the population. The widespread use of technologies may translate into reduced effectiveness: the more we use the technologies, the less effective they may become if they are used for groups of patients beyond the initial indications for which they were designed. While this may not harm patients, and may even produce marginal health benefits in terms of quality of life, this certainly can harm the patients' purse, or at least their insurers' or the public finances, who will in return require higher premiums or taxes.

The results of the Ageing-Related Disease study generally support the view that supply-side incentives play a key role in terms of the availability and the use of costly technologies that "create" the expenditures in modern health care systems: for example, MRIs, lasers, mammography machines, PTCA, catheterisation laboratories. However, the results in relation to health outcomes deserve careful examination to obtain a full understanding of performance.

2.2. *Demand and supply led economic incentives*

Health care systems involve a complex interaction of demand and supply led economic incentives. Demand side incentives include copayments, and listing and prescription policies for ambulatory care drugs; while supply side incentives include planning and regulating special care facilities, assessing health technologies and paying providers. How the various demand and supply side components interact is often intrinsically linked with the structure of a given health care system. We introduce here a broad distinction between two families of health systems, which will inform the analysis of the interactions between demand and supply led incentives and treatment patterns.

A distinction can be made between an "integrated public model" and an "insurance system". These broad categories are important since they were found to have a strong influence on patterns of care, and performance achievements:

- The "integrated public model" primarily includes public hospitals for the delivery of acute care. In this case there is strict planning of facilities and generally a use of global budgets to reimburse hospitals and other providers of acute care. This system is generally found in the United Kingdom, in Nordic countries, and in some Mediterranean countries such as Italy and Spain.

- The "insurance" model is another type of system, which includes both social or private insurance models. In these systems, a certain among of hospital care is reimbursed either through fee-for-service or through case-based payment systems, such as Diagnosis Related Groups. These systems generally rely less on planning and overall regulation, and more on reimbursement systems for patients and providers. These systems exist under the form of a social insurance system for the elderly in the United States and for the general population in continental Europe, in countries such as Belgium, France, Germany, and the Netherlands. In other cases, such as for the working age population in the United States, or in Switzerland for the general population, a market-based insurance system is used with some regulation.

With this distinction in mind, we now consider two of the diseases included in the study, ischaemic heart disease (IHD), and breast cancer. The discussion addresses the interrelationship between demand and supply incentives, and treatment patterns. At the same time, we also analyse the links between the treatment patterns and the availability and use of facilities.

i) *The case of* IHD

Demand constraints generally play a small role in IHD-related care provided in acute care settings, but can be significant for ambulatory care drugs. The exception is the United States where studies have shown the uninsured have less access to expensive elective procedures (Wenneker *et al.*, 1990; Hadley *et al.*, 1991). More recent studies that have controlled for patient's insurance status, found similar results for access to emergency intensive cardiac procedures for Acute Myocardial Infarction (AMI), but found no differences in outcomes by insurance status (Sada *et al.*, 1998; Canto *et al.*, 2000). However, the impact of restricted coverage in the US for IHD related health care is limited because the bulk of health care for IHD is delivered to older persons, for whom there is near universal coverage through Medicare and Medicaid.

Even where universal coverage exists, it is not without some form of restriction. Universal coverage for health care is defined within the parameters of what may be considered as "medically necessary", a definition which varies by country. This definition entails the strongest evidence of implicit demand-side constraints, as it reflects priorities. For some countries this definition limits coverage to providers employed by or contracted to the public system, thus limiting choice of provider. The option to choose a private provider is thus available to those who can afford the option by paying out-of-pocket, or as is more common, through private or supplemental health insurance. The potential impact is greatest in countries such as Greece and the United Kingdom where longer waiting times for invasive interventions in the public sector can be eased by choosing a private provider with shorter waiting times.

Demand side incentives are more important with respect to prescription drugs delivered outside the acute care hospital setting, since health insurance generally covers drugs within hospitals. Our

169

analysis of drug consumption refers primarily to the consumption of drugs in the ambulatory care sector: the data collected on drug consumption concern the consumption of ambulatory drugs related mostly to primary and secondary preventive care of IHD. However, we note from our results that the countries with lower levels of drug consumption have universal coverage, while countries with non-universal coverage, or coverage limited through copayments, experience higher rates of consumption. The role of prescription patterns, and possibly the budgeting of physician prescriptions in some countries (Jacobzone, 2000), may play a greater role for overall levels of consumption, suggesting that variations across countries in patterns of drug consumption may result from a mix of demand and supply-side constraints.

More comprehensive results can be obtained from a study linked to the ageing-related disease project (Dickson and Jacobzone, 2002). The results suggest associations between use of diuretics (C03) and beta blockers (C07) with IHD mortality, where these drugs are relatively cheap and old, while being effective. However, for "newer" pharmaceutical agents (calcium channel blockers, ACE inhibitors, and serum lipid reducers), the study found that the use is higher among those countries that spend a greater percentage of GDP on health. These drugs being usually more expensive, the study formulates the hypothesis that countries that spend more on health might have an implicit preference for these newere and more costly therapies (see Charts A1 and A2 in the annex).

Overall, supply-side constraints exert a strong influence on treatment patterns. Supply-side constraints reflect a complex interaction between payment methods, availability and constraints on technology that determine utilisation levels. For example, supply-side factors appear to be important in determining utilisation levels for the more resource intensive procedures of Percutaneous Transluminal Coronary Angioplasty (PTCA) and Coronary Artery Bypass Graft (CABG), relative to drug therapy. These procedures have diffused rapidly over the 1980s and the 1990s across OECD countries, with PTCA introduced after CABG but with a more rapid growth (Chart A3).

Utilisation of PTCA and CABG procedures requires that the proper human[3] and physical resources are available. We find a positive relationships between the availability of cardiac surgery facilities and utilisation of CABGs, and between the number of catheterisation laboratories and utilisation of PTCAs (see Chart A4 and A5 in the annex) . However, these charts reveal even more information if interpreted as illustrating the various "production functions" across countries. Countries above the trend line tend to produce relatively more CABGs per facility. We observe that production levels for CABG in Denmark, Italy and Sweden for instance, are lower than the level in the United States, or to a lesser extent Canada (Ontario), Germany or Australia. One very important feature separates countries above the line from those below: in the countries above the line, physicians operating in hospitals are paid fee-for-service, whereas in all the countries at or below the line, physicians operating in hospitals are paid on a salaried basis with hospitals financed with global budgets. Generally, the health care systems for the countries above the line are organised on an "insurance" model, whereas the health care systems of the countries below the line are more of the "integrated public" model.

The analysis is similar for catheterisation laboratories, with an even stronger link between utilisation levels and the availability of facilities. The distribution of countries is slightly different with the United States, Canada (Ontario), Norway, Greece and Australia being above the line, Germany and Canada being on the line, and Denmark, Sweden and Finland being clearly below the line. There are some slight differences in the link between physician payment methods and production levels, Norway for example has a relatively high production level of PTCA. The reader should bear in mind a caveat regarding this analysis. This production level analysis is limited to "throughputs", that is we cannot draw conclusions from this in terms of the adequacy of care delivered with regard to potential needs, and no conclusions in terms of the effectiveness of the care delivered.

These relationships have been further explored using multivariate panel data analysis (Table 1). Our initial analysis shows that, across 11 countries, utilisation of these procedures is income elastic. That is, for each 1 per cent increase in income (expressed as GDP per capita) utilisation of CABG or PTCA increases by more than 1 per cent. The regression analysis also indicates that "need", as proxied through mortality, is a statistically significant determinant of the use of revascularisation procedures,

Table 1. **Analysis of the determinants of CABG and PTCA utilisation**

Regressions with CABG per 100 000 population aged 40 and over as the dependent variable

Share of health expenditure in GDP				GDP per capita			
Share of health expenditure	++	+		GDP per capita	++	++	
Mortality	n.a.	++	++	Mortality	n.a.	++	++
Hospital constraints	+	++	++	Hospital constraints	++	++	++
Facility constraints			+	Facility constraints	+	+	+
Yearly dummies 91-97		n.a.	++	Yearly dummies 91-97		n.a.	++
Constant	> 0	++	++	Constant	++	++	++
Observations	81	81	81	Observations	81	81	81
Percentage of variance explained	55	65	79	Percentage of variance explained	63	71	79

Regressions with PTCA per 100 000 population aged 40 and over as the dependent variable

Share of health expenditure in GDP				GDP per capita			
Share of health expenditure	++	++	+	GDP per capita	++	++	++
Mortality	n.a.		++	Mortality	n.a.	+	
Hospital constraints	+	+	++	Hospital constraints	++	++	++
Facility constraints	+	+	++	Facility constraints	++	++	++
Yearly dummies 91-97		n.a.	++	Yearly dummies 91-97		n.a.	++
Constant			++	Constant		++	++
Observations	85	85	85	Observations	85	85	85
R-squared	57	57	81	R-squared	80	81	87

++ denotes significant at 1%; + denotes significant at 5%; others significant at 10%.
n.a. Not included in the model.

Note: The constant term is negative except for where it is denoted by (> 0).
Endogenous variable: Number of CABG (PTCA) per 100 000 population aged 40 and over.
Exogenous variables:

Share of health exp.	Ln(Share of Health Expenditure/GDP)
GDP per cap.	Ln(GDP/capita) (GDP in US $ PPP)
Mortality	Ln(Number of IHD deaths per 100 000 population aged 40+)
HOSPCON	Hospital payment constraints: 1: mainly global budget
	2: mixed financing or DRG
	3: mainly FFS
FACCON	Macroregulation of facilities: 1: explicit constraints and targeted funding
	2: explicit constraints or targeted funding
	3: no constraints

Source: Moise and Jacobzone (2002) for definition of constraints per country.

the relationship being stronger for CABG than for PTCA. The latter result can be looked on as successful "needs-based planning" for CABG: many of the countries that rely heavily on public planning of cardiac surgery facilities, combined in some cases with regulation on the number of CABG performed, also tend to have a high burden of ischaemic heart disease. The positive, but statistically weaker relationship between PTCA and needs probably reflects the effect of fee-for-service payment for physicians and lower fixed costs, both of which will favour the use of PTCA over CABG. In both cases, the payment mechanisms for hospitals (HOSPCON) and the facility constraints or physician reimbursement systems play a significant role in the utilisation of these procedures.[4] Without including time variables (which depict the diffusion of these technologies over time), these variables explain between 70 to 80 per cent of the variance using GDP per capita as a independent variable (the results for health expenditure as a percentage of GDP are similar, but not as strong). With the time variables the results explain even more of the variation. It is quite clear that economic variables, including both the level of income and payment mechanisms play a key role in determining utilisation levels of revascularisation procedures, while the role of "health needs" have a lesser influence.

Payment mechanisms can also influence the mix of care, in this case the proportion of CABG in the total number of revascularisations. Chart A6 presents the use of CABG as a proportion of total revascularisations. First, the data clearly show that for all countries CABG as a means of revascularization is losing ground to PTCA. Since the rate of CABG use per 100 000 persons has been increasing during this period (see Moise and Jacobzone, 2002), PTCA use is growing even faster. In addition, we see that the insurance countries (Belgium, Germany and the US), rely far less on CABG as a means of revascularisation than PTCA. These three countries have in common fee-for-service arrangements for paying hospitals and physicians (in Germany physicians are not paid exclusively fee-for-service). In an environment where both hospitals and physicians are paid fee-for-service, there are several factors that make PTCA more financially attractive: on the cost side, the procedure is not as intensive and requires less fixed capital costs; in terms of financial benefits for physicians, it is fixed fees combined with a lower risk of complications during the production process (the operation itself). It is the combination of these factors that makes PTCA the more attractive alternative for revascularization under a fee-for-service regime for both hospitals and physicians.

The impact of payment mechanisms can be felt in other ways as well, not just in creating a higher propensity to use more intensive and costly procedures. Open-ended financing of hospitals creates the incentive for keeping patients in hospital longer. This is the case for Belgium and Japan, which have much longer lengths of stay than other countries, even after controlling for patient homogeneity in terms of age groups (although in the case of Japan, this also reflects a substitution of acute care beds for use as long-term care beds).

ii) The case of breast cancer

There is little evidence of any constraint on the demand for health care related to breast cancer. The one exception is the United States where14% of individuals have no health care coverage. These are mainly the working poor and the young. There are some studies showing evidence of the detrimental effect of the lack of coverage on middle-aged uninsured women. However, this seems to be due to a lack of access to early screening, and results in more severe cases and worse outcomes (Decker and Rappaport, 2001). The US evidence shows that differential access to mammography screening results in initial diagnosis taking place at more severe stages for the uninsured (Osteen et al., 1994). However, in spite of being conditional on stage and age, the uninsured receive about the same proportion of care as the better insured patients, which reflects the absence of demand-side incentives in the acute phase of treatment, even in the United States. The poor outcomes observed for the uninsured are the result of the lack of a proactive preventive approach for these groups within a fragmented system. However, the impact of restricted coverage in the US for care related to breast cancer is limited because the bulk of health care for breast cancer is provided to older persons, for whom there is universal coverage through Medicare. Some UK studies reported that lower socio-economic status can also result in a lower rate of breast-conserving surgery (Albain et al., 1996).

In terms of screening, available data show a weak link between the number of women undergoing a mammography and the availability of mammography machines (Chart A7). Although fully comparable data for the rate of women receiving a mammography in the past year are difficult to assemble, some countries, and particularly the Nordic countries, achieve a fairly high rate of screening, although they have fewer machines than countries such as France or the United States. These findings are consistent with the overall epidemiological trends and the high incidence observed in those countries. In addition, countries with integrated public systems achieve high rates of screening as part of organised programs, whereas insurance countries such as France do not achieve such a high rate even if they have more machines. In the insurance countries, the primary role devolved to opportunistic screening tends to distribute this screening unevenly and is not necessarily the most cost-effective use of the technological resources available. In the integrated public system countries, the organised screening programs, when they cover the relevant population, are efficient tools in ensuring high rates of screening for a relatively limited stock of mammography machines.

In terms of treatment, supply-side constraints exert a strong influence. In some countries, supply-side factors appear to be important in determining levels of radiotherapy for older people (Charts A8 and A9 in the annex). The combination of age and economic factors makes it difficult to disentangle the two. The two most important supply-side factors are the methods used for paying for inpatient treatment, and how strictly facilities are regulated. Providing care requires proper facilities, but aside from radiotherapy, the surgical facilities used for breast cancer surgery are not defined. The relative availability across countries of radiation therapy appear important, but more so for older patients. An additional consideration is the lack of qualified personnel. The information provided by national reports points to potential shortages of qualified oncologists in a number of countries, for example the United Kingdom.

The previous section has investigated the links between treatment patterns and economic incentives. This addresses implicitly one dimension of performance, which is the relationships between system design and the quantity of care delivered. The following section takes the discussion a step further in investigating the links with value for money.

2.3. Do we get value for money ? Improving health system performance, systems design and patterns for prevention and care

Policy makers are generally interested not only in the relationship between incentives and throughputs, but also in what happens to patients and how much does this cost. This means that research needs to be informative in terms of the links between actual resources and outcomes. The current study has gathered some evidence in this area. We have analysed disease-related outcomes in a cross country perspective, and scrutinised any evidence of a correlation between outcomes and interventions. In addition, we have analysed unit expenditure per intervention. However, prevention is also very important for population health outcomes. Therefore, we also give attention to specific aspects of medical prevention, either of the disease itself, or of its disabilitating consequences. The global picture can be obtained from making the general link between resources, including both prevention, medical intervention and the associated unit expenditures, and overall results in terms of the available outcome indicators. The analysis considers ischaemic heart disease, breast cancer and stroke.

i) The case of IHD

The easiest and perhaps best population-based aggregate measure of health outcomes for IHO is the trend in mortality rates. Since the 1970s age-standardised mortality rates have been on the decline in the majority of OECD countries, but at different rates (see Moise and Jacobzone, 2002). How much of a role has the health care system played in bringing about these reductions? The three countries that achieved the greatest reductions in IHD mortality, Australia, Canada and the United States, differ from each other in the mix of health care services used to treat IHD. The US has the highest use of intensive procedures among these countries, followed by Australia and then Canada, yet the reductions in IHD mortality were roughly similar. On the other hand, both Belgium and Germany, two countries with similar utilisation levels for intensive procedures as the US and Australia, had lower reductions in IHD mortality. The United Kingdom, which has the lowest utilisation rates of intensive treatments for IHD, also saw mortality from IHD decline. Putting aside any causal implications, we find that at an aggregate level the countries with the highest activity rates, in terms of utilisation of medically intensive procedures, do not necessarily achieve the steepest reductions in IHD mortality.

While health care treatments may certainly explain some of the success in reducing IHD mortality rates, there must be other contributing factors. As evidence from other studies shows, especially the WHO-MONICA study, it appears important to investigate the reductions in underlying risk factors. Perhaps the most cited example of this is the change in smoking patterns since the 1970s. For example, Australia, Canada and the United States not only saw the largest reductions in IHD mortality during this period, but they also saw the largest reductions in tobacco consumption. Germany, Sweden and the UK had lower declines in IHD mortality as well as lower declines in tobacco consumption. Conversely, tobacco consumption increased in Denmark, Finland, Italy and Norway at the same time that IHD mortality rates were decreasing.

The discussion in the previous paragraph was based on aggregate mortality data. However, the impact of intensive treatment can best be observed at the micro-level, with patient-based data (Chart A10). Based on the materials collected as part of this project,[5] we have provided a graphical depiction showing jointly treatment trends in terms of the proportion of AMI patients receiving a

173

revascularisation procedure (CABG + PTCA) within 90-days from the initial admission and outcomes, in terms of the proportion of patients who died within one-year from the initial admission on the y-axis.

The most obvious depiction from these charts is that they clearly separate the countries with a higher propensity to use revascularisation as a means of treating AMI, the US and to a lesser extent Australia (Perth), from the countries that rely less on this method, Canada (Ontario), Finland and Sweden. What is also clear is that, within each country, there was generally an increase over time in the proportion of patients receiving revascularisation procedures and an accompanying declining case fatality. Modest increases in revascularisation rates in Ontario and Sweden have been accompanied by significant declines in case fatality for the elderly. The United States seems to be on a different "production function", with much higher increases in revascularisation rates but similar declines in mortality. For the younger age groups, the pattern is more mixed, with some declines in case fatality in Finland, Sweden and Ontario, and a mixed picture for the United States.

From these charts we see that persons aged 40-64 in the US do not fare as well in terms of case fatality relative to the other countries as their older fellow citizens. Since we have not controlled for case-mix or socioeconomic status, the poorer results for the younger age group in the US likely reflect the inclusion of individuals with no health insurance, which is not a problem for Americans aged 65. These charts tend to support the view that Ontario, Perth, Finland and Sweden are more or less on the same production function. The United States is either on a different production function, or on the part of the same production function exhibiting decreasing marginal returns to health interventions: the US also experiences reductions in case fatality, but these do not seem to be in line with the additional amount of resources invested.

Any assessment regarding "value for money" requires that we make a link between outcome indicators and some notion of expenditure, keeping in mind that expenditure reflects both volume of activity and prices. The health care expenditure patterns of OECD countries are well documented. The United States stands alone as the largest overall spender on health care. A second group of countries including Australia, Belgium, Canada and Germany tend to spend more than the average of OECD countries, while the lowest spenders include countries such as Finland, Spain and the United Kingdom. The study as a whole found a general link between activity levels as reported above and trends in expenditure. In order to forge a stronger link, we examined per-unit expenditure on IHD-related care. Our study shows that the United States spends more than other countries per unit of input (see Moise and Jacobzone, 2002). Therefore, the gap in expenditure between the United States and other countries with similar volumes of activity for intensive procedures, such as Belgium and Germany, can be further explained through higher per-unit expenditures.

Since the United States is such an outlier, it is difficult to have a discussion on spending on health care among OECD countries without the US experience dominating. Based on the data we collected on overall spending and per-unit expenditures, combined with at best marginally better health outcomes, it is hard not to conclude that the marginal returns to spending in the US appear to be modest relative to other countries.

However, the question remains open whether other technologically intensive countries, such as Germany and Belgium, with cheaper inputs than the US get as much value for their money compared with countries such as Australia and Canada, which use technology but to a more moderate extent. For the time-being, our ability to examine this issue is restricted by the lack of longitudinal data in many countries. At the other end of the health expenditure spectrum lies the UK, for which we did not, at this point,[6] have information linking interventions, costs and outcomes since we did not have data on case fatality or readmissions. We do know that the UK is among the countries that rely the least on technologically intensive treatments, which is probably attributable to the lower levels of health expenditures in the UK. Furthermore, we know that the long-run decline in IHD mortality in the UK was not as great as in other countries with a similar burden of the disease. Thus, we could hypothesise an indirect link between the lower levels of spending in the UK, the consequent lower level of utilisation of invasive cardiac procedures and the weaker declines in IHD mortality in this country.

ii)   The case of breast cancer

Assessing performance is a complex task in the case of breast cancer, which ideally would involve multivariate analysis of variations in survival. Currently, there is a limitation because severity cannot be fully controlled for across countries. The available data in terms of aggregate survival offer only mixed evidence. Gatta, Capocacccia, Coleman *et al.* (2000) compare trends in survival between American and European cancer patients: survival rates are higher in the United States than in Europe, particularly for those cancers, such as breast cancer, where treatment and screening can make a difference. However, the conclusions based on cancer-registry data remain very limited, as they cannot adjust for stage and disentangle the relative roles of treatment *versus* screening. Evidence exists that shows that generally screening is very intensive in the United States, and that, as a result the cases are on average less severe.

In terms of the links with technologies, one of the paths for analysis is to explore any correlation between patterns of survival, and the availability of mammography and radiotherapy machines (Charts A11. and A12 in the annex). No general conclusion can be drawn from these exploratory charts: the regions with the highest survival rates, including Sweden, the United States, Japan and Manitoba, have either a high or low availability of mammography machines. The UK has a poor level of survival, although it has a few more machines than Manitoba. Again, in terms of the availability of radiotherapy machines, no conclusions can be draw, except for the UK which has fewer machines and poorer survival. However, one would need to better understand the use of these machines, either in terms of screening or treatment.

Screening seems to be part of the explanation for why some countries have a higher survival rate than others. However, use of screening cannot be approximated by the availability of the technology only, as demonstrated in Chart A11. Therefore the study has gathered some evidence on the participation in screening, either as part of organised screening programmes implemented in a number of countries, or opportunistic screening, outside an organised program. The rate of mammography screening displayed in Chart A13 can be considered as an "intermediate output", and in itself as a measure of performance, since it shows how successful organised screening programs have been in reaching their goals.

This study has also gathered data on standardised breast cancer mortality as shown in Chart A14 (see also Jacobzone and Jee-Hughes, 2001 for more detail, including relevant data by age groups).

In terms of trends in mortality, countries can be included in four groups:

- Countries with a reduction in mortality, and relatively low levels (Sweden, Australia, Italy, Manitoba, United States, Canada);
- Countries with an increase in mortality and relatively low levels (Japan, France, Norway);
- Countries with an increase in mortality, at relatively high level (Belgium, Hungary, Ontario);
- Countries with a reduction in mortality, at relatively high levels (United Kingdom).

Countries in the first group include Sweden, which had the lowest rate of mortality in 1995, and the strongest reduction. Australia, Italy Manitoba, the United States and Canada can also be added to this group. All these regions experienced a reduction in mortality and relatively low levels, very close to 60 per 100 000 women aged 40 and over. Canada and its Manitoba province, and Sweden, have experienced clear reductions in mortality for the 50-69 age groups, which are the target age groups for screening programs,[7] while the reduction is not clear for Italy. The hypothesis could be formulated that these results may be reflective of the specific implementation of the screening programs in the corresponding age groups. On the other hand, the United States experienced a decrease in mortality for all age groups, and screening is mainly opportunistic in the US.

In the second group, Japan experiences a very low mortality rate, which is maybe due to differing underlying epidemiological patterns for this country. France also experienced an increase between 1985 and 1990, although these data remain too limited to permit meaningful conclusions. The same applies for Norway.

The third group includes Ontario in Canada, which has significantly higher mortality rates than the rest of the country, as well as Hungary and Belgium. These entities do not generally have organised screening programs for the population as a whole (Belgium, Hungary), and may also suffer some restrictions in supply (Hungary). Belgium has experienced an increase in spite of its generally aggressive treatment practices. Ontario has an organised screening program, but the rates of organised screening remain apparently low.

The fourth group includes the United Kingdom (for a more detailed previous account, see Quinn and Allen, 1995). The data is now becoming dated, but it could be hypothesised that these reductions reflect the introduction of organised screening in this country at the end of the 1980s following the Forrest report in 1986 (Moss *et al.*, 1995; Blanks *et al.*, 2000). The program detected more carcinoma *in situ* at the beginning (1988-1993) but less invasive cancers than expected. The efficiency of the program in detecting more invasive cancers has improved at a later stage. It has been estimated that the program has been responsible for a third of the fall in the death rate from breast cancer among women aged between 55 and 69 years (Patnick, 2000). This introduction would have allowed some reduction in mortality, in spite of the lack of financial resources for technologically intensive treatments. The early uptake of Tamoxifen has certainly had significant benefits (Quinn and Allen, 1995). A debate has taken place following publications in the UK in 1999 (Sikora, 1999) on the evidence of lower survival: from the available evidence, it seems that the financial constraints in terms of treatment may have had an impact on outcomes given restrictions in terms of the availability of qualified medical staff, screening equipment, and funds for radiation and chemotherapy.

For breast cancer, performance seems to be achieved through a mix of rigorously organised population-based breast cancer screening programs, combined with the availability of treatment protocols able to follow the most recent clinical guidelines, and not too constrained by economic considerations. However, a strategy relying on prevention only, or on treatment only is not sufficient to achieve performance. In addition further data needs to be developed, for better assessing the efficacy of screening programs across countries, and evaluating the severity of stages in a consistent way at the international level.

iii) Stroke and the case of stroke units

Stroke is an acute event, for which few direct cures are available but which has long-term implications. Treatment results from a combination of appropriate diagnosis, involving high technology, such as Magnetic Resonance Imaging (MRI), or CT Scanning (CT). In addition, a systematic review of over 20 trials shows that specialised stroke units can make a difference in terms of performance showing benefit both in terms of survival and reduced disability. There are a number of different models for organising the care, and some have been demonstrated in a randomised control trial to be both effective and cost-effective. Stroke units have been shown to benefit a wide range of stroke patients (Stroke Units Trialists Collaboration, 1997*a*; Stroke Units Trialists Collaboration, 1997*b*; Indredavik *et al.*, 1999; Jorgensen *et al.*, 1999; Jorgensen *et al.*, 2000).

The studies that have examined the benefits of stroke units use a clear definition of a stroke unit; although, a standard definition has not yet emerged. Aspects of these definitions in some of these studies include:

- multidisplinary staffing (such as a mix of doctors, nurses, physiotherapists, speech therapists);
- access to technology such as CT scanners;
- organised care usually in a dedicated unit with dedicated staff;
- usually includes both acute and rehabilitation care.

Stroke units appear to have primarily developed in the Nordic countries, where long-term care is fully funded from the public purse, (public funding accounts for as much as 3 per cent of GDP against 1 per cent or less in other European or OECD countries (Jacobzone, 1999). This may be linked with the fact that disability is a costly outcome for these health and social systems, which as a result has more

Table 2. **Available information on stroke units in a subset of countries**

	Year	Stroke units (per 100 000)	Stroke unit beds (per 100 000)	% of patients care for in stroke unit	Comments
Denmark	1998	0.93	10.39		49 hospitals with 550 beds
Netherlands	2000	0.42	1.69		67 hospitals with 268 beds
Sweden	1998	0.78	5.8	70%	SU at 70 of 84 hospitals, 518 beds, % patients cared for in SU rose from 54% to 70% between 1995 and 1998
Hungary	2000	0.15		Approx. 15%	4 SU in 1992, 15 in 2000
United Kingdom				26% at least ½ admission	1999, 45% of trusts had SU
Norway				Approx. 60%	

Source: Moon *et al.* (forthcoming).

incentive to develop cost effective care aimed at reducing disability, compared to other countries relying more on informal care.

Definitional aspects are an issue when comparing the use of stroke units in data collection undertaken for this study. Nevertheless, it is still valuable to make general comparisons between the use of stroke units in the various countries with available data. Information is available on the use of stroke units in six of the countries participating in this study, and is summarised in Table 2.

These results show that stroke units are being implemented in many countries, and the use of organised stroke units tends to increase over time. However, the extent to which stroke units are used differs between countries. A crude measure of the supply of stroke units, the number per 100 000 population, shows variation from 0.15 in Hungary to 0.93 in Denmark. The percentage of stroke patients receiving care in a stroke unit also differed markedly between countries, ranging from 15 per cent in Hungary to 70 per cent in Sweden.

However, despite their proven efficacy in treating stroke patients, and their wide use in Nordic countries such as Sweden, few guidelines exist regarding the planning, establishment or utilisation of dedicated stroke units. Where guidelines do exist, they tend to be local guidelines, products of the efforts of health professionals who regularly treat stroke patients and realise the potential of stroke units in improving outcomes for stroke patients.

If stroke units are as efficient as studies seem to show, why then are they not a part of the regular organisation of hospitals? Among the several possible explanations might be a lack of common definition from country to country and between jurisdictions, which hampers measurement and improving of performance. There are at least two consequences of not having a standard definition for a stroke unit. The first consequence may simply be that the number of stroke units are underestimated in most countries. It is possible that, because there is no standard definition of what stroke units are, there are no variables in hospital administrative databases that identify them. Furthermore, various regular surveys of health care institutions may not include questions on stroke units due to the lack of a standard definition. Therefore, the actual number of stroke units may be underestimated because they have not all been identified. The other consequence of not having a standard definition is that it complicates the planning process for creating stroke units.

177

A second possible explanation for why stroke units are not more common is that the concept of a stroke unit is still at an early stage of evolution. In the 1970s it was recognised that organised stroke care, from acute care to rehabilitation, could result in beneficial outcomes for stroke patients (Indredavik *et al.*, 1999). Since then the development of stroke units has been slow to take root. It is only within the last few years, as evidence continues to mount supporting the efficacy of stroke units, that we have witnessed a significant growth in them, particularly in the Nordic countries of Europe.

A third possible explanation why stroke units apparently are not part of the regular organisation of hospitals is the lack of an established "evidence base", in countries beyond the Nordic countries (Wolfe, 2001). Practice in the United Kingdom, Wolfe states, focuses on "evidence from clinical trials and meta-analysis", which is in contrast to continental Europe which puts more emphasis on "physiological observation". The studies that have demonstrated the efficacy of stroke units have been observational studies of individual stroke units, there is little trial evidence in existence and only one known meta-analysis (Stroke Units Trialists Collaboration, 1997*a*). If the proliferation of stroke units in the UK has been retarded by a lack of trial evidence, then this may explain the lack of stroke units. However, this slow development in the "information infrastructure", may also result in lower levels of performance. This may also be linked with the types of "outcomes" which can be measured for stroke. In our study, we found relatively high, but similar case fatality rates, for those countries for which information was available.

3. What is to be maximised: different perspectives on improving performance

3.1. *Understanding variations in outcomes in relation to treatment and environmental factors*

This paper provides just a few key highlights from a study which represents one of the first full-scale attempts at comparing the performance of health care systems using a comprehensive disease-based framework, utilising large hospital administrative databases based on individual medical records, supplemented with other sources of relevant information. We hope this study can serve as a useful reference and starting point for understanding patterns of prevention, screening and treatment in relation to the health care system environment. Of course, this study has many limitations, which we need to draw to the reader's attention. First, this is not a clinical study, and therefore the analysis of medical interventions remains fairly crude from a clinical perspective. In the interests of time and comparability, we were often unable to use detailed information on clinical status, comorbidities and follow-up drug therapy treatments available in some of these large administrative data sets. In addition, we were not able to fully reflect patients' episodes of care through lack of information on ambulatory care practices. Finally, it was not possible to address the issue of quality of life. Collecting such data was beyond the scope of the current study, but would certainly represent a good direction for future research.

3.2. *From health system performance to patient's satisfaction and improved quality of life*

When assessing performance, various stakeholders have different parameters in mind that they wish to evaluate. Patients and physicians tend to focus on the "clinical" success of health interventions, which is likely to remain limited to the inpatient episode of care. In addition, patients often focus on other issues associated with the episode of care: length of waiting time, availability of nurses and support staff and quality of life, including suffering and physical aspects. At the aggregate level, health care system administrators are likely to have more interest in the general health system variables: overall activity rates, mortality rates and costs. The ARD project is an attempt at bridging the micro-macro gap in knowledge in understanding the broad effects of health systems, representing an example of how the various stakeholder perspectives can be reconciled. However, we acknowledge that further efforts will be needed to fully reconcile the perspectives of the various stakeholders.

The strength of this study is the demonstration of the link between health care system supply-side incentives and the level and diffusion of various key procedures reflecting the use of technology. We found that universal coverage does not necessarily guarantee that utilisation rates for treatments would be the same across countries, since OECD countries devote very different levels of resources to health care, each within their own "universal system". However, higher "activity rates" observed in some countries do not necessarily translate into improvements in outcomes that parallel the investment in resources, as some lower-spending countries are able to achieve similar or even better results for IHD or breast cancer. What higher activity rates do is to exert pressures on the financing side. However, it seems to be clear that significant results can be achieved through a proactive population-based approach including prevention, screening and proper follow-up treatments. Standing apart from most other countries, the financers of health care in the United States pay more per unit of treatment than in other OECD countries. From our results, we could conclude that an effective health care system would be one where expenditures are sufficient to avoid excessive resource restrictions, and where these resources are optimised, for example through rational and cost-effective use of modern technologies.

Finally, this study shows the irreplaceable value of information systems for evaluating health care systems. We have taken advantage of an enormous wealth of information sources to provide an extensive analysis of how health care systems treat these diseases, yet the assessment remains incomplete since not all data were available in all participating countries. Improvements in these information systems require long-term investments, as well as the goodwill and participation of patients and physicians. These are more likely to participate if we can demonstrate that the information these resources have to offer can be used to improve health care systems in the long run. It is the final hope of the authors of this report that it demonstrates the value of using a disease-based approach for cross-national studies for improving health care system performance.

NOTES

1. The views expressed here are solely the authors' responsibility. We first wish to thank Melissa Jee-Hughes for her critical contribution to the project during the launching phase and for the breast cancer component. This work has benefited from inputs from Mark McClellan while at Stanford University, David Wise and David Cutler at Harvard University. Finally, we especially wish to acknowledge the comments and advice of the researchers from all the participating countries, without whom this project could not have succeeded. In some cases, this report still reflects work in progress. We would also like to thank Pr. Isabelle Durand-Zaleski for her medical advice throughout the study, Veronique De Fontenay for her wonderful assistance with the data, Marianne Scarborough and Victoria Braithwaite for helping us with the text and editing. We thank our colleagues Michael Dickson, Jeremy Hurst and Peter Scherer for their comments, as well as participants in the NBER 2001 Summer Institute and in the IHEA 2001 International Health Economics Conference. This work benefited from a strong collaboration from the TECH Research Network, from the EUROCARE and EUROPREVAL networks, from the WHO MONICA and MONICA stroke networks, from the collaboration with the International Agency for Research on Cancer. Finally, we especially wish to acknowledge the comments and advice of all the researchers from the participating countries, without whom this project could not have succeeded. The study has received support from the United States National Institute on Aging, and from the Japanese Ministry of Health, Labour and Welfare.

2. Risk adjustment for case-mix and severity can be an important concern. However, the diagnoses have been carefully selected for acute conditions, and for very large samples of patients, often at the country or state level.

3. The availability of specialised human resources as well is likely important, but the data we collected do not allow us to draw any meaningful conclusions with respect to utilisation levels of PTCA and CABG.

4. The physician payment variable was found to be highly correlated to the facility constraint, making the joint use of both variables impossible in the regression due to multicollinearity problems.

5. And in collaboration with the TECH research network.

6. Although further data might be coming for a revised version of this paper.

7. There seems to have been a significant debate in Sweden, as some authors have argued that screening had not in fact reduced morality whereas this was apparently strongly disputed by the head of the national assessment authority and the board of health and welfare. However, this debate was published only in Swedish which limits our ability to fully report on it. [See Sjönell, G. and Ståhle, L. (1999), "Mammographic Screening Does Not Reduce Breast Cancer Mortality" (in Swedish), *Läkartidningen*, Vol. 96, pp. 904-913; and Rosen, M. and Stenbeck, M. (2000), "The Debate on Mammography", the National Board of Health and Welfare is answering Sjonell and Stahle, *Läkartidningen*, Vol. 97, No. 8, pp. 859-860]. This debate continues for other countries in year 2000, following the publication of results by the Cochrane review on screening in the *Lancet* (Olsen Gotzsche 2001). However, these results remain themselves highly debated in the Cancer research field.

REFERENCES

ALBAIN, K.S. *et al.* (1996),
"Breast cancer outcome and predictors of outcome: are there age differentials?", *Monogr. Natl Cancer Inst.*, Vol. 16, pp. 35-42.

ANDERSON, G. (1997),
"In search of value: an international comparison of cost, access, and outcomes", *Health Affairs*, Nov./Dec., pp. 163-171.

ATC (2000),
Anatomical Therapeutic Chemical Classification Index with Defined Daily Doses, World Health Organisation, Collaborating Centre for Drug Statistics Methodology, Oslo, Norway.

AUSTRALIAN INSTITUTE OF HEALTH AND WELFARE (AIHW) (2000),
Australia's Health 2000: the seventh biennial health report of the Australian Institute of Health and Welfare, AIHW, Canberra.

BLANKS, R.G., MOSS, S.M. and PATNIK, J. (2000),
"Results from the UK NHS breast screening programme 1994-1999", *Journal Medical Screening*, Vol. 7, No. 4, pp. 195-198.

CANTO *et al.* (2000),
"Payer status and the utilization of hospital resources in AMI: a report from the National Registry of AMI", *Arch Intern Med*, Mar. 27, Vol. 160, No. 6, pp. 817-823.

CUTLER, D. and McCLELLAN, M. (1996),
"The determinants of technological change in heart attack treatment", NBER Working Paper No. 5751.

DECKER, S.L. and RAPPAPORT, C. (2001),
Medicare and Disparities in Health: The Case of Breast Cancer, International Longevity Center, Mount Sinai School of Medicine, Federal Reserve Bank of New York, NBER Summer Institute.

DICKSON, M. and JACOBZONE, S. (2002),
"Trends in cardiovascular drug use in 12 countries: 1989 to 1999", OECD Ageing-Related Diseases Project, technical paper.

EVANS, R.G. and STODDART, G.L. (1990),
"Producing health, consuming health care", *Soc Sci Med*, Vol. 31, No. 12, pp. 1347-1363.

GATTA, G. *et al.* (2000),
"Toward a comparison of survival in American and European cancer patients", *Cancer*, Vol. 89, pp. 893-900.

HADLEY, J. *et al.* (1991),
"Comparison of uninsured and privately insured hospital patients. Condition on admission, resource use, and outcome", *Journal of the American Medical Association*, Vol. 265, No. 3, pp. 374-379.

HURST, J. and JEE-HUGHES, M. (2001),
"Performance measurement and performance management in OECD health systems", Labour Market and Social Policy Occasional Papers No. 47, OECD, Paris.

INDREDAVIK, B., BAKKE, F., SLORDAHL, S., ROKSETH, R. and HAHEIM, L. (1999),
"Treatment in a combined acute and rehabilitation stroke unit: which aspects are most important?", *Stroke*, Vol. 30, pp. 917-923.

JACOBZONE, S. (2000),
"Pharmaceutical policies in OECD countries: reconciling social and industrial goals", Labour Market and Social Policy Occasional Papers No. 40, OECD, Paris.

JACOBZONE, S. (forthcoming),
"Healthy ageing and the challenges of new technologies – Can OECD social and health care systems provide for the future?", OECD Healthy Ageing and Biotechnology, Proceedings of the conference held in Tokyo in 2000.

JEE-HUGHES, M. and JACOBZONE, S. (forthcoming),
"OECD study of cross-national differences in the treatment, costs and outcomes of breast cancer", OECD, Paris.

JORGENSEN, H., KAMMERSGAARD, L., NAKAYAMA, H. *et al.* (1999),
"Treatment and rehabilitation on a stroke unit improves 5-year survival", *Stroke*, Vol. 30, pp. 930-933.

JORGENSEN, H. *et al.* (2000),
"Who benefits from treatment and rehabilitation in a stroke unit?", *Stroke*, Vol. 31, pp. 434-439.

MCCLELLAN, M. and KESSLER, D. (1999),
"A global analysis of technological change in health care: the case of heart attack: Preliminary report from the TECH network", *Health Affairs*, May/June, pp. 250-255.

MCKINSEY GLOBAL INSTITUTE with assistance from ARROW, K., BAILY, M., BÖRSCH-SUPAN, A. and GARBER, A. (1996),
Health Care Productivity, McKinsey Health Care Practice, Los Angeles.

MOISE, P. (2001),
"Using hospital administrative databases for a disease-based approach", OECD Ageing-Related Disease project, Technical Paper, Paris.

MOISE, P. and JACOBZONE, S. (2002),
"Comparing treatments, costs and outcomes for ischaemic heart disease", Labour Market and Social Policy Occasional Papers No. 58, OECD, Paris.

MOON, L., MOISE, P. and JACOBZONE, S. (forthcoming),
"OECD study of cross-national differences in the treatment, costs and outcomes of stroke", OECD, Paris.

MOSS, S.M., MICHEL, M., PATNICK, J., JOHNS, L., BLANKS, R. and CHAMBERLAIN, J. (1995),
"Results from the NHS breast screening programme 1990-1993", *Journal Med Screen*, Vol. 2, No. 4, pp. 186-190.

NEWHOUSE, J.P. (1992),
"Medical care costs: how much welfare loss?", *Journal of Economic Perspectives*, Vol. 6, No. 3, pp. 3-21.

OLSEN, O. and GØTZSCHE, P.C. (2001),
"Cochrane review on screening for breast cancer with mammography", *Lancet*, Vol. 358, No. 9290, pp. 1340-1342.

OR, Z. (2001),
"Exploring the effects of health care on mortality across OECD countries", Labour Market and Social Policy Occasional Papers No. 46, OECD, Paris.

OECD (1992),
The Reform of Health Care Systems: A Comparative Analysis of Seven OECD Countries, Paris.

OECD (1994),
The Reform of Health Care Systems, A Review of Seventeen OECD Countries, Paris.

OSTEEN, R.T., WINCHESTER, D.P., HUSSEY, D.H. *et al.* (1994),
"Insurance coverage of patients with breast cancer in the 1991 commission on cancer patient care evaluation study", *Annals Surgial Oncology*, Vol. 1, pp. 462-467.

PATNICK, J. (2000),
"Breast and cervical screening for women in the United Kingdom", *Honk Kong Medical Journal*, Vol. 6, No. 4, pp. 409-411.

PHELPS, C.E. (1997),
"Good technologies gone bad: How and why the cost-effectiveness of a medical intervention changes for different populations", *Med Decis Making*, Jan.-Mar., Vol. 17, No. 1, pp. 107-117.

QUINN, M. and ALLEN, E. (1995),
"Changes in incidence of and mortality from breast cancer in England and Wales since introduction of screening", *British Medical Journal*, Vol. 311, pp. 1391-1395.

SADA, M.J. *et al.* (1998),
"Influence of payor on use of invasive cardiac procedures and patient outcome after myocardial infarction in the United States. Participants in the national registry of myocardial infarction", *Journal of the American College of Cardiology*, June, Vol. 31, No. 7, pp. 1474-1480.

SIKORA, K. (1999),
"Cancer survival in Britain is poorer than that of her comparable European neighbours", *British Medical Journal*, Vol. 319, No. 21, pp. 461-462.

STROKE UNIT TRIALISTS' COLLABORATION (1997a),
"Collaborative systematic review of the randomised trials of organised inpatient (stroke unit) care after stroke", BMJ, Vol. 314, pp. 1151-1159.

STROKE UNIT TRIALISTS' COLLABORATION (1997b),
"How do stroke units improve patients outcomes?", *Stroke*, Vol. 28, pp. 2139-2144.

TECH – THE TECHNOLOGICAL CHANGE IN HEALTH CARE RESEARCH NETWORK (2001),
"Technological change around the world: Evidence from heart attack care", *Health Affairs*, Vol. 20, No. 3, pp. 25-42.

TU, J., NAYLOR, D., KUMAR, D., DEBUONO, B., McNELL, B. and HANNAN, E. (1997a),
"Coronary artery bypass graft surgery in Ontario and New York state: which rate is right?", *Annals of Internal Medicine*, Vol. 126, pp. 13-19.

TU, J., PASHOS, C.L., NAYLOR, C.D., CHEN, E., NORMAND, S.L., NEWHOUSE J., MCNEIL B. (1997b),
"Use of cardiac procedures and outcomes in elderly patients with myocardial infarction in the United States and Canada", *New England Journal of Medicine*, Vol. 336, pp. 1500-1505.

WEISBROD, B. (1991),
"The health care quadrilemma", *Journal of Economic Literature*, Vol. 29, No. 2, pp. 523-552.

WENNEKER, M.B. *et al.* (1990),
"The association of payer with utilization of cardiac procedures in Massachusetts", *Journal of the American Medical Association*, Vol. 264, No. 10, pp. 1255-1260.

WOLFE, C. (2001),
"Taking acute stroke care seriously", *British Medical Journal*, Vol. 323, pp. 5-6.

XIANGLIN, D., JEAN, L., FREEMAN, J.S. and GOODWIN (1999),
"Information on radiation treatment in patients with breast cancer: the advantages of the linked Medicare and SEER data", *Journal of Clinical Epidemiology*, Vol. 52, pp. 463-470.

Annex

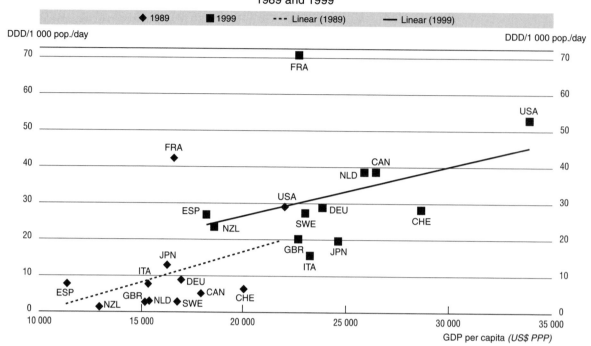

Chart A1. **Serum lipid reducer (C10) consumption and national income**
1989 and 1999

Note: The code C10 refers to the World Health Organization's ATC classification for drugs. See ATC (2000).
In 1989, the R^2 is around 15%. In 1999, it is a bit more than 13%.
Source: Dickson and Jacobzone (2002).

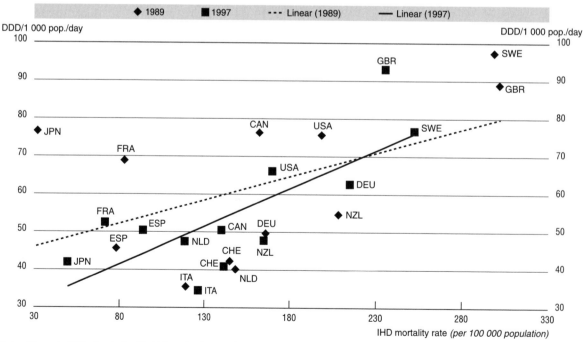

Chart A2. **Diuretic (C03) consumption and mortality**
1989 and 1997

Note: The code C03 refers to the World Organization's ATC classification for drugs. See ATC (2000).
In 1989, the R^2 is a bit more than 25%. In 1997, it is close to 57%.
Source: Dickson and Jacobzone (2002).

Chart A3. **Utilisation rates for PTCA procedures**

Number per 100 000 inhabitants aged 40 and over
1990-1998

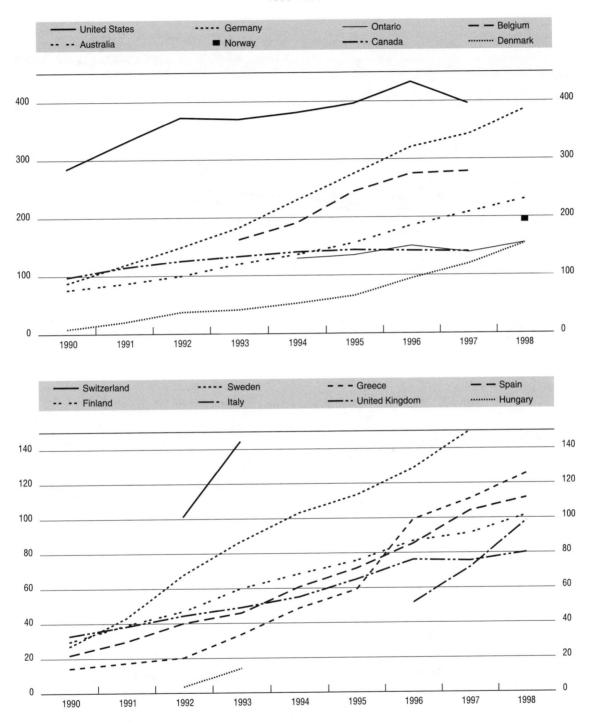

Note: The two charts use different scales for the number of PTCA per 100 000 inhabitants. Greece: After 1996 only includes 17 out of possible 24 hospitals.

Source: Moise and Jacobzone (2002).

Chart A4. **Rate of CABG procedures and cardiac surgery units**

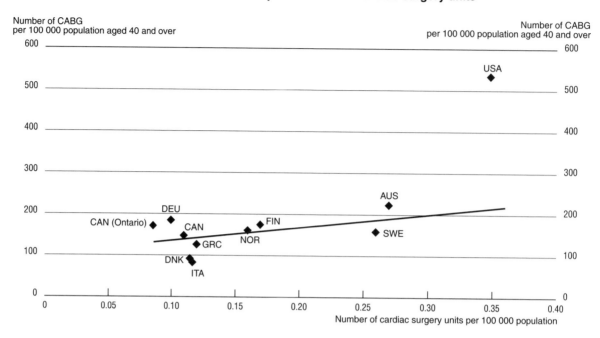

Note: Canada, Denmark, Sweden (1995); United States (1996); Italy (1997); Australia (1998). For Ontario, Finland, Greece and Norway: CABG (1998), cardiac surgery units (2000). The regression does not take the United States into account.
Source: Moise and Jacobzone (2002).

Chart A5. **Rate for PTCA procedures and catheterisation laboratories**

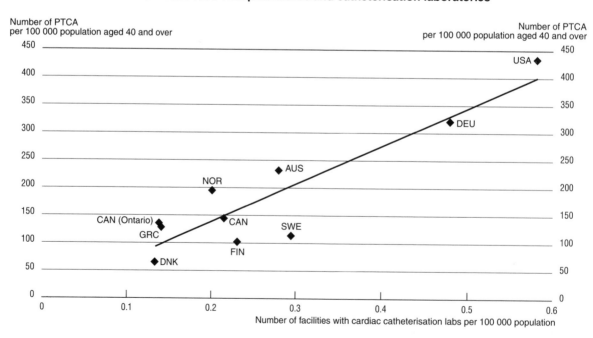

Note: Canada, Ontario, Denmark, Sweden (1995); Germany, United States (1996); Greece (1999). For Australia, Finland and Norway: PTCA (1998), catheterisation laboratories (2000). The figures for facilities includes all facilities able to do cardiac catheterisation due to the difficulty of separating these facilities from those additionally equipped to do PTCA.
Source: Moise and Jacobzone (2002).

Chart A6. **Utilisation of CABG as a proportion of total revascularisation procedures**

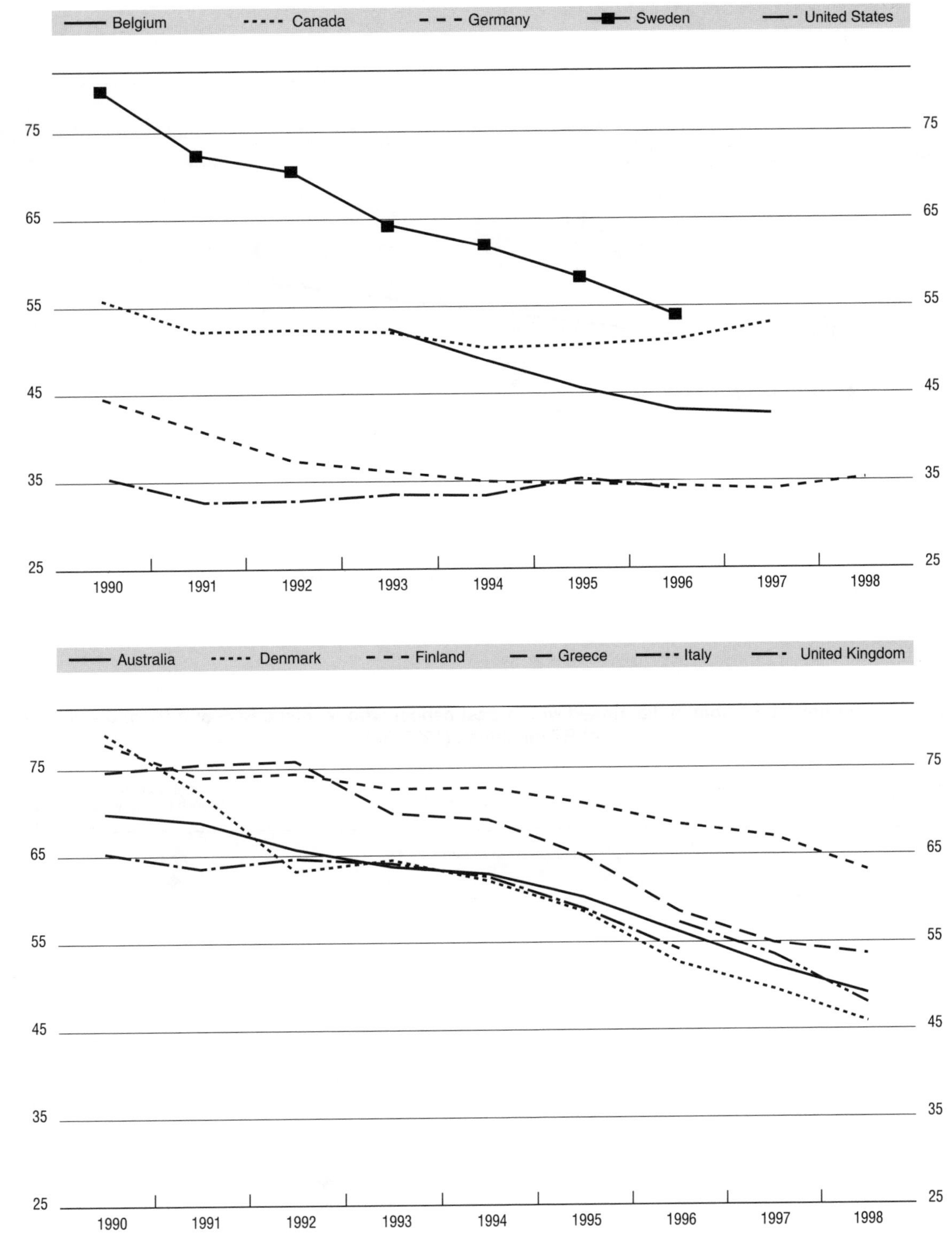

Note: Numerator (CABG per 100 000 inhabitants aged 40 and over). Denominator (CABG per 100 000 inhabitants aged 40 and over + PTCA per 100 000 inhabitants aged 40 and over).
Source: Moise and Jacobzone (2002).

189

Chart A7. **Proportion of women undergoing a mammography and availability of mammography machines (1995-99)**

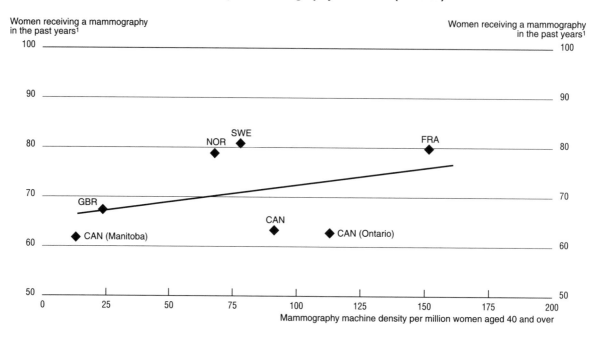

Note: For the United Kingdom, proportion of English women aged 50 to 64 receiving a mammography in the past years.
Source: Jee-Hughes and Jacobzone (forthcoming).

Chart A8. **Proportion of women diagnosed with breast cancer who received BCS and RT and availability of RT machines (1995-99)**

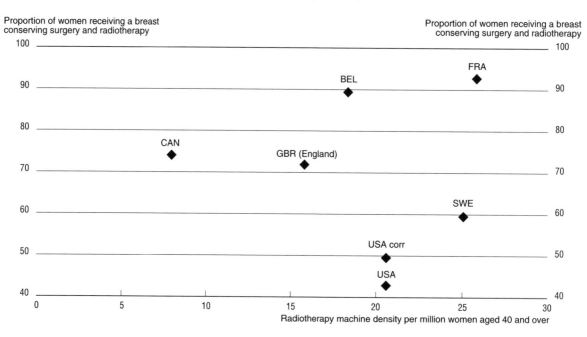

Note: A corrected point has been inserted for the USA (+16%). See Xianglin *et al.* (1999).
Source: Jee-Hughes and Jacobzone (forthcoming).

Chart A9.   **Proportion of women aged 70-79 diagnosed with breast cancer who received BCS and RT and availability of RT machines**

1995-99

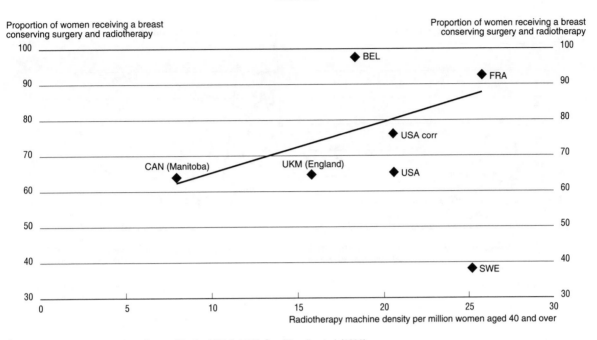

Note: A corrected point has been inserted for the USA (+16%). See Xianglin *et al.* (1999).
Source: Jee-Hughes and Jacobzone (forthcoming).

Chart A10. **One-year case fatality rates and utilisation of revascularisations for 90-day episode of care**

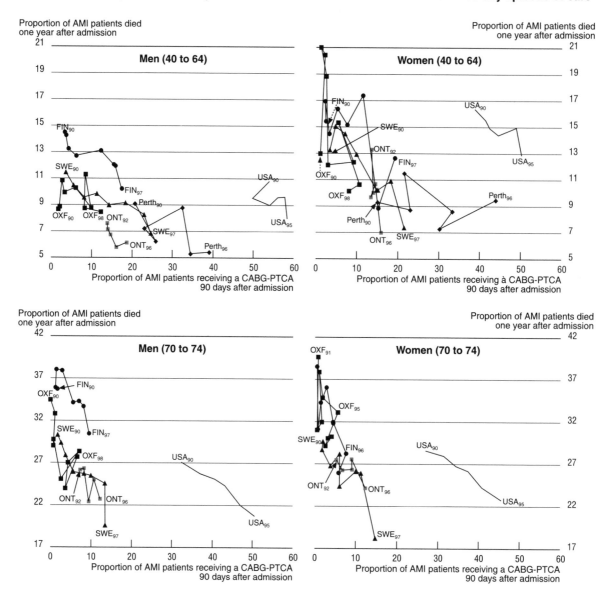

Note: Australia, Perth (1990-1995); Canada, Ontario (1992-1996); Sweden (1990-1997); USA (1990-1995).
Source: Moise and Jacobzone (2002).

Chart A11.   **5-year relative survival rate and availability of mammography machines in a recent year**

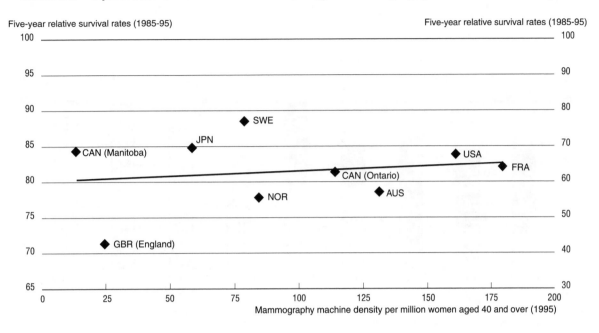

Source: Jee-Hughes and Jacobzone (forthcoming).

Chart A12.   **5-year relative survival rate and availability of radiotherapy machines in a recent year**

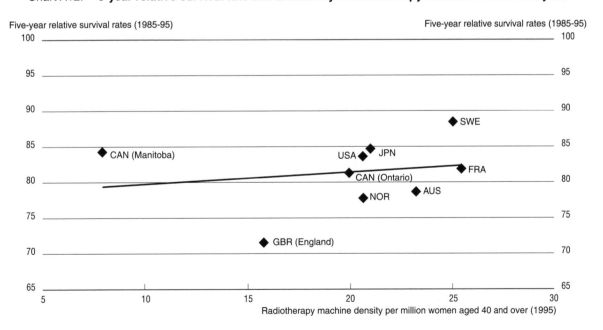

Source: Jee-Hughes and Jacobzone (forthcoming).

Chart A13. **Participation in mammography, organised and overall across countries**

As a percentage of eligible women, 1995-97

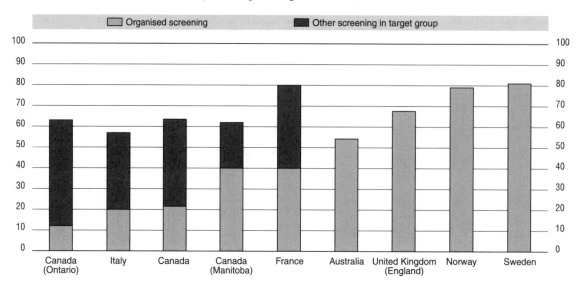

Notes: For United Kingdom, data refer to women aged 50 to 64. Rates for organised screening have been gathered for a number of countries. For United Kingdom, Sweden and Norway, it can be hypothesised that this represents most screening. For other countries, we have also displayed estimates of overall screening rates, including in dark the difference between organised screening and overall rates which is due to opportunistic screening.

Source: Health interview surveys, experts submissions, Health Canada 2001. For Australia, opportunistic screening is significant, but the data were missing. See also Jee-Hughes and Jacobzone (forthcoming).

Chart A14. **A cross-sectional perspective on mortality rates for breast cancer**

Per 100 000 women aged 40 and over

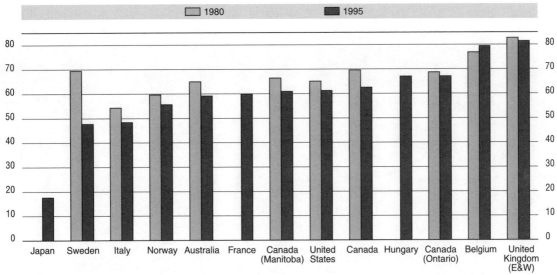

Note: 1990 for France, Hungary, Japan, Norway and the United Kingdom (E&W); 1983 and 1996 for Australia; 1996 for Italy.
Source: Jee-Hughes and Jacobzone (forthcoming).

Chapter 9

THE EVOLUTION OF WHO'S APPROACH
TO HEALTH SYSTEM PERFORMA3NCE ASSESSMENT

by

David B. Evans[*]

Abstract

Policy makers have long been concerned with improving the performance of their health systems with reforms targeting all system functions – financing, provision, stewardship and resource generation (Maynard and Bloor, 1995; Collins *et al.*, 1999). Yet the evidence of what types of changes to health systems improve their performance is limited, inconsistent and inconclusive. Accordingly, WHO has developed a wide ranging work plan to develop the scientific basis to ensure that its technical advice on health system development is based on the best available evidence. One component of this work was to summarise and disseminate the available evidence on the links between health policy, system design and system performance in the *World Health Report* 2000 (WHO, 2000) and the Executive Board of WHO has committed the Organization to report on the health system performance of all WHO Member States regularly.

The first section of this paper summarizes the framework used as the basis for the first round of performance assessment undertaken in 2000. The next section considers two issues that have emerged from the subsequent discussion and debate. The first makes the point that much of the health and health system related survey data commonly collected is not comparable across populations within or across countries, and suggests ways of solving this problem. The second argues that there is value in measuring the outcome of interest (*e.g.* health inequality) and then trying to identify the determinants rather than focusing on some part of the outcome that is believed *a priori* to be associated with a particular determinant (*e.g.* only measuring health inequalities associated with socioeconomic differences).

1. A framework for health system performance assessment

The *World Health Report* 2000 proposed a framework to assess performance in a consistent manner over time and across populations. It was based on the principal that a clear focus on outcomes is required if the potential of health systems is to be fully realised. This required defining a parsimonious set of goals to which the system should contribute. It required defining indicators of the extent to which the system was contributing to these goals and testing and validating measures for these indicators. It required evaluating the role of key health system functions in contributing to goal attainment.

Full details of the framework can be found elsewhere (WHO, 2000; Murray and Frenck, 2001) and some of the debate since October 2000 is reported on the WHO site on the world wide web (*www.who.int/ health-systems-performance*). An essential feature is that the health system was defined to include all

---

[*] Director, Global Programme on Evidence for Health Policy, WHO on behalf of the Cluster on Evidence and Information for Policy. This paper reports on the work of many people in the Cluster on Evidence and Information for Policy in WHO.

actors, institutions and resources that undertake health actions – *i.e.* all actions whose primary intent is to improve health. It is a broader definition than the health actions typically under the direct control of a Ministry of Health but stops short of defining all actions that might improve health as being part of the system.

The health system contributes towards many outcomes that are socially desirable, including improving health, educational attainment, and the incomes of individuals and households. To ensure that monitoring performance does not impose too great a burden on health information systems, a set of criteria were used to determine which goals are intrinsically valued and which of those should be measured routinely.

A goal is intrinsically valued if:

- It is possible to raise the level of attainment of the goal while holding the level of all other intrinsic goals constant – *i.e.* an intrinsic goal must be at least partially independent of all others.

- Raising the level of attainment of an intrinsic goal is always desirable – *e.g.* more is always better than less. If the levels of attainment of other intrinsic goals are kept constant and raising the level of attainment of a given goal is not necessarily desirable, it is probably an instrumental goal.

An instrumental goal is something that is desirable because it contributes to attainment of an intrinsic goal. More is not necessarily better than less, holding attainment of the intrinsic goals constant.

To justify measuring attainment of an intrinsic goal regularly, two additional criteria were used. The health system must be able to make a large enough contribution to the goal to warrant the expense of measuring it regularly and it must be feasible to measure the health system impact on a regular basis.

Using these criteria, three intrinsic goals were identified. The defining goal of a health system is to improve health, where there are two components. The system should seek to improve the average level of population health as well as to reduce health inequalities in the population. The second intrinsic goal was to enhance the responsiveness of the health system to the legitimate expectations of the population for the non-health improving dimensions of their interaction with the health system. Responsiveness does not include expectations for the health improving dimensions of their interactions which are fully reflected in the first goal. "Legitimate" was used to recognise that some individuals may have frivolous expectations for the health system which should not be part of the articulation of this goal. Responsiveness has two key sub-components: respect of persons and client orientation. Again, concern lies not just with the average level of responsiveness, but also with inequalities in responsiveness.

The third intrinsic goal was the fairness in financial contributions to the health system. To be fair, household contributions to finance the health system should represent an equal sacrifice. Fairness would mean that no household would become impoverished or pay an excessive share of their income to finance the health system. Equal sacrifice also means that the poor households should contribute a smaller share of their income than rich households.

The WHR2000, therefore, measured five components of the three intrinsic goals (Table 1). Each intrinsic goal meets the criteria established above. More health (more responsiveness and more fairness of financial contributions) is always better than less holding attainment on the other goals constant, for example.

The annex tables included in the WHR2000 reported attainment on each of the five components for all 191 Member States, as well as attainment on a composite index – a weighted sum of attainment on the five components. Although a number of instrumental goals, such as the coverage of health services, were discussed in the WHR2000, attainment of these goals was not measured or reported.

The WHR2000 also defined four basic functions which contribute to determining observed levels of goal attainment – financing, service provision, resource generation, and stewardship. They will not be discussed further here.

Table 1.   **Intrinsic goals to which the health system contributes**

	Health System Goals		
	Level	Distribution	
Health	✔	✔	Efficiency
Responsiveness	✔	✔	
Financial contributions		✔	
	Quality	Equity	

2.   Selected measurement issues relating to health systems performance

Since publication of the WHR2000 there has been wide debate at various conferences, seminars and in the scientific literature. In addition, WHO has sought the opinions of scientists and policy makers through six regional consultations and eight technical consultations on specific technical topics, including stewardship, responsiveness, fairness of financial contributions and health inequalities. Valuable comments and suggestions have been made on all aspects of HSP – inputs, functions, intrinsic and intermediate goals, outcomes and ways of increasing its relevance to decision-makers.

Here I focus on two issues which have emerged from the discussion which are critical to increasing the policy relevance of HSP. The first is the need to ensure validity, reliability and comparability of any measures that are routinely made. The second is the value of measuring key outcomes of interest, then disaggregating them into components as a means of understanding causation. The alternative approach would be to measure only those components of the final outcome which are perceived to be of interest. Questions of measurement are illustrated with respect to health and responsiveness. Understanding causality is illustrated using health inequalities as an example.

2.1. Measurement issues – Cross-population comparability

The need to ensure that measures are valid and reliable has been well discussed in the literature and is widely understood. The question of comparability is less well understood. Measures used to monitor the performance of a given system must be comparable over time, otherwise it is not possible to be sure if attainment has improved. Measures must be comparable across populations in a given setting to allow national aggregates to be computed. They must be comparable across settings if the international evidence-base of what works and what does not work is to be improved.

It is well known that self-report categorical responses are often not comparable between groups of people with different cultural or demographic characteristics (i.e., the data exhibit what is known as *differential item functioning*). As part of its Multi-country Survey Study 2000-2001 (Ustun *et al.*, 2001), WHO developed and tested novel ways of adjusting for differential item functioning. Part of this was a new common survey instrument with a modular structure for use in nationally representative general population samples. The main purpose was to develop the methods and instruments necessary to measure key indicators in a way that is valid, reliable and comparable. Method development included comparison of survey modes, questionnaire design, and issues dealing with cross-population comparability.

The survey instrument was developed in multiple languages using cognitive interviews and cultural applicability tests, stringent psychometric tests for reliability (*i.e.* test-retest reliability to demonstrate the stability of application) and most importantly utilizing novel psychometric techniques for cross-population comparability. Seventy-one surveys were carried out in 61 countries – different modes were used for comparison purposes in ten countries. The modes included face-to-face personal interviews in households; brief face-to-face interviews; computerized telephone interviews; and postal surveys.

Figure 1. **Response category cut-point shifts**

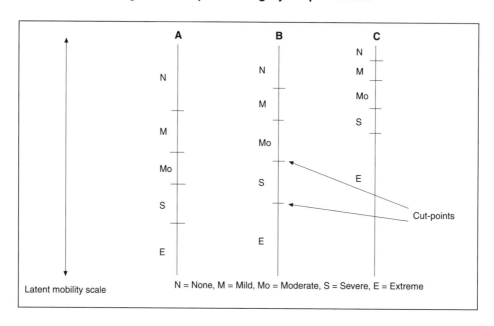

Latent mobility scale

N = None, M = Mild, Mo = Moderate, S = Severe, E = Extreme

All samples were designed to be selected from nationally representative sampling frames with a known probability so as to make estimates based on general population parameters. More than 188 000 responses were received.

The question of cross-population comparability was important particularly for health and responsiveness. For example, to estimate the prevalence of non-fatal health outcomes, people are commonly asked to report their current health by domain, according to a limited number of categories of possible response. Figure 1 illustrates the main challenge of using self-reported levels on a domain even when reliability and within-population validity have been well established. For each domain, there is some true or latent scale. Figure 1 shows the latent scale for mobility. A survey might include a general question on mobility such as "do you have any difficulties walking up stairs" and provide five possible responses of "no difficulty", "mild difficulty", "moderate difficulty", "severe difficulty", and "extreme/cannot do". The second column in Figure 1 shows for population A, the response category cut-points.

Cut-points for populations B and C are also shown. For any point on the latent mobility scale, population C is likely to rate that point as being of a higher level of difficulty than population A. Cut points can vary between populations because of different cultural or other expectations for domains of health or responsiveness. Cut-points might also vary within a particular group – for example, cut-points may shift as expectations for a domain diminish with age.

To ensure that measurements are comparable across populations, the same questions or items must be included in surveys. Comparability also requires explicit strategies to measure the response category cut-points of each item in different populations and socio-demographic groups. One way of establishing cross-population comparability is to fix the level of health or responsiveness on a domain and assess variation in the response categories across individuals, groups, and populations. A series of vignettes were included in the Multi-country Study for this purpose covering health and responsiveness (Sadana, Salomon *et al.*, 2001; Tandon *et al.*, 2001; Salomon, Tandon and Murray, 2001; Valentine *et al.*, 2001). They described a concrete level of ability or responsiveness on a given domain that individuals were asked to evaluate and this was compared to their self-report on that domain.

For health, calibration tests which capture a domain and which can be implemented in different settings without systematic bias were also used to establish a comparable scale for a domain. They

Figure 2. **Unadjusted and adjusted mobility scores by age, Colombia**

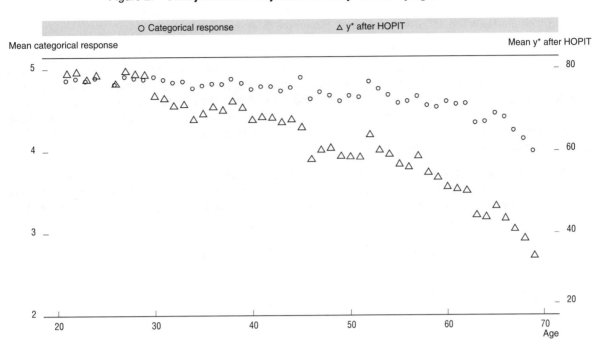

were used for mobility, vision, hearing, and cognition. For example, for a given level of visual acuity measured using the Snellen's eye exam, some people classify themselves as having moderate difficulty, some as severe, and some extreme difficulty. The self-reports can be adjusted for these apparent cut-point shifts using the hierarchical ordered probit (HOPIT) model developed by WHO for this purpose.

HOPIT uses information from vignettes and/or measured tests to calibrate self-report responses to make them cross-population comparable (Tandon, Murray and Salomon, 2001). The model is a variant of the standard ordered probit model in that cut-points are allowed to be functions of explanatory variables and maximum likelihood methods are used for estimation.

The effect of using vignettes and the hierarchical ordered probit model is illustrated for the health domain of mobility in Figure 2. In this survey in Colombia respondents were asked whether they had any difficulties moving around over the last 30 days and the possible responses were no difficulty, mild difficulty, moderate difficulty, severe difficulty or extreme/unable. The circles show the mean response by age. There is only a slight decrease in average mobility with age when responses are not adjusted. Once the way in which respondents use the categorical scale is taken into account, the drop-off in mobility with age is more pronounced.

Respondents in the household or postal surveys were asked to rate their current health according to six key domains based on the International Classification of Functioning, Disability and Health which was ratified at the World Health Assembly in 2001 (Sadana, Tandon *et al.*, 2001). More detailed surveys in 10 countries asked about another 15 domains. All responses on these domains need to be adjusted to ensure comparability.

These data can then be used to estimate the prevalence of non-fatal health outcomes in different groups and populations. They can be combined with mortality estimates to produce summary measures of population health such as healthy life expectancy (HALE) (Mathers *et al.*, 2001). To do this requires valuing non-fatal health outcomes. This was done using information obtained from the full-length household surveys in 10 countries. The valuation function constitutes an empirical means of mapping between multiple domains of health and a scalar index of the level of health measured on a cardinal scale anchored by perfect health and death. The valuation function was estimated based on individual descriptions of domain levels.

Each respondent was asked to value 10 hypothetical health states from a panel of 34 as well as their own health. Different sets of health states were assigned to different people to ensure that all 34 state were covered. The methods are described elsewhere (Salomon, Murray *et al.*, 2001).

Figure 3 shows the mean visual analogue scale (VAS) results by country for each of the health states provided as stimuli to the respondents. While there is some variation for any given state across countries, there is substantial consistency across countries. It is also important to note that in this study, individuals were asked to provide their own descriptions of how they imagined each state in terms of the core domains of health, so that in fact, the label "QUA" (quadriplegia) represents not a single defined set of domain levels across all respondents but a range of different states depending on how each respondent described quadriplegia.

New estimates of HALE (for 2000) using the valuation functions suggest that new-borns could expect to live more than 70 years in equivalent good health in some countries, but on the other hand, children in other countries can expect to live less than 35 healthy years. Figure 4 shows that HALE at

Figure 3. **Average VAS scores by country and state**

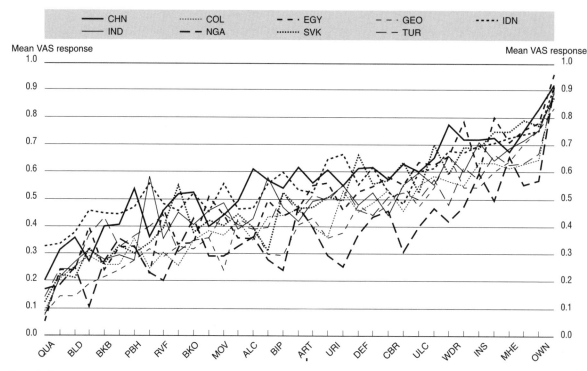

Note: Only every second health state is labelled in the graph.

Country Code	Condition Code	
CHN – China	QUA – quadriplegia	ART – arthritis
COL – Colombia	BLD – total blindness	URI – urinary tract infection
	BKB – below the knee amputation	
EGY – Egypt	in both legs	DEF – deafness
GEO – Georgia	PBH – paralysis in both hands	CBR – chronic bronchitis
IDN – Indonesia	RVF – recto–vaginal fistula	ULC – pain in stomach, as in ulcer
	BKO – below the knee amputation	
IND – India	in one leg	WDR – watery diarrhoea
NGA – Nigeria	MOV – movement disorder	INS – insomnia
SVA – Slovakia	ALC – alcohol dependence	MHE – mild hearing problems
TUR – Turkey	BIP – bipolar depression	OWN – overall health

Figure 4. **Life expectancy minus healthy life expectancy at birth plotted against life expectancy at birth, by sex**

191 WHO Member States, 2000

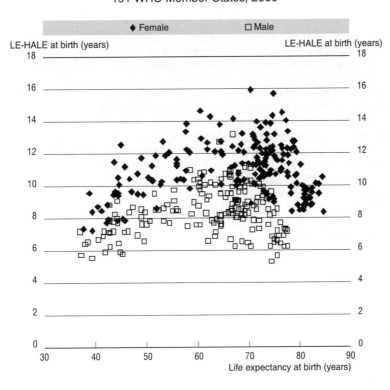

birth and life-expectancy at birth is highly correlated across countries – the simple correlation coefficient is 0.98. However, the difference between life expectancy and HALE (measured on the vertical axis) can be substantial at any given level of life expectancy (on the horizontal axis). At a life expectancy of approximately 70 years, HALE is only five years lower than life expectancy for males in some countries while it is as much as 16 years lower for females in other countries. The gap between HALE and life expectancy increases up to a life expectancy of 68 for males and 72 for females. Above that level of life expectancy, the gap between HALE and life expectancy declines. This appears to confirm the compression of morbidity hypothesis (Fries, 1980; Robine *et al.*; 1996).

The problem of cross-population comparability applies to responsiveness as well. Responsiveness is an intrinsic goal because the way people are treated when they come in contact with the system can improve or reduce well-being independent of health outcomes. Responsiveness is concerned with what actually happens to people when they come in contact with the system rather than their expectations or opinions about their experiences that is measured in patient satisfaction surveys (Blendon and Kim Benson, 2001; Murray *et al.*, 2001). The domains of responsiveness included in the Multi-country Survey Study were dignity, autonomy, communication, confidentiality, and prompt attention (collectively called respect for persons) and access to social support, quality of basic amenities and choice (called client orientation).

The survey instrument asked respondents to rate their last contact with the health system on different domains of responsiveness using five response categories – very good, good, moderate, bad and very bad. For any given level of autonomy, for example, people categorise their experiences in different ways, implying that their cut-points between the possible categorical responses differ (as explained earlier with respect to self-reported health).

To establish how individuals use the categorical responses very good to very bad, a series of vignettes were devised for each domain covering the entire range of the latent or unobserved variable. For each vignette, respondents were asked to rate the experience described using the same categories.

Figure 5. **Levels of prompt attention (inpatient) after adjustment**
World standardized population distribution

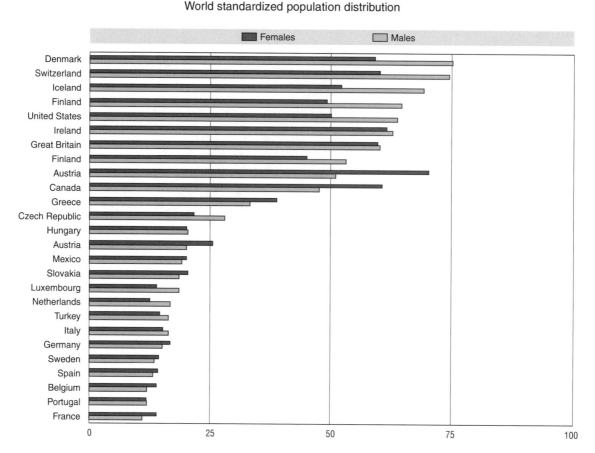

The responses on their own experiences with the system were then adjusted using the information about how people categorised the set of vignettes for each domain, using the hierarchical ordered probit model. This adjusted for the way cut-points on the latent scale systematically varied across groups (Valentine, Da Silva *et al.*, 2001; Valentine, Ortiz *et al.*, 2001; Valentine and Salomon, 2001).

Figures 5 and 6 show reported levels of prompt attention for inpatient and outpatient care after adjusting for cut-point differences across countries. These are very much preliminary results from a survey study designed to test the methods and the instruments. They also compare across different modalities of surveys so they might not be strictly comparable.

It is clear that the way people classify their health and rate the responsiveness of health systems varies systematically within countries according to different socioeconomic characteristics and across countries. Some way of adjusting survey responses for this is required before survey results can be aggregated at a country level or compared across countries. The approach of using vignettes and measured tests (for health) appears promising.

2.2. Attribution and measurement

Many of the consultations pointed out that goal attainment is not only influenced by health actions but also by many non-health system actions. Multivariate statistical analysis allows the concept of outcome measurement to be separated clearly from the assessment of causal attribution. Overall mortality and changes in it, for example, can be measured and then the causes explored using multivariate statistical analysis. This allows all possible hypotheses of causation to be tested.

Figure 6. **Levels of prompt attention (outpatient) after adjustment**
World standardized population distribution

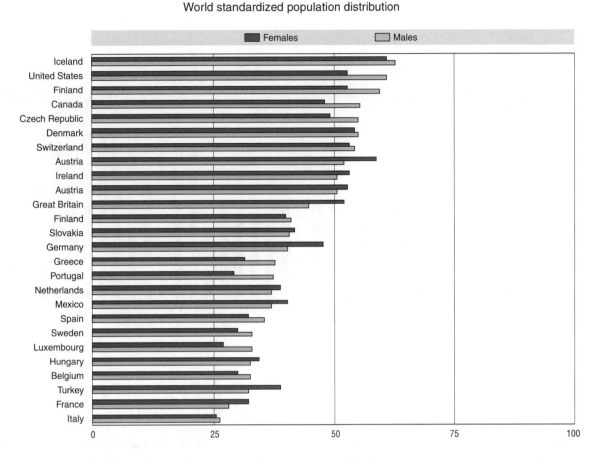

An alternative approach implicit in many of the comments received since the publication of the WHR2000 is to define partial indicators of overall goal attainment which are believed to be determined largely by the activities of the Ministry of Health. In this approach, mortality due to medical errors would be measured in preference to overall mortality because the Ministry of Health can reduce medical errors but cannot control the fact that some people die from war and violence.

This approach focuses attention only on determinants that are identified *a priori*, rather than allowing analysts to explore all possible causes. We argue that some of these indicators might be useful to measure in different settings, but not at the expense of measuring the system's contribution to goal attainment. This can be illustrated using health inequalities as an example.

In the WHR2000 inequality in the probability of child survival was reported although the eventual aim was to measure inequality in healthy life expectancy. Details of this estimation have been presented elsewhere (Gakidou *et al.*, 2000). This allows for the quantification of the existing inequalities in health and the subsequent exploration of all potential determinants (Gakidou and King, 2001) rather than focusing on one or two factors which are believed *a priori* to be correlated with the health inequalities. To do this, the child survival equality index has been decomposed into the contribution of different factors. The Demographic and Health Surveys provide information on some socioeconomic variables such as household assets and mother's education, and several variables that together can be considered as a proxy for access to the health system – including antenatal visits, measles immunisation, BCG immunisation and births attended by a nurse or doctor.

To study the effects of these covariates a counterfactual analysis was performed in which the inequality index was recalculated assuming first that there were no inequalities in assets, then that

Figure 7. **Decomposition of child survival inequality**

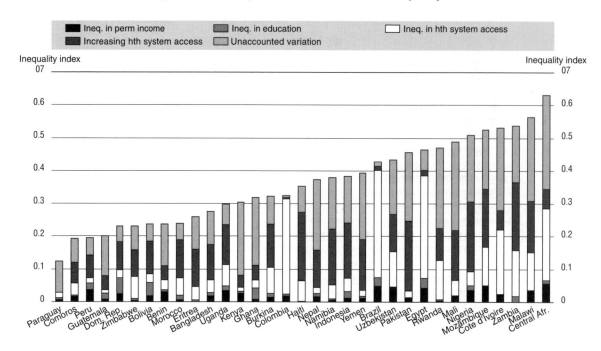

there were no inequalities in education and third that there were no inequalities in access to the health system. For assets and education, this was done by substituting for each child the mean value for all children and recalculating the inequality index. For access, it was assumed that all children had access to the recommended level of services, rather than to the mean level, and the inequality index recalculated. The reduction in the index that resulted at each step corresponded to the effect of removing inequalities in each variable. This analysis is path dependent but we find that, at least for these data, the order in which the counterfactual scenarios are applied does not materially influence the results.

This analysis suggests that reducing inequalities in assets and education would reduce inequalities in child mortality to some extent in all countries (Figure 7). Reducing inequalities in access to health systems would reduce inequalities in child survival in all countries. On average the contribution of inequalities in access to inequalities in child survival appears to be larger than the contribution of reducing income or education inequalities. This is as yet exploratory. However, it suggests that if we had focused only on assets or education, we would have missed the chance to consider other possible determinants such as access. Of course policy makers may well be interested in measuring inequality in health across socioeconomic groups. But this analysis implies that measuring pure inequalities in health allows disaggregation by all possible determinants.

3. Conclusion

The Director-General of WHO and the Executive Board have committed the Organization to measuring and reporting on the performance of the health systems of all 191 Member States at regular intervals. This required development of a framework for defining and measuring performance that could be used across populations within countries, across countries, and over time. The methods that were developed and reported in the WHR2000 have since benefited from increased international debate and the regional and technical consultations described earlier. They will continue to develop over time, as is customary with scientific endeavours.

The debate, discussion and consultations after the release of the report have provided many useful ideas on ways to develop the work, and the Director-General has appointed a Scientific Peer Review Group to advise on methods to be used in subsequent rounds. In this paper I focused on two of the many issues that have emerged from the discussions, both relating to the need to ensure that the measurement associated with the analysis of the performance of health systems is directly relevant to the needs of policy-makers. The first is that indicators should be measured in a way that is valid, reliable and comparable. Without adjustment for different cut-points, for example, self-report data cannot be aggregated across groups or over time. WHO has embarked on a process aimed at ensuring that the indicators it proposes to use can be measured in ways that are valid, reliable and comparable. The approach of using vignettes and measured tests in questionnaires is promising.

The second issue concerned the value of measuring the outcome of interest and then seeking to determine causation, rather than focusing only on a part of the outcome which is believed, *a priori*, to be controllable. The former approach allows all possible hypotheses of causation to be tested while the latter explores only a limited set of possible determinants.

REFERENCES

BLENDON, R. and KIM BENSON, J.M. (2001),
"The Public versus the World Health Organization on Health System Performance: who is better qualified to judge health care systems: public health experts or the people who use the healthcare?", Health Affairs, Vol. 20, No. 3, pp. 10-20.

COLLINS, C., GREEN, A. and HUNTER D. (1999),
"Health sector reform and interpretation of policy context", Health Policy, Vol. 47, No. 1, pp. 69-83.

FRIES, J.F. (1980),
"Aging, natural death, and the compression of morbidity", New England Journal of Medicine, Vol. 303, No. 3, pp. 130-135.

GAKIDOU, E.E. and KING, G. (2001),
"Determinants of inequality in child survival: results from 40 countries", WHO, EIP Discussion Paper, Geneva.

GAKIDOU, E.E., MURRAY, C.J.L. and FRENK, J. (2000),
"Defining and measuring health inequality: an approach based on the distribution of health expectancy", Bulletin of the World Health Organization, Vol. 78, No. 1, pp. 42-54.

MATHERS, C., SADANA, R., SALOMON, J.A., MURRAY, C.J.L. and LOPEZ, A.D. (1999),
"World Health Report 2000: Healthy life expectancy in 191 countries", Lancet, Vol. 357, pp. 1685-1691.

MAYNARD, A. and BLOOR, K. (1995),
"Health care reform: informing difficult choices", International Journal of Health Planning and Management, Vol. 10, No. 4, pp. 247-264.

MURRAY, C.J.L. and FRENK, J. (2001),
"A framework for assessing the performance of health systems", Bulletin of the World Health Organization, Vol. 78, No. 6, pp. 717-732.

MURRAY, C.J.L., VALENTINE, N. and KAWABATA, K. (2001),
"People's experience versus people's expectations. Satisfaction measures are profoundly influenced by people's expectations, say these WHO researchers", Health Affairs, Vol. 20, No. 3, pp. 21-24.

ROBINE, J.M., MATHERS, C. and BROUARD, N. (1996),
"Trends and differentials in disability-free life expectancy: concepts, methods and findings", in Caselli, G. and Lopez, A.D. (eds), Health and Mortality among Elderly Populations, Clarendon Press, Oxford, pp. 182-201.

SADANA, R., SALOMON, J.A., TANDON, A., CHATTERJI, S. and MURRAY, C.J.L. (2001),
"Health state vignettes: design, empirical analysis and critical assessment", WHO, EIP Discussion Paper, Geneva.

SADANA, R., TANDON, A., CHATTERJI, S., USTUN, B. and MURRAY, C.J.L. (2001),
"Describing population health in six domains: comparable results from 65 household surveys", WHO, EIP Discussion Paper, Geneva.

SALOMON, J.A., TANDON, A. and MURRAY, C.J.L. (2001),
"Using vignettes to improve cross-population comparability of health surveys: concepts, design and evaluation techniques", WHO, EIP Discussion Paper, Geneva.

SALOMON, J.A., MURRAY, C.J.L., USTUN, B. and CHATTERJI, S. (2001),
"Health state valuations in summary measures of population health", WHO, EIP Discussion Paper, Geneva.

TANDON, A., MURRAY, C.J.L. and SALOMON, J.A. (2001),
"Statistical models for enhancing cross-population comparability", WHO, EIP Discussion Paper, Geneva.

TANDON, A., CHATTERJI, S., USTUN, B., SALOMON, J.A. and MURRAY, C.J.L. (2001),
"Cross-validation of cutpoint estimation using measured tests and vignettes: the case of vision", WHO, EIP Discussion Paper, Geneva.

USTUN, B., CHATTERJI, S., VILLANUEVA, M., BENDIB, L., CELIK, C., SADANA, R., VALENTINE, N., MATHERS, C., ORTIZ, J.P., TANDON, A., SALOMON, J.A., CAO, Y., WAN JUN, X. and MURRAY, C.J.L. (2001),
"The WHO multicountry household survey on health and responsiveness 2000-2001", WHO, EIP Discussion Paper, Geneva.

VALENTINE, N. and SALOMON, J.A. (2001), "Weights for Responsiveness domains: analysis of country variation in 57 national country surveys", WHO, EIP Discussion Paper, Geneva.

VALENTINE, N., DE SILVA, A., SALOMON, J.A., MURRAY, C.J.L., KAWABATA, K. and ORTIZ, J.P. (2001), "Responsiveness vignettes: design and empirical assessment", WHO, EIP Discussion Paper, Geneva.

VALENTINE, N., ORTIZ, J.P., LIU, B., TANDON, A., KAWABATA, K., POE, R. and MURRAY, C.J.L. (2001), "Levels of responsiveness in eight domains for outpatient and inpatient experiences in 60 national country surveys", WHO, EIP Discussion Paper, Geneva.

WHO (2000), *The World Health Report 2000. Health systems: improving performance*, the World Health Organization, Geneva.

Chapter 10

MEASURING AND IMPROVING PATIENTS' EXPERIENCES: HOW CAN WE MAKE HEALTH CARE SYSTEMS WORK FOR PATIENTS?

by

Angela Coulter[*] and Paul Cleary[**]

Abstract

This paper focuses on the patient's perspective on health care quality. We look first at data on patients' experience of hospital care in five countries: United States, United Kingdom, Germany, Sweden and Switzerland. Having identified the extent and nature of the problems from the patient's point of view, we then describe various policy initiatives that have been taken in the United States and the United Kingdom to try to improve the patient's experience, looking at research evidence on the actual and likely impact of these.

One of the conclusions of the paper is that even though the hospitals studied are not necessarily representative of all hospitals in the study countries, the results offer compelling evidence that there are major deficits in the quality of care in all the countries studied and wide variations between countries that might provide evidence about how organisations and providers in different countries could meet patient needs most effectively.

It is extremely difficult to interpret the differences among countries for both methodological and substantive reasons. For example, one might argue that patients' views of appropriate care might differ substantially among the countries studied. Care needs to be taken to verify that the questions asked are salient and important in each of the countries studied. Nevertheless, we think systematically studying and trying to understand the system differences that might account for the differences observed can be productive.

The traditional approach of feeding back patient survey results to providers has produced some successes in the United States and the United Kingdom, but lack of clear incentives to use the data, and perhaps lack of knowledge about how to improve the processes asked about, have limited the effectiveness of this strategy.

Public disclosure looks more promising. It has had only limited effect to date, but there are signs that patients are becoming more sophisticated as consumers of health services and are increasingly willing to select care givers who provide the "best" quality. Measures of patient experience may prove easier for patients to interpret than other measures of performance such as mortality rates. Even so, it will be important to ensure that these measures are valid, reliable and comprehensible to those for

[*] Chief Executive, Picker Institute Europe, King's Mead House, Oxpens Road, Oxford OX1 1RX, UK and Visiting Professor of Health Services Research, University of Oxford. *angela.coulter@pickereurope.ac.uk.*

[**] Department of Health Care Policy, Harvard Medical School, 180 Longwood Avenue, Boston MA, 02115-5899, USA. *cleary@hcp.med.harvard.edu.*

Acknowledgements: We are very grateful to Steve Bruster, Crispin Jenkinson, Michael Massagli, and Kathi Rossi-Roh for assistance with data management and analysis.

whom they are intended. Awareness that these data are publicly available may prove to be an effective incentive for providers to ensure that their services are truly patient-oriented.

Introduction

There are many views and perspectives on what constitutes high quality health care and most definitions reflect different perspectives on this complex question. These have been summarised as follows:

- Quality from the *professional* perspective includes adherence to professional standards, ensuring technical competencies, achieving desired clinical outcomes and striving to expand medical knowledge.

- Quality from a *management* perspective incorporates factors such as appropriate use of resources, ensuring compliance with organisational standards, identifying and managing risks, and facilitating service developments.

- Quality from a *patient* perspective includes fast access to care, responsiveness and empathy, good communication, clear information provision, appropriate treatment, relief of symptoms and improvement in health status (Birch *et al.*, 2000).

In this paper we focus on the patient's perspective, which is increasingly being recognized as essential in quality assessment and improvement efforts. Having outlined the case for obtaining feedback from patients, we look at how this can best be done. Drawing on data from surveys of patients' experience of hospital care in five countries: the United States, the United Kingdom, Germany, Sweden and Switzerland, we describe the extent and nature of the problems from the patient's point of view. Expanding on an earlier paper which included summary data from Picker Surveys (Coulter and Cleary, 2001), we provide a detailed analysis of patients' responses to 44 questions about their experience of a hospital episode. We then go on to describe various policy initiatives that have been taken to try to improve the patient's experience.

1. Why patient feedback is important

Improving responsiveness to patients has been a goal of health policy in many countries for several decades, but the results have often been disappointing. The harsh realities of budgetary pressures, staff shortages and other managerial imperatives tend to displace good intentions about informing and involving patients, responding quickly and effectively to their needs and wishes, and ensuring that they are treated in a dignified and supportive manner. Patient surveys can help to refocus managers' and staff attention on the patient's experience and can galvanise them into action to improve quality standards.

The high cost of health care has led to pressure for greater public accountability, resulting in the publication of performance indicators designed to enable comparison between health care facilities. As well as providing an indication of the results of public expenditures, these are intended to provide information for quality improvement purposes. In the United States, the Consumer Assessment of Health Plans Survey (CAHPS®) is used by purchasers, accreditors and consumers to make comparisons between different health plans (Zaslavsky *et al.*, 2001). In England the government has announced its intention to include measures of patient and carer experience in the next set of national performance indicators (Secretary of State for Health, 1998). It is therefore incumbent on providers to gather feedback from their users and provide detailed reports for use in performance assessment.

Public access to data on quality of care among different providers has developed much further in the United States than in Europe, but hospital report cards and physician profiles are now being promoted widely and the new emphasis on internet information is boosting these efforts. Recent developments among commercial websites, such as Dr Foster in the United Kingdom (*www.drfoster.com*) and its many US equivalents (*www.medicare.gov/mphCompare/home.asp*), are encouraging patients to seek and use systematic information on health care quality. The establishment in the United Kingdom of new mechanisms for promoting involvement and choice, such as Patient Forums and the requirement to publish a Patient Prospectus for each hospital and primary care Trust, will add a further boost to these efforts (Secretary of State for Health, 2000). Providers cannot ignore this trend.

2. Measurement issues

If we want to centre quality improvement efforts on the needs and wishes of patients, we must first understand how things look through their eyes and those of their carers. Health care providers in Europe and the United States have been measuring patient satisfaction for many years, but often these surveys have been conceptually flawed and methodologically weak (Draper and Hill, 1995). There has been a tendency to focus on issues important to managers or clinicians rather than on the topics which are most important to patients. Patient surveys have often been used simply as marketing tools, with providers making claims on the basis of poorly designed and badly conducted surveys that "95 per cent of our patients are satisfied". Furthermore, few surveys have been designed to produce actionable results. It is difficult to identify problems with specific processes of care by asking global rating questions or by focussing solely on food and amenities while ignoring patients' concerns about their illness and clinical care.

More rigorous methods are required if quality improvement efforts are to become truly patient-centred. A more valid approach is to ask patients to report in detail on their experiences by asking them specific questions about whether or not certain processes and events occurred during the course of a specific episode of care (Cleary and Edgman-Levitan, 1997). Building on extensive qualitative research to determine which aspects of care are important to patients, standardised instruments have been developed to measure the quality of care in relation to particular domains (Clearly et al., 1993).

The advantage of asking specific factual questions about detailed aspects of patients' experience is that answers to such questions are easier to interpret than the rating questions commonly included in patient satisfaction surveys. Knowing that, say, 15 per cent of your patients rated their care as "fair" or "poor" doesn't give a manager or clinician much clue about what they need to do to improve the quality of care in their hospital. On the other hand, knowing the proportion of patients who felt they had to wait too long for the call button to be answered, and monitoring trends in these indicators over time, is much more useful when it comes to setting priorities for quality improvement. Focusing on the details of patients' experience can help to pinpoint the problems much more precisely.

The ubiquitous nature of satisfaction surveys leads many people to underestimate the complexities of the process of obtaining reliable feedback from patients. This is a specialist task. Both qualitative and quantitative methods can be used, but it is important to be aware of the advantages and disadvantages of each method. Postal surveys are commonly used because they are a relatively efficient way of obtaining data from patients after a hospital admission or an episode of care. Organising a successful postal survey requires meticulous attention to detail. The design must comply with local ethical and data protection requirements. Questionnaires must be carefully drafted, tested for comprehensibility and relevance, and piloted in realistic settings. Sampling frames must be accurate and sampling procedures must be designed to minimise biases. Mailing must be carried out efficiently and at least two reminders should be sent in order to maximise the response rate. Data entry, analysis and reporting must be carried out to the highest standards. Finally, and most importantly, health care providers must be willing and able to learn from and use the results.

3. Patient surveys in Europe and the United States

The Picker Institute has extensive experience of organising surveys of patients' experience of health care in different countries. Picker surveys have been used since 1987 in hospitals in the United States and since 1997 in Germany, Sweden, Switzerland and the United Kingdom. Below we present recent data from Picker surveys of hospital in-patients in each of these five countries.

The conceptual basis and design of the Picker questionnaires has been described elsewhere (Coulter and Cleary, 2001; Gerteis et al., 1993; Cleary et al., 1992). Building on initial qualitative studies to determine patients' priorities, the questionnaires were designed to cover seven dimensions of care: information and education, coordination of care, respect for patients' preferences, emotional support,

213

Table 1. **Samples and response rates for each of the countries**

	Year surveyed	Number of hospitals	Total sample size	Exclusions (returned undelivered)	Response (completed questionnaires received)	Response rate
Switzerland	1999	9	13 939	83	7 163	52%
Germany	1999/2000	6	3 716[1]	96	2 663	74%
Sweden	1999/2000	9	5 306	104	3 274	63%
United States	1998/1999	272	103 426[2]	4 212	47 576	46%
United Kingdom	1999	4	3 590	146	2 249	65%

1. Only includes those patients who agreed to be surveyed.
2. Data on exclusions not available in the United States, total eligible sample and exclusions estimated.
Source: Picker Institute.

physical comfort, involvement of family and friends, and continuity and transition. A total of 32 items make up these dimensions, with each item coded as a dichotomous "problem score", indicating the presence or absence of a reported problem. Each dimension is scored from 0 (no reported problems) to 100 (all items coded as a problem). Patients who undergo surgical procedures are asked to respond to four additional questions, and eight other questions elicit views on patients' overall impression of their care.

Data presented here came from mail surveys carried out by the Picker Institute in acute care hospitals in the United States, the United Kingdom, Germany, Sweden and Switzerland. The analysis was restricted to data collected from inpatients over a 12 month period in each of the countries. Table 1 details the data sources, sample sizes and response rates from each of the countries. Due to the longer establishment of the Picker Institute in the United States, the data set for the selected year was much larger there than in the European countries where the organisation has commenced work relatively recently.

Summary results have been published previously (Coulter and Cleary, 2001). This paper includes hitherto unpublished detailed breakdowns for all questions, showing the proportion of respondents indicating problems in response to each item.

4. Survey results

Characteristics of the samples are shown in Table 2. There was a greater proportion of younger people in the samples for Switzerland and Germany than in the other three countries and it is known that younger people are more likely to report problems than older people (Sitzia and Wood, 1997). We therefore used direct standardization to adjust the results for age and sex differences.

The problem scores shown in Table 3 indicated that in all countries the most commonly reported problems concerned communications about clinical issues:

- didn't have enough say about treatment;
- insufficient information in emergency room;

Table 2. **Characteristics of samples in each of the countries**
Key characteristics as proportion (%) of patients in sample

		Switzerland (n = 7 163)	Germany (n = 2 663)	Sweden (n = 3 274)	United States (n = 47 576)	United Kingdom (n = 2 249)
Sex	Female	51.5	53.1	49.6	55.1	53.5
Age	Under 65	58.4	58.2	43.8	49.7	51.2
Hospital type	Admitted to teaching hospital	93.3	45.2	34.4	53.7	100.0
Hospital size	Admitted to large hospital (> 250 beds)	72.8	37.5	55.1	66.1	50.0
Type of admission	Non-emergency (planned)	54.8	61.7	38.5	50.2	50.4

Source: Picker Institute.

Table 3. **Problem scores and dimension scores for each country**

Age and sex adjusted rates

	Switzerland	Germany	Sweden	United States	United Kingdom
Information and education					
Insufficient information in A&E/ER	28.3	32.4	25.8	39.7	52.3
Delay to go to room/ward not explained	7.6	7.4	9.6	9.9	5.7
Doctors answers to questions not clear	10.7	17.1	21.9	21.2	27.7
Nurses answers to questions not clear	10.6	12.9	15.7	28.9	23.6
Test results not clearly explained	26.2	32.1	44.0	26.2	34.0
Dimension score	**16.7**	**20.4**	**23.4**	**25.2**	**28.7**
Coordination of care					
Emergency care not well organised*	18.6	20.5	n/a	26.4	37.0
Admission process not well organised*	15.3	23.4	n/a	21.2	20.1
Long wait to go to ward/room	13.0	18.0	28.6	26.8	15.0
No doctor in overall charge of care	7.1	10.4	28.8	11.4	15.1
Staff gave conflicting information	13.6	14.6	19.1	18.0	22.9
Scheduled tests or procedures not done on time	10.7	16.7	16.7	26.3	21.4
Dimension score	**13.1**	**17.2**	**n/a**	**21.7**	**21.9**
Physical comfort					
Didn't get help to go to bathroom/toilet	5.5	4.4	5.0	20.3	15.0
Had to wait too long after pressing call button	0.6	0.6	0.4	4.1	0.9
Had to wait too long for pain medicine	0.8	14.8	2.1	3.9	4.5
Staff did not do enough to control pain	4.9	11.4	8.9	16.2	14.6
Given too little pain medicine	1.1	2.4	3.7	5.9	6.5
Dimension score	**2.6**	**6.7**	**4.0**	**10.1**	**8.3**
Emotional support					
Doctor didn't discuss anxieties or fears	17.3	23.4	36.2	23.7	34.1
Didn't always have confidence in doctors	10.4	19.1	19.7	15.8	18.7
Nurse didn't discuss anxieties or fears	18.5	25.8	31.0	32.4	32.3
Didn't always have confidence in nurses	10.2	13.2	13.9	28.6	19.8
Not easy to find someone to talk to about concerns	17.1	28.0	29.0	33.7	30.3
Dimension score	**14.7**	**21.9**	**26.0**	**26.8**	**27.1**
Respect for patient preferences					
Doctors sometimes talked as if I wasn't there	11.3	10.0	13.0	12.5	29.4
Nurses sometimes talked as if I wasn't there	7.0	3.2	5.8	12.8	14.6
Didn't have enough say about treatment	35.7	46.1	53.8	37.0	59.4
Not always treated with respect and dignity	8.4	12.3	12.3	17.4	19.5
Dimension score	**15.6**	**17.9**	**21.2**	**19.9**	**30.7**
Involvement of family and friends					
Family didn't get opportunity to talk to doctor	13.8	17.0	13.8	22.8	32.3
Family not given enough info about condition	3.9	5.2	7.5	9.3	11.6
Family not given info needed to help recovery	16.9	27.6	22.4	25.9	38.5
Dimension score	**11.5**	**16.6**	**14.6**	**19.3**	**27.5**
Continuity and transition					
Purpose of medicines not fully explained	13.1	23.3	18.9	14.8	23.1
Not told about medication side effects	36.1	43.7	51.3	31.5	36.0
Not told about danger signals to watch for at home	33.5	43.9	47.7	32.3	60.3
Not told when to resume normal activities	37.3	51.5	43.0	35.2	60.9
Dimension score	**30.0**	**40.6**	**40.2**	**28.4**	**45.1**
Surgery specific					
Explanation of risks and benefits not clear	12.6	14.3	30.3	12.3	21.9
Answers to questions about surgery not clear	11.6	14.5	23.4	14.1	17.2
Not told accurately how could feel after surgery	40.4	56.9	33.9	40.5	49.0
Results of surgery not well explained	19.0	28.9	27.8	19.2	30.9
Dimension score	**20.9**	**28.7**	**28.8**	**21.5**	**29.7**
Overall impression					
Courtesy of admissions staff not good	2.7	4.4	6.1	5.7	2.5
Courtesy of doctors not good	2.8	6.1	8.4	4.7	6.9
Availability of doctors not good	3.8	5.3	27.3	11.9	30.0
Courtesy of nurses not good	2.6	4.9	4.4	7.6	5.6
Availability of nurses not good	1.5	2.3	16.3	14.1	29.8
Doctor/nurse teamwork not good*	3.9	6.1	n/a	7.5	8.1
Overall rating of care "fair" or "poor"	3.7	6.6	7.4	8.1	8.5
Would not recommend this hospital to friends/family	3.6	5.0	2.8	4.8	7.8

*   Questions not included in Swedish surveys.
Source: Picker Institute.

215

- tests results not clearly explained;
- not told about medication side-effects;
- not told accurately how could feel after surgery;
- not told about danger signals to watch for at home; and
- not told when to resume normal activities.

In many cases the level of reported problems was high. For example, inadequate post-discharge information was a significant problem in each of the countries. More than a third of surgical patients in all countries felt inadequately prepared for how they would feel after the operation. Patients were also concerned about organisational issues, such as coordination of their care and delays in accessing tests and treatment, but these topics received fewer complaints on the whole. Patients in the United Kingdom and Sweden were more likely to report problems due to staff shortages than those in the other countries, possibly reflecting differences in resource levels. On the other hand, the questions to elicit overall impressions tended to receive quite favourable responses, with the exception of those relating to the availability of doctors and nurses.

These results offer compelling evidence that, in general, patients have unacceptably high rates of problems with selected issues, such as emergency care, explanations of test results and treatment options, opportunity to discuss anxieties with doctors or nurses and to have a say in their treatment, and information about treatment outcomes and follow-up care (e.g. after surgery or discharge from hospital). In the face of the common perception that patients' concerns centre on waiting times and hospitals, hotel, facilities, it is worth noting that these survey results indicate greatest concern about clinical issues.

The difficulties of interpreting international comparisons are well known (Ovretveit, 1998). When considering these data, it is important to be aware of demographic differences, translation problems, cultural and health system differences. Nevertheless, we think the differences between the countries are very suggestive. Swiss patients reported markedly fewer problems than those in the other countries, producing the lowest (best) dimension scores for all except the *continuity and transition* dimension in which the United States had the lowest score. The UK sample produced the worst scores on every dimension except *physical comfort* in which more problems were identified by US patients. These findings do not necessarily mean the average Swiss patient gets better care than the average UK patient. However, they do show that the study hospitals in Switzerland seem to do a better job in certain areas than the UK study hospitals.

Patient feedback surveys such as these provide a snapshot of the quality of care through the patient's eyes which can be used as the first step in a change programme. The findings can be used to prioritise areas where improvement is needed. Comparison against national and international benchmarks can be helpful for persuading staff that better care is possible. Studying survey results over time within one provider can be a useful way of monitoring the effectiveness of quality improvement initiatives. Further examination of the procedures and processes used in different hospitals could provide useful insights on how to improve certain aspects of care.

5. Using the findings

Having established that quality standards in hospitals in the United States and the United Kingdom fall considerably short of the ideal and that patients in both countries reported considerably more problems than those in Switzerland or Germany, what can be done at a policy level to raise standards?

5.1. *Provider feedback*

The most common use of quality information has involved feedback to clinicians and managers to motivate improvements. Traditionally, physicians review either cases in which problems arose (e.g. morbidity and mortality conferences) or randomly selected cases to assess how care was provided and what could have been done better. This approach is appealing because it is consistent with the way physicians receive their initial training and receiving feedback and advice from professional colleagues is consistent with their professional norms and expectations. Patient feedback can be considered alongside the information from clinical notes to provide a more rounded picture.

Until recently, attempts to understand the patient's perspective on care depended on the efforts of a few enthusiasts. In hospitals or other care facilities were there was strong leadership and committed staff there have been good examples of improvements as a direct result of feeding back results from surveys documenting patients' experience. For example, the Beth Israel Hospital in Boston used regular patient surveys to identify the need to improve the quality of their discharge planning process, particularly in patient education (Reiley *et al.*, 1996). They asked recently discharged patients to help them develop interventions to improve patient care. A discharge teaching package was designed and distributed to every unit in the hospital. On re-surveying patients one year after implementation they found statistically significant decreases in the frequency of problems related to discharge and an overall improvement in the continuity and transition dimension of the survey. Similar initiatives using systematic patient feedback to stimulate quality improvements have been reported from a number of hospitals in the United States and Europe.

Our survey results show that patients want to be confident that their doctors are acting in their best interests, but nurses also play a very important role in ensuring the quality of patient care. Nurses who are enthusiastic about patient feedback can make an important difference. For example, a nurse-led unit in the University Hospital of Umeå in Sweden commissioned a patient survey in 1997 and used the results to initiate change in three key areas: admission routines, ward organisation, and pain relief (Frantzen and Hoglund, 2001). In the 1997 survey 29 per cent of patients with pre-booked admissions reported a long wait before they were allocated a bed. Staff discussed the problem and decided to reorganise the admissions process. When a second survey was carried out in 2000, the proportion of patients reporting long waits was down to 14 per cent. Similar improvements were achieved in the proportion of patients who said there were insufficient opportunities to talk to a nurse when necessary – down from 19 to 10 per cent following staff training and reorganisation into smaller work groups – and in pain relief, where the proportion of patients reporting a problem was reduced from 15 per cent to 6 per cent following retraining, reorganisation and provision of self-medication facilities.

In spite of the intuitive and professional appeal of this approach to data use, many think that traditional methods of monitoring quality have not resulted in the consistent and high levels of quality we would hope for, given what is now known about medical care (Schuster *et al.*, 1998). There are several reports in the literature of positive benefits arising from feedback of patient survey data (Cleary *et al.*, 1991; Wedderburn *et al.*, 1995) but little systematic evidence that provider feedback on its own, without additional incentives to use the information to make changes, will be sufficient to stimulate large-scale quality improvements.

Although many clinicians are given the results of patient surveys, little is known about how commonly this is done, how formalised the processes used are, and what is the impact on behaviour. One recent study found that in a sample of physicians who had received reports of ambulatory patient satisfaction data, only 23 per cent found the reports useful for improving patient care and only 7 per cent reported actually using the reports to change the way they provided care (Rider and Perrin, 2000).

The trend is towards a more systematic approach to incorporating patients', users' and carers' views into quality assessment. Voluntary accreditation schemes, such as that operated by the Health Quality Service in the United Kingdom (Health Quality Service, *www.hps.org.uk*) require evidence that providers have sought the views of users. The new Commission for Health Improvement, an independent statutory body established and funded by the British government, is responsible for carrying out regular reviews of NHS Trusts (Secretary of State for Health, 1998). Their review programme is still under development but it is intended that it will include measures of patients' experience derived from patient surveys, as well as patients' diaries, an audit of the environment and access issues from the patient's perspective, structured observation of interactions between patients and staff, and meetings with local stakeholders including individual patients and patients' groups.

5.2. Purchaser feedback

In the United States there has been an increasing emphasis on the role of health care purchasers, such as employers, in monitoring quality and stimulating improvements. The most prominent example of this approach in the United States is the work of the National Committee for Quality Assurance (NCQA, 1998). NCQA is the largest accreditor of managed care health plans. NCQA works closely with companies and government agencies that pay for health care [e.g. The Centers for Medicare and Medicaid Services (CMS), formely the Health Care Financing Administration] to develop standardized measures of quality and requires use of those measures as part of their accreditation process. The measures that NCQA requires plans to collect are collectively called HEDIS (Health Plan Employer Data and Information Set) and include the Consumer Assessment of Health Plans Study (CAHPS®) survey.

The NCQA work is probably the best example of providing standardized indicators of ambulatory care quality to plans and employers to stimulate quality improvements. It is not clear, however, how much of an impact on quality these efforts have generally. For example, in spite of the almost universal awareness of NCQA's efforts among health services researchers, many companies are not even aware of HEDIS. A study by Gable and colleagues found that 31 per cent of the companies offering managed care plans were unaware of HEDIS and only 6 per cent used HEDIS data for selecting health care plans (Gable et al., 1998).

The most common finding in previous studies of health plan choice is that price negatively affects the likelihood of choosing a particular plan (Royalty and Solomon, 1999; Barringer et al., 1994; Scanlon et al., 1997). Studies suggest that choice of plans and providers is related to satisfaction (Kao et al., 1998a and 1998b; Schoen and Davidson, 1996; Davis et al., 1995; Schmittdiel et al., 1997; Ullman et al., 1997), but because standardized survey data have only recently become available to the public, there is much less work on the impact of reports of consumer surveys on choice than the effects of premiums. Some studies suggest that patients will select better providers (Rice et al., 1991; Luft et al., 1990; Chernew et al., 1998) but early direct tests of the hypothesis that information about quality influences choices have yielded negative results (Schneider and Epstein, 1998; Chernew and Scanlon, 1998; Knutson et al., 1998).

Purchasing is organised very differently in the United Kingdom, where health care is more centrally organized and funded out of taxation. Purchasers are part of the National Health Service (NHS) which covers the entire population of England, Scotland, Wales and Northern Ireland. The term purchaser came into use in the United Kingdom along with changes introduced in 1991 by the Conservative government then in power but the current Labour government prefers the term commissioner. UK purchasers or commissioners include health authorities, who purchase health services on behalf of a geographical population and the new primary care trusts, who are responsible for purchasing services on behalf of a defined group of general practices and their registered patients. Commissioners make service agreements with health care providers specifying the volume of services they wish to purchase, their cost and agreed quality standards.

When the purchaser-provider split was introduced into the NHS, the government hoped that the introduction of a competitive internal market would help to raise quality standards, but achieving cost-efficiencies took precedence over quality improvements in purchasers' priorities. Evaluations of the introduction of the purchasing system into the British NHS have so far failed to find evidence of a beneficial impact on the quality of patient care (Goodwin, 1996).

5.3. Public disclosure

A further way in which information can be used is to make it publicly available. The premises underlying this approach, sometimes referred to as the consumer choice model, are that lay persons will use the information to select high quality providers and the selection process will motivate providers to improve the quality of care.

These premises underlie the CAHPS project (Veroff et al., 1998). For this approach to work, the information provided must be perceived to be valid, salient to the choice of health care providers, presented in a useful format, must be read and understood, must influence, or be perceived to influence, health plan choices, and providers with poor quality must fail and/or improve in response to this process (Cleary and Edgman-Levitan, 1997).

The balance of financial and quality issues related to health plan choice has shifted dramatically in the past few years and new consumer assessment surveys and reports are now available (Cleary, 1999). Thus, few available studies are applicable to decisions currently being made by consumers (Scanlon *et al.*, 1997). The CAHPS project was developed to assist consumers in their choice of ambulatory care providers. Early evaluations of this survey suggest that consumers attend closely to the survey results and that the results can have an important influence on decisions (Veroff *et al.*, 1998). When state employees in the State of Washington were asked what source provided the most important information about health plan, the CAHPS report was the most frequently mentioned source. More than 70 per cent of respondents said that the CAHPS report was helpful for deciding whether to switch health plan (Guadagnoli *et al.*, 2000). Another study in Denver and St. Louis evaluating a report including consumer ratings of plans found that 82 per cent of respondents found the report useful in learning about quality and 66 per cent found it useful in deciding about whether to change health plans (Fowles *et al.*, 2000).

Although there is not a standard survey for US hospital patients, most hospitals conduct surveys. An example is the data from the Picker Institute presented here. There is increasing interest in reporting such data publicly to stimulate and facilitate quality improvement efforts. One such example in the United States is the Massachusetts Health Quality Partnership (MHQP). MHQP is a coalition of hospitals, businesses and the state Medical Society that conducted Picker surveys in 51 hospitals and health systems. The hospitals that voluntarily participated cared for about 80 percent of the state's medical and surgical adult patient discharges and 90 per cent of childbirths. Results were released publicly and anecdotal evidence suggests that the reports generated a great deal of quality improvement activity (Rogers and Smith, 1999; Smith *et al.*, 2000).

In recent policy statements the Department of Health for England has placed considerable emphasis on the publication of a detailed set of performance indicators, including measures of patient experience derived from the National Surveys of NHS Patients which were launched in 1998 (Airey and Erens, 1999; Airey *et al.*, 2001). Two surveys have been completed – a general practice survey (sample size 100 000, response rate 65 per cent) and a survey of patients with coronary heart disease (sample size 112 000, response rate 74 per cent) – and a third survey, of patients with cancer, is in progress. Newspapers regularly publish a selection of performance indicators and these have also been placed on open access websites, but little is known as yet about whether or how patients have made use of these.

Well-designed national surveys have the great advantage of providing standardised results for comparative purposes, but the turn-around time is slow. In England it has recently been decided that all hospitals and primary care trusts will be required to perform their own local surveys, which would include standard questions that could be used for national performance monitoring and benchmarking. The requirements of top-down performance assessment and bottom-up quality improvement are hard to reconcile. Nationally-organised surveys can be implemented centrally and the results fed back to providers. In this way methodological quality can be assured and consistency in data analysis ensures that performance indicators derived from the surveys are valid and comparable. However, there may be no local "ownership" of an externally-imposed survey and hence less inclination to act on the findings. National surveys also take a long time to organise, with resulting loss in timeliness of the results. Local surveys can be carried out much more quickly and providers are more likely to "own" the results, but methodology and data quality is likely to be poor and inconsistent, with the result that performance indicators will be unreliable. Probably the best way forward is to promote national methodological standards and a core set of questions for use in centrally coordinated, but locally implemented, surveys.

A recent review concluded that consumers and purchasers rarely seek performance information and do not understand or trust it, but there is some evidence that its influence on their behaviour, though small, is increasing (Marshall *et al.*, 2000). Publication of performance data does appear to have an effect on providers themselves, however, and several studies have found an association with improved health outcomes (Davies, 2001; Schneider and Lieberman, 2001). Public disclosure of information about health care quality is a trend that seems set to continue. The inclusion of patient feedback among the performance indicators may serve to increase interest among members of the public and may prove to be less controversial than mortality rates and other clinical indicators.

5.4. Direct financial and other incentives

Financial incentives are increasingly being used in both the United States and the United Kingdom in an attempt to increase the efficiency and quality of care. Data from the US Community Tracking Study (St. Peter et al., 1999) indicates that about 75 per cent of practicing physicians receive at least some of their reimbursement in the form of capitated payments. However, most of these receive only a minority of their reimbursement this way and an even smaller proportion receive capitated payments that are adjusted based on various performance indicators, including the results of patient surveys. Almost no hospital revenue comes from capitated payments that are based on performance data.

In his plan for modernising the NHS in England published in July 2000, the Secretary of State for Health announced his intention to use "earned autonomy" and direct enhancements to financial allocations as incentives to improve standards of care (Secretary of State for Health, 2000). A new performance rating system identifies the best performing organisations, those meeting most but not all of the national standards, those who meet some but not enough of the standards, and those whose performance is poor according to the national performance framework (Department of Health, 2001). The best performing provider organisations are rewarded with greater autonomy, less frequent monitoring and national recognition as beacons of good practice. They also receive automatic access to a new National Health Performance Fund which can be used to buy new equipment, improve facilities for staff or as cash incentives for individuals and teams. Provider units which perform less well can also apply for this additional funding but they have to jump through many more bureaucratic hoops to get it. It will be very interesting to see if this new approach involving the use of direct financial incentives and regulatory freedom will have a greater impact on the quality of patient care than previous initiatives.

6. Conclusion

Even though the hospitals studied are not necessarily representative of all hospitals in the study countries, the findings from our analysis of data from the Picker surveys offer compelling evidence that there are major deficits in the quality of care in all the countries studied. Further study of the causes of the wide variations between countries could provide evidence about how organisations and providers in different countries could meet patient needs most effectively.

Patient satisfaction is determined by expectations. The Picker surveys of patients' experience aim to collect factual reports of processes and events and are, arguably, less subject to variations in expectations. Nevertheless, it is possible that patients' views of appropriate care could differ substantially among the countries studied. Those involved in the development of these surveys, however, have verified that the questions asked are salient and important in each of the countries studied. Furthermore, a recent study in the United Kingdom, Norway, Sweden, Denmark, the Netherlands, Germany, Portugal, and Israel found that although patients in different cultures and health care systems have different views on certain aspects of care, many expectations and values are very similar, particularly with respect to doctor-patient communication and accessibility of services (Grol et al., 1999).

There are undoubtedly other important differences between the countries that may cause different reactions to comparable experiences. Nevertheless, we think systematically studying and trying to understand the system differences that might account for the differences observed could be productive. The data demonstrate that some hospitals do dramatically better than others at meeting patient needs. Identifying the most effective strategies for doing this is a challenge we think that all hospitals should accept.

The traditional approach of giving patient survey results to providers has produced some successes, but lack of clear incentives to use the data, and lack of knowledge about to improve the processes asked about, have limited the effectiveness of this strategy. For the most part, the successes have resulted from the efforts of individual enthusiasts. These can have considerable impact but on their own they are unlikely to produce significant system-wide change.

Purchaser feedback has been used more in the United States than in the United Kingdom, probably because of the very different nature of health care purchasing in the two countries. Nevertheless, US purchasers do not appear to be making purchasing decisions based on the data and there are no evaluations demonstrating that other strategies have been effective at improving quality of patient-centered care. This is especially true for hospital care, where purchasers have less of a say in facility choice than providers and health plans. Purchasers in the UK's "internal market" were relatively weak and reluctant to use their financial muscle to stimulate quality improvements (Light, 1998). The internal market has now been officially abolished and the new strategy places much greater emphasis on direct incentives for providers to raise standards.

Public disclosure has had only limited effect to date but there are signs that patients are becoming more sophisticated as consumers of health services and are increasingly willing to shop around to secure the "best" quality. Measures of patient experience may prove easier for patients to interpret than other measures of performance such as mortality rates. Awareness that these data are publicly available may prove to be an effective incentive for providers to ensure that their services are truly patient-centred.

The initiatives recently announced in *The* NHS *Plan* mark a new departure for the health service in England. The plan places patients firmly at the centre of the government's attempt to modernise the health service and, as such constitute the first really concerted attempt to align a number of incentives – provider feedback, public disclosure, and financial incentives – to improve patients' experience. These new incentive systems, coupled with the announcement that funding will be increased to match levels in other European countries, offer a real opportunity for improvement. If the roll out of these new policy initiatives is rigorously evaluated, they will also offer an unprecedented opportunity to learn more about the mechanisms for achieving system-wide change and the problems that have to be overcome if health care systems are to work really well for patients.

As difficult as inter-country comparisons are to interpret, we think the data show that we have a great deal to learn from each other. Developing strategies for doing this could result in important new insights that world benefit patients throughout the world.

REFERENCES

AIREY, C. and ERENS, B. (eds) (1999),
National Survey of NHS Patients, General Practice 1998, Department of Health, London.

AIREY, C., BRUSTER, S., CALDERWOOD, L., ERENS, B., PITSON, L., PRIOR, G. and RICHARDS, N. (2001),
National Survey of NHS Patients, Coronary Heart Disease 1999. Summary of key findings, Department of Health, London.

BARRINGER, M.W. et al. (1994),
"Workers' preferences among company-provided health insurance plans", Industrial Labor Relations Review, Vol. 48, pp. 141-152.

BIRCH ,Q., FIELD, S. and SCRIVENS, E. (2000),
Quality in General Practice: Radcliffe Medical Press, Abingdon, pp. 27-28.

CHERNEW, M. and SCANLON, D.P. (1998),
"Health plan report cards and insurance choice", Inquiry, Vol. 35, pp. 9-22.

CHERNEW, M. et al. (1998),
"Insurance type and choice of hospital for coronary artery bypass graft surgery", Health Services Research, Vol. 33, pp. 447-466.

CLEARY, P.D. (1999),
"The increasing importance of patient surveys", British Medical Journal, Vol. 319, pp. 720-721.

CLEARY, P.D. and EDGEMAN-LEVITAN, S. (1997),
"Health care quality: incorporating consumer perspectives", JAMA, Vol. 278, pp. 1608-1612.

CLEARY, P.D., EDGEMAN-LEVITAN, S., McMULLEN, W. and DELBANCO, T.L. (1992),
"The relationship between reported problems and patient summary evaluations of hospital care", Quality Review Bulletin, February, pp. 53-59.

CLEARY, P.D., EDGEMAN-LEVITAN, S., WALKER, J.D., GERTEIS, M. and DELBANCO, T.L. (1993),
"Using patient reports to improve medical care: a preliminary report from 10 hospitals", Quality Management in Health Care, Vol. 2, pp. 31-38.

CLEARY, P.D., EDGEMAN-LEVITAN, S., ROBERTS, M., MOLONEY, T.W., MCMULLEN, W., WALKER, J.D. and DELBANCO, T.L. (1991),
"Patients evaluate their hospital care: a national survey", Health Affairs, Vol. 10(4), pp. 254-267.

COULTER, A. and CLEARY, P. (2001),
"Patients' experience with hospital care in five countries", Health Affairs, Vol. 20 (3), pp. 244-252.

DAVIS, K. et al. (1995),
"Choice matters: enrollees' views of their health plans", Health Affairs, Vol. 14, pp. 99-112.

DAVIES, H.T.O. (2001),
"Public release of performance data and quality improvement: internal responses to external data by US health care providers", Quality in Health Care, Vol. 10, pp. 104-110.

Department of Health (2001),
NHS Performance Ratings: Acute Trusts 2000/01, London, September.

DRAPER, M. and HILL, S. (1995),
The Role of Patient Satisfaction Surveys in a National Approach to Hospital Quality Management, Australian Government Publishing Service, Canberra.

FOWLES, J.B. et al. (2000),
"Consumer responses to health plan report cards in two markets", Med Care, Vol. 38, pp. 469-481.

FRANTZEN, K. and HOGLUND, E. (2001),
Learn from Your Patients!, Poster at European Forum for Quality in Health Care conference, Bologna, March.

GABLE, J.R. et al. (1998),
"When employers choose health plans: Do NCQA accreditation and HEDIS data count?", KPMG Peat Marwick Report, September.

GERTEIS, M., EDGMAN-LEVITAN, S., DALEY, J. and DELBANCO, T.L. (eds) (1993),
Through the Patient's Eyes, Jossey-Bass, San Francisco.

GOODWIN, N. (1996),
"GP Fundholding: a review of the evidence", *Health Care* UK 1995/96, King's Fund, London, pp. 116-130.

GROL, R. *et al.* (1999),
"Patients' priorities with respect to general practice care: an international comparison", *Family Practice*, Vol. 16, pp. 4-11.

GUADAGNOLI, E. *et al.* (2000),
"Providing consumers with information about quality of health plans: The consumer assessment of health plans demonstration in Washington State", *Joint Comm J. on Qual. Imp.*, Vol. 26, pp. 410-420.

KAO, A. *et al.* (1998a),
"Patients' trust in their physicians: effects of choice, continuity and patient perceptions of physician payment method", J *Gen Int Med.*, pp. 681-686.

KAO, A. *et al.* (1998b),
"The relationship between method of physician payment and patient trust", JAMA, Vol. 280, pp. 1708-1714.

KNUTSON, D.J., ADLIS, S. *et al.* (1998),
"Impact of report cards on employees: A natural experiment", *Health Care Financing Review*, Vol. 20, pp. 3-27.

LIGHT, D.W. (1998),
"Is NHS purchasing serious?", *British Medical Journal*, Vol. 316, pp. 217-220.

LUFT, H.S. *et al.* (1990),
"Does quality influence choice of hospital?", JAMA, Vol. 263, pp. 2899-2906.

MARSHALL, M.N., SHEKELLE, P.G., LEATHERMAN, S. and BROOK, R.H. (2000),
"The public release of performance data: what do we expect to gain? A review of the evidence", JAMA, Vol. 282, pp. 1866-1874.

NCQA. Accreditation 99 (1998),
Standards for the Accreditation of Managed Care Organizations, National Committee for Quality Assurance, Washington, D.C.

OVRETVEIT, J. (1998),
Comparative and Cross-cultural Health Research, Radcliffe Medical Press, Abingdon.

REILEY, P., PIKE, A., PHIPPS, M., WEINER, M., MILLER, N., STENGREVICS, S., CLARK, L. and WANDEL, J. (1996),
"Learning from patients: a discharge planning improvement project", *Quality Improvement*, Vol. 22(5), pp. 311-322.

RICE, T. *et al.* (1991),
"The effectiveness of consumer choice in the Medicare supplemental health insurance market", *Health Serv Res.*, Vol. 26, pp. 223-246.

RIDER, E.A. and PERRIN, J. M. (2002),
"Performance profiles: the influence of patient satisfaction data on physicians' practice", *Pediatrics*, in press.

ROGERS, G. and SMITH D.P. (1999),
"Reporting comparative results from hospital patient surveys", Int J *Quality Health Care*, Vol. 11, pp. 251-259.

ROYALTY, A.B. and SOLOMON, N. (1999), "Health plan choice: Price elasticities in a managed competition setting", *Journal of Human Resources*, Vol. 34, pp. 1-41.

SCANLON, D.P. *et al.* (1997),
"Consumer health plan choice: current knowledge and future directions", *Annual Review of Public Health*, Vol. 18, pp. 507-528.

SCHMITTDIEL, J. *et al.* (1998),
"Choice of a personal physician and patient satisfaction in a health maintenance organisation" [published erratum appears in JAMA, March 4, Vol. 279(9), p. 656], JAMA, Vol. 278, pp. 1596-1599.

SCHNEIDER, E.C. and EPSTEIN, A.M. (1998),
"Use of public performance reports: a survey of patients undergoing cardiac surgery", JAMA, Vol. 279, pp. 1638-1642.

SCHNEIDER, E.C. and LIEBERMAN, T. (2001),
"Publicly disclosed information about the quality of health care: response of the US public", *Quality in Health Care*, Vol. 10, pp. 96-103.

SCHOEN, C.A. and DAVIDSON, P. (1996),
"Image and Reality: Managed-care experiences by type of plan", *Bull NY Acad Med.*, Vol. 73, pp. 506-531.

SCHUSTER, M.A., MCGLYNN, E.A., BROOK, R.H. (1998), "How good is quality of health care in the United States?", *Milbank Quarterly*, Vol. 76, pp. 517-563.

SECRETARY OF STATE FOR HEALTH (1998),
A *First Class Service: quality in the new NHS*, HMSO, London.

SECRETARY OF STATE FOR HEALTH (2000),
The NHS Plan, HMSO, London.

SITZIA, J. and WOOD, N. (1997), "Patient satisfaction: a review of issues and concept", Social Science and Medicine, Vol. 45, pp. 1829-1843.

SMITH, D. et al. (2000), "Balancing accountability and improvement: a case study from Massachusetts", Joint Comm J Quality Imp, Vol. 26, pp. 299-312.

ST. PETER, R.F. et al. (1999),
"Changes in the scope of care provided by primary care physicians", N Engl J Med, Vol. 341, pp. 1980-1985.

ULLMAN, R. et al. (1997),
"Satisfaction and choice: a view from the plans", Health Aff (Millwood), Vol. 16, pp. 209-217.

VEROFF, D.R. et al. (1998),
"Effective reports for health care quality data: lessons from a CAHPS demonstration in Washington State", Int J Qual Hlth Care, Vol. 10, pp. 555-560.

WEDDERBURN TATE, C., BRUSTER, S., BROADLEY, K., MAXWELL, E. and STEVENS, L. (1995),
"What do patients really think?", Health Service Journal, 12th January, pp. 18-20.

ZASLAVSKY, A.M., ZABORSKI, L.B., DING, L., SHAUL J.A., CIOFFI, M.J. and Cleary, P.D. (2001),
"Adjusting performance measures to ensure equitable plan comparisons", Health Care Financing Review, Vol. 22 (3), pp. 109-126.

Chapter 11

EQUITY IN THE USE OF PHYSICIAN VISITS IN OECD COUNTRIES: HAS EQUAL TREATMENT FOR EQUAL NEED BEEN ACHIEVED?

by

Eddy van Doorslaer[*], Xander Koolman[*] and Frank Puffer[**]

Abstract

This paper uses methods proposed by Wagstaff and Van Doorslaer (2000) to generate new international comparative evidence for 1996 on the degree of horizontal equity achieved in health care utilisation in 14 OECD countries. The index of horizontal inequity used measures deviations in the degree to which the use of doctor visits is distributed according to need. The data for the 12 European Union member states are taken from the third wave of the *European Community Household Panel*, the data for Canada are from the second wave *National Population Health Survey* and the US data stem from the first wave of the *Medical Expenditure Panel Survey*. We find that in all countries physician visits tend to be significantly more concentrated among the worse-off. After standardising for need differences across the income distribution, significant horizontal inequity in total physician visits emerges in only four of the countries studied: Portugal, the United States, Austria and Greece. However, disaggregating by general practitioner and specialist visits reveals that this is the net effect from quite diverging patterns in the type of doctor consulted by income level: in all countries (except Luxembourg) the rich see a medical specialist more often than expected on the basis of need, while the use of GP visits is fairly closely related to need and in several countries even distributed somewhat pro-poor. The degree and distribution of private health insurance coverage and regional disparities seem to have the expected effect on inequity but in most countries their contribution is rather small. Only in the United States, the effect of private insurance cover is quite large. The results suggest that even in countries which have long achieved fairly universal and comprehensive degrees of health insurance coverage, some differential patterns of doctor utilization remain: higher income individuals are more likely to receive specialist services whereas lower income individuals are more inclined to use general practitioner care. To the extent that these differential use patterns result in differences of quality of treatment, persons in equal need cannot be said to receive equal treatment at all income levels.

Introduction

Most OECD Member states have long achieved close to universal coverage of their population for a fairly comprehensive package of health services. There are exceptions, but in most of these countries,

[*] Department of Health Policy and Management, Erasmus University, 3000 DR Rotterdam, The Netherlands.

Corresponding author: Eddy van Doorslaer Tel. +31 10 4088555. E-mail: *vandoorslaer@bmg.eur.nl*. This paper derives from the project "Economic determinants of the distribution of health and health care in Europe" (known as the ECuity II Project), which is funded in part by the European Community's Biomed II programme (contract BMH4-CT98-3352). We are grateful to the EC for financial support and to Stéphane Jacobzone, Peter C. Smith and discussants and participants at the OECD Health Conference "Measuring up", Ottawa, 5-7 Nov, for helpful comments on an earlier version.

[**] Department of Economics, Clark University, Clark, MA 01610, USA.

access to good quality physician services is ensured at relatively low and sometimes at zero financial cost, even for low-income groups. This is mainly the result of a variety of public insurance arrangements aimed at ensuring equitable access. Equity in access is also regarded as a key element of health system performance by the OECD (Hurst and Jee-Hughes, 2001). The question that arises is to what extent OECD countries have achieved the goal of equal access or utilisation for equal need, irrespective of other characteristics like income, place of residence, ethnicity, etc.? As in our previous cross-country comparative work (Van Doorslaer *et al.*, 1992, 1993 and 2000) we will focus here on the principle of *horizontal* equity – *i.e.* that those in equal need ought to be treated equally – and test for the extent of any systematic deviations from this principle by income level. Van Doorslaer *et al.* (2000) concluded that both in the United States and in several European countries some systematic deviation of the horizontal equity principle could be detected, *i.e.* that persons in equal need be treated equally, irrespective of their income. In particular, we found that often the rich tend to be more intensive users of medical specialist services than one would expect on the basis of differences in need for care.

This earlier work was based on secondary analysis of existing national health interview surveys or general purpose surveys (like the *General Household Survey* for the UK) and – despite great efforts at maximizing data comparability – it was still hampered by cross-country comparability problems of self-reported utilisation and health data. Since 1994, the European Statistical Office (Eurostat) has started the *European Community Household Panel* which collects longitudinal data on the socio-economic characteristics, self-reported health status and annual health care utilisation of representative samples of the populations of all EU member states. For the first time, very comparable survey data have become available which enable the cross-European comparison of levels and patterns of health care utilisation. Here we use the 1996 data wave which provides comparable data for 12 EU member countries.[1] In North-America, the 1996 US *National Medical Expenditure Panel* and the Canadian 1996 *National Population Health Survey* collect utilisation data which are very comparable to the European data. This paper provides the first comparative analysis of the use of physician services in those European and North-American datasets with the objective of determining the degree to which the 14 countries included in the analysis have been able to achieve an equitable distribution of physician services.

The paper starts by defining our equity measurement instruments in Section 1. Section 2 contains a summary of the salient features of the health care systems in the 14 countries which may affect the degree to which systematic deviations of an equitable distribution may occur by income status. Section 3 provides a description of the data and estimation methods used and Section 4 presents the main results. We conclude with a discussion in Section 5.

1. Horizontal inequity in health care delivery

1.1. *Defining horizontal inequity*

Many OECD countries have explicitly included equity in access to health care as one of the main objectives in policy documents (Van Doorslaer *et al.*, 1993; Hurst and Jee-Hughes, 2001). In most European countries and in Canada, an egalitarian viewpoint of social justice seems to have been an important source of inspiration for these positions with respect to health care access. This is not true of the United States, where the (more libertarian) viewpoint that access ought to be guaranteed to a minimum standard of health care appears to have been one of the driving forces behind the introduction and expansion of public programmes like Medicaid and Medicare. But also in many other countries, traces of both viewpoints can be found. In Ireland and the Netherlands, for instance, health care systems have only aimed to equalize access for the lower income parts of the population. Usually, the horizontal version of the egalitarian principle is interpreted to require that people in equal need of care are treated equally, irrespective of characteristics such as income, place of residence, race, etc.[2] It is this principle of horizontal equity that the present study uses as the yardstick for the international comparisons. This yardstick is obviously only useful for performance measurement to the extent that this principle is in accordance with a country's policy objectives. For countries not subscribing to this principle, the methods may still be useful for comparison with others but not for internal performance measurement.

The method we use in this paper to measure the degree of horizontal inequity in health care delivery is conceptually identical to the ones used in Wagstaff and Van Doorslaer (2000a) and Van Doorslaer *et al.* (2000). It proceeds by comparing the actual observed distribution of medical care by income with the distribution of need. Because a measure of the need for medical care is obtained by the method of indirect standardization, it does assume implicitly that "on average, the system gets it right" or that the average treatment differences between those in unequal need are appropriate. This means that in order to statistically equalize needs for the groups or individuals to be compared, we are using the average relationship between need and treatment for the population as a whole as the vertical equity norm. In other words: on the assumption, that the average relationship can be used as the (country specific) norm, we will investigate to what extent there are any systematic deviations from this norm by income level.

1.2. *Measuring inequity*

Let m_i denote the amount of medical care received by individual i in a given period. The inequality in the distribution of medical care by income is captured by the medical care *concentration curve* L_M (R) in Figure 1, which graphs the cumulative proportion of medical care against the cumulative proportion R of the sample, ranked by income. The concentration index, C_M, corresponding to L_M(R) indicates the degree of *inequality* in the distribution of medical care and can be measured as twice the area between L_M(R) and the diagonal, or equivalently as:

(1) $$C_M = 1 - 2\int_0^1 L_M(R)\mathrm{d}R,$$

But the degree of *inequality* in utilization of medical care will tell us something about the degree of *inequity* only in the unlikely event that need for medical care does not vary with income. If this is not the case, it needs to be compared to the degree of inequality in need. Using the method of indirect standardization (see below) we can generate a predicted value m_i^* for each individual i indicating the amount of medical care she would have received if she had been treated as others with the same need characteristics were, on average, treated by the system.[3] We interpret this as her need for medical care, N. By analogy, we can then define a concentration index of need (*i.e.* indirectly standardized medical care) C_N based on the concentration curve of need, labeled L_N(R), as follows:

(2) $$C_N = 1 - 2\int_0^1 L_N(R)\mathrm{d}R,$$

The extent of horizontal equity can then be assessed by comparing each income group's share of "need" (or need-expected utilization) with its share of medical care (or unstandardized utilization). If horizontal equity obtains, each group's medical care share will equal its share of need. The degree of horizontal inequity can be measured by comparing the curves L_M(R) and L_N(R) in Figure 1: if the latter lies above (below) the former, the higher income groups obtain a higher (lower) share of medical care than their share of need, and we say there is horizontal inequity favoring the better-off (worse-off). The proposed measure of horizontal inequity HI_{WV} is defined as twice the area between the need and medical care concentration curves and can simply be computed as the difference between C_M and C_N:

(3) $$HI_{WV} = 2\int_0^1 \left[L_N(R) - L_M(R)\right]\mathrm{d}R = C_M - C_N$$

A positive (negative) value of HI_{WV} indicates horizontal inequity favoring the better-off (worse-off). A zero index value indicates no horizontal inequity, *i.e.* that medical care and need are proportionally distributed across the income distribution. It is worth emphasizing that coinciding concentration curves for need and actual use provide a sufficient but not a necessary condition for no inequity. Even with crossing curves, one could have zero inequity if, for example, inequity favoring the poor in one part of the distribution exactly offsets inequity favoring the rich in another.[4]

Figure 1. **Concentration curves for actual and need-expected medical care**

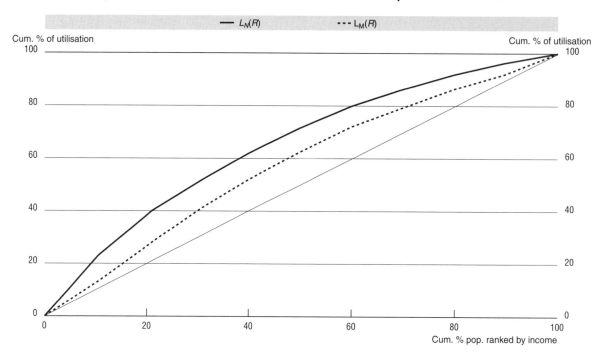

1.3. Explaining horizontal inequity

Obviously, if any inequitable pattern of utilisation is observed, the interesting question is why it arises. There are several ways in which one can try to go beyond measurement and towards explanation of inequity findings.[5] One straightforward – albeit indirect – method of assessing to what extent any observed inequity patterns are due to the distribution of other (*i.e.* non-need) factors which may have an impact on the demand for care is by including such additional determinants in the need standardization process. Even if such determinants clearly do not belong in a vector of need adjusters, it allows to assess indirectly to what extent the observed degree of inequity is affected by the inclusion of such non-need determinants. This approach resembles the assessment of the role of "intermediary factors" and "confounders" in the analysis of any association. In this case, the question is to what extent the association between an individual's health care use and his or her relative rank in the income distribution is mediated or confounded by variables other than acceptable proxies for "need" such as demographics and self-reported morbidity.

In this paper, we will briefly explore the role of just two other possible access determinants: private health insurance coverage and regional access differences. Obviously, the inclusion of a dummy variable indicating that the individual (or household) has private coverage allows for the estimation of an insurance effect, but it does not enable us to distinguish between the *moral hazard effect* (those with insurance are likely to have higher use) and the *selection effect* (those with higher expected use are more likely to buy cover). Because the voluntary purchase of such cover is related to the likelihood of (future) consumption, in principle the insurance coverage variables ought to be treated as endogenous. We do not attempt such an investigation here. The sole purpose of this exercise is to ascertain to what extent the existence and unequal distribution of such coverage affects the degree of measured inequity. Similarly, the question to what extent income-related differences in physician utilisation rates are driven by regional differences in availability ideally ought to be examined using the appropriate variables capturing regional characteristics like GP and specialist densities, mean distances to facilities, etc. In the absence of such regional data, the regional dummies inevitably only capture inter-regional differences in utilisation but do not allow to attribute these differences to specific regional characteristics. Still, because of their policy relevance, it seems worth exploring to what extent our inequity findings are affected by the insurance and regional factor.

2.   Differences in equity-relevant health care delivery system characteristics

While all of the countries included in this analysis – except for the United States[6] – had by 1996 achieved close to universal coverage of their population for the majority of physician services, important other between-country differences remain with respect to potentially equity-relevant features of their financing and delivery systems. In Appendix Tables A1 and A2 we have summarized some of the salient system characteristics which may have an impact on any differential utilisation of the general practitioner or medical specialist by income level. In a number of countries, there are different groups of insured with often varying degrees of coverage or rules of reimbursement at different levels of income. This is the case for rather small numbers of high income earners with private coverage in Denmark and Germany, but it concerns sizeable portions of the population in Ireland and the Netherlands. Some countries' public insurance rules, like Portugal, France and Belgium, still require their citizens to pay substantial copayments while in many other countries (like Denmark, Canada, Germany, Spain, Portugal and the United Kingdom) visits to public sector doctors are free at the point of delivery. In some countries, notably Denmark, Canada, Ireland, Italy, The Netherlands, Portugal, Spain and the UK, the primary care physician acts as a "gatekeeper" referring to secondary care provided by medical specialists, whereas in other countries, there is direct access to all physicians. Some countries pay their general practitioners mainly by capitation (Denmark, Italy, Netherlands) or salary (Greece, Portugal, Spain) whereas others rely mainly on fee-for-service payment. Although this summary is by no means complete in the sense that it provides a full picture of the diversity represented by these systems characteristics, it does serve to illustrate which factors may help to account for any regularities found in the cross-country differences in horizontal equity.

3.   Data and estimation methods

3.1. Data

The data for the European Union (EU) member countries are taken from the third wave (held in 1996) of the *European Community Household Panel* (ECHP) conducted by Eurostat, the European Statistical Office.[7] The ECHP is a survey based on a standardised questionnaire that involves annual interviewing of a representative panel of households and individuals of 16 years and older in each EU member state (Eurostat, 1999). It covers a wide range of topics including demographics, income, social transfers, health, housing, education, employment, etc. We use data for the following twelve member states of the EU: Austria, Belgium, Denmark, Germany, Greece, Ireland, Italy, Luxembourg, Netherlands, Portugal, Spain and the United Kingdom. The three missing member states are France, Finland and Sweden.[8] The Canadian data are taken from the 1996 wave of the *National Population Health Survey* (NPHS) conducted by Statistics Canada.[9] A total of 73 402 individuals aged 12 years or older were selected for an in-depth interview, but we have only included individuals of 16 and older. The survey includes questions on health care utilization, health status, risk factors, and demographic and socio-economic information. The data are weighted using the survey weights to adjust for the complex multi-cluster sample design of the NPHS. The US data are taken from the *Medical Expenditure Panel Survey* (MEPS) conducted by the Agency for Healthcare Research and Quality (AHRQ)[10] It is a nationally representative survey that collects detailed information on the health status, access to care, health care use and expenses, and health insurance coverage of the civilian noninstitutionalized population of the United States. Analysis was restricted to individuals over the age of 16. Some summary information on all surveys is presented in Table 1.

The ECHP income measure (*i.e.* our ranking variable) is disposable (*i.e.* after-tax) household income per equivalent adult, using the modified OECD equivalence scale.[11] Total household income includes all the net monetary income received by the household members during the reference year (which is 1995 for the 1996 wave). It includes income from work (employment and self-employment), private

Table 1. **Details of surveys and samples**

	Year	Survey	Age limits	Sample size	Recall period doctor visits	Income variable	Equivalence scale
Canada	1996	National Population Health Survey	16+	55 249	12 months	Before tax household income, per equiv adult, midpoints 11 classes	Modified OECD
12 EU member states	1996	European Community Household Panel	16+	105 889	12 months	Disposable household income per equiv adult	Modified OECD
United States	1996	Medical Expenditure Panel Survey	16+	15 973	12 months	Net hh income after federal tax, estimated using TAXSIM	Modified OECD

income (from investments and property and private transfers to the household), pensions and other direct social transfers received. No account has been taken of indirect social transfers (*e.g.* reimbursement of medical expenses), receipts in kind and imputed rent from owner-occupied accomodation. Income information was more limited in the Canadian survey. Respondents are only being asked for their best estimate of total income, before taxes and deductions, of all household members from all sources in the past 12 months in eleven income categories. We assigned $2 500 to the lowest income category, $87 500 to the highest income category and midpoints to the remaining categories. These assigned income values were equivalised using the "modified OECD scale". The US before-tax household income measure recorded in the survey was adjusted to a net household income using estimates of the federal tax paid per household, which was obtained with the NBER TAXSIM model. Insufficient information was available to estimate state taxes.

Measurement of utilisation of general practitioner (GP) and medical specialist services in the ECHP is based on the question "During the past 12 months, about how many times have you consulted a GP/ medical specialist?" Similar questions referring to a 12 month reference period were used in Canada and the United States, though the US MEPS survey does not distinguish between GP and specialist visits. The measurement of health was based on two types of questions. Respondents' categorical responses to a question on self-assessment of their general health status in the ECHP could be "Very good, good, fair, bad or very bad" while the analogous five response options in the NPHS and MEPS are "Excellent, very good, good, fair or poor". A further health related question in the ECHP is: "Do you have any chronic physical or mental health problem, illness or disability? (yes/no)" and if so "Are you hampered in your daily activities by this physical or mental health problem, illness or disability? (no; yes, to some extent; yes, severely)". We used two dummies to indicate the degree of limitation. Similar but not quite identical questions were used in the NPHS and MEPS. The exact wording and definition is presented in Table 2.

The survey information used on health insurance coverage is described in Table 3. The available information in the ECHP is fairly limited and not very specific. The few questions are insufficiently tailored to specific countries to be always meaningful. The question was "Are you (also) covered by *private* medical insurance, whether in your own name or through another family member?" This variable for many countries may be an indicator of a mixture of various different types of (additional) coverage. It can be the *main* source of cover (as for higher income groups in The Netherlands), it can be complementary cover (for copayments or for things *not* covered in the public scheme, as in *e.g.* Austria, Denmark, Ireland, Luxembourg, Spain) or it can be supplementary or "double cover" (for things already covered in the public sector, as *e.g.* in the United Kingdom). In several countries, this variable can refer to various types at the same time. For example, in Belgium, it can be the coverage for "normal physician services" for self-

Table 2. **Details of health questions**

Country and survey	Wording of general self-assessed health question and response categories	Wording of question on chronic ill-health
European ECHP	"How do you rate your health in general?" very good, good, fair, bad or very bad	"Do you have any chronic physical or mental health problem, illness or disability? (yes/no)" and if so "Are you hampered in your daily activities by this physical or mental health problem, illness or disability? (no/ yes, to some extent/ yes, severely)".
Canadian NPHS	In general would you say your health is excellent/very good/good/fair/poor?	Because of any condition or health problem, do you need the help of another person in preparing meals/in shopping for groceries or other necessities/in doing normal everyday housework/in doing heavy household chores such as washing walls or yard work/in personal care such as washing, dressing or eating/in moving about inside the house? (yes/no).
US MEPS	In general, compared to other people of [one's] age, would you say your health is excellent/very good/good/fair/poor?	Combination of a number of questions asking whether respondent is limited in any way in the ability to work at a job, do housework or go to school because of an impairment of a physical or mental health problem (yes/no).

Table 3. **Details of insurance and region variables**

Country survey	Wording of private health insurance question	Regional dummies
European ECHP	"Are you (also) covered by *private* medical insurance, whether in your own name or through another family member?"	Regional dummies for Belgium (2), Ireland (1), Austria (2), UK (10), Italy (10), Greece (3), Spain (6), Portugal (7)
Canadian NPHS	Four questions: "Do you have insurance that covers all or part of the cost of your prescription medications? (Include any government or employer-paid plans) (yes/no)"	10 provinces
US MEPS	Constructed from a series of detailed questions about insurance status. Indicates whether or not the individual had any private insurance during the year	Four large census regions: Northeast, Midwest, South and West

employed (who do not have compulsory cover), it can be complementary cover for hospital public copayments or it can be supplementary cover. In the MEPS, the variables relating to (private) health insurance coverage were far more detailed. For the sake of comparability, we nevertheless only used a simple 0/1 indicator of the presence of private coverage without specifying further detail of type and degree of coverage. Similarly, for the NHPS, we only used whether or not the individual had private coverage for prescription drugs. Whatever the type and level of private coverage, in virtually all countries for which the variable is available, the uptake of private cover generally tends to rise with income level.

The information available in the ECHP regarding the region of residence of the respondents was very limited. Mostly for privacy reasons, either no information was provided (as in Denmark, Germany, Luxembourg, Netherlands) or only at a very broad regional level (all other countries). Also the MEPS public use files only contain the four large US Census regions. Only in the NPHS, some more detailed regional disaggregation below provincial level was available but for comparative purposes we only used the provincial level. As such, the regional fixed effects on physician visits can only pick up variations across some large regions in the various countries and cannot really be assumed to pick up local circumstances in supply of and demand for such care. The information we could use is presented in Table 3.

3.2. Estimation methods

Health care utilisation data like physician visits are known to have a very skewed distribution with typically the large majority of survey respondents reporting zero or few visits and only a very small proportion reporting frequent use. Various specifications of two-part models have been proposed in the literature, distinguishing between the probability of positive usage and the conditional amount of usage given positive use in the reference period (cf. e.g. Pohlmeier and Ulrich, 1995; or Jones, 2000, for a review). The choice depends on both theoretical and statistical considerations regarding the utilization process. The two-part model we have used to predict "needed" health care use is based on a logit specification for the first part and a truncated negative binomial count model for the second (conditional) part. This version resembles the hurdle model proposed by Mullahy (1986) and used before by e.g. Gerdtham (1997) and Wagstaff and Van Doorslaer (2000b) to analyze equity in the utilisation of physician visits.

The logit model estimates the probability of any positive use in the reference period as

(4) $$Prob(y = 1|x) = \Lambda(x\beta)$$

where $\Lambda(.)$ is the cumulative density function of the logistic distribution and β is the estimated parameter vector. For the second part we use a truncated negative binomial model with the truncation at zero (cf. e.g. Greene, 1997). The expected value of positive consumption with this model, conditional on consumption being positive, is

(5) $$E(y_i|y_i > 0, x) = \exp(x\beta)(\frac{1}{1 - P_0})$$

where β is the estimated coefficient vector and P_0 is the probability of observing zero counts. $1/(1-P_0)$ is an adjustment factor to ensure that the probabilities of positive counts sum to one (Pohlmeier and Ulrich, 1995). The combined two-part model predictions of overall utilization are obtained by multiplying the predictions from equations 4 and 5. For all countries and surveys, cross-sectional sample weights were used in all computations in order to make the results more representative of the countries' populations.[12] Robust standard errors were obtained by applying White's correction for heteroskedasticity. Huber's correction for cluster sampling was applied for countries where cluster sampling had been used and primary sampling unit information was made available.[13]

4. Results

4.1. Quintile distributions of health care utilisation

Tables 4-7 present unstandardized and need-standardized quintile distributions of GP and specialist visits for the EU countries and Canada. Standardized distributions were obtained by adding the difference between the observed and standardized (or expected) means per quintile to the overall country sample mean. Expected means were obtained using a simple (one-part) OLS model for convenience. European quintile rates have to be interpreted with caution as they were computed as population-weighted averages of country-specific quintiles.[14] Simple difference and ratio measures for

Table 4. **Mean number of GP visits by income quintile (unstandardised)**

	Austria	Belgium	Denmark	Germany	Greece	Ireland	Italy	Luxem-bourg	Nether-lands	Portugal	Spain	United Kingdom	EU-12	Canada
Bottom 20%	6.02	6.47	3.41	5.53	2.96	4.75	4.76	3.70	3.10	4.27	4.19	4.90	4.83	4.07
20-40%	6.00	6.51	3.47	5.69	2.37	4.87	5.20	4.01	3.25	3.71	4.37	4.51	4.87	3.54
40-60%	5.21	4.84	3.31	5.08	2.27	3.37	4.63	3.40	3.00	3.62	4.23	3.64	4.29	3.13
60-80%	4.74	3.94	2.77	4.86	1.71	2.86	4.43	3.17	2.69	3.45	3.24	3.22	3.88	2.83
Top 20%	4.97	4.26	2.35	4.08	1.65	2.59	3.51	2.37	2.56	2.88	2.66	2.74	3.30	2.72
Mean	5.39	5.21	3.06	5.05	2.19	3.69	4.51	3.33	2.92	3.59	3.74	3.80	4.23	3.26
Q1/Q5	1.21	1.52	1.45	1.36	1.80	1.83	1.35	1.56	1.21	1.48	1.58	1.79	1.46	1.50
Q1-Q5	1.05	2.21	1.06	1.45	1.31	2.16	1.25	1.33	0.55	1.39	1.53	2.16	1.52	1.35
N	6 446	5 928	4 978	8 510	11 258	7 363	17 434	1 898	9 111	11 577	15 283	6 103	105 889	55 249

Note: EU-12 rates computed as weighted average of country-specific rates.

Table 5. **Mean number of GP visits by income quintile**

OLS standardised for age, sex and morbidity

	Austria	Belgium	Denmark	Germany	Greece	Ireland	Italy	Luxem-bourg	Nether-lands	Portugal	Spain	United Kingdom	EU-12	Canada
Bottom 20%	5.09	5.33	2.92	5.00	2.16	4.12	4.57	3.36	2.83	3.23	4.01	4.02	4.29	3.44
20-40%	5.49	5.68	3.07	5.23	2.22	3.83	4.72	3.61	2.94	3.43	3.90	3.92	4.39	3.33
40-60%	5.47	5.09	3.37	5.12	2.39	3.47	4.46	3.43	2.98	3.77	3.87	3.71	4.26	3.23
60-80%	5.14	4.86	3.11	5.20	2.04	3.49	4.50	3.22	3.02	3.83	3.49	3.79	4.23	3.10
Top 20%	5.77	5.08	2.84	4.67	2.10	3.51	4.22	3.02	2.82	3.67	3.42	3.59	3.99	3.19
Q1/Q5	0.88	1.05	1.03	1.07	1.03	1.17	1.08	1.11	1.00	0.88	1.17	1.12	1.08	1.08
Q1-Q5	−0.68	0.25	0.07	0.33	0.05	0.61	0.35	0.33	0.01	−0.44	0.59	0.44	0.31	0.25
N	6 446	5 928	4 978	8 510	11 258	7 363	17 434	1 898	9 111	11 577	15 283	6 103	105 889	55 249

Note: EU-12 rates computed as weighted average of country-specific rates.

Table 6. **Mean number of specialist visits by income quintile (unstandardised)**

	Austria	Belgium	Denmark	Germany	Greece	Ireland	Italy	Luxem-bourg	Nether-lands	Portugal	Spain	United Kingdom	EU-12	Canada
Bottom 20%	2.65	2.21	0.98	2.95	1.89	0.53	1.14	2.81	1.68	1.22	1.45	1.32	1.83	1.18
20-40%	2.91	1.93	0.96	3.45	1.63	0.58	1.31	2.52	2.07	1.07	1.64	1.12	1.99	1.19
40-60%	2.65	1.70	1.05	3.52	1.78	0.57	1.24	1.97	1.82	1.21	1.58	1.14	1.98	1.10
60-80%	2.62	1.58	1.17	3.07	1.60	0.70	1.29	2.41	1.76	1.54	1.58	0.98	1.84	1.16
Top 20%	3.39	2.04	0.98	3.48	1.56	0.74	1.34	1.99	1.61	1.80	1.70	1.14	2.03	1.20
Mean	2.84	1.89	1.03	3.29	1.69	0.62	1.26	2.34	1.79	1.37	1.59	1.14	1.93	1.17
Q1/Q5	0.78	1.08	1.00	0.85	1.21	0.72	0.85	1.41	1.04	0.68	0.85	1.16	0.90	0.98
Q1-Q5	−0.74	0.17	0.00	−0.53	0.33	−0.21	−0.20	0.82	0.07	−0.58	−0.26	0.18	−0.20	−0.02
N	5 578	5 801	4 980	8 485	11 257	7 361	17 428	1 898	9 125	11 574	15 283	6 104	104 875	55 249

Note: EU-12 rates computed as weighted average of country-specific rates.

Table 7. **Mean number of specialist visits by income quintile**

OLS standardised for age, sex and morbidity

	Austria	Belgium	Denmark	Germany	Greece	Ireland	Italy	Luxem-bourg	Nether-lands	Portugal	Spain	United Kingdom	EU-12	Canada
Bottom 20%	2.40	1.87	0.92	2.64	1.32	0.44	1.05	2.48	1.45	0.90	1.34	1.06	1.60	0.99
20-40%	2.75	1.78	0.84	3.21	1.47	0.46	1.20	2.32	1.81	0.98	1.49	0.91	1.81	1.13
40-60%	2.68	1.74	1.05	3.57	1.83	0.58	1.24	2.01	1.81	1.22	1.48	1.15	1.99	1.13
60-80%	2.66	1.84	1.25	3.24	1.81	0.78	1.31	2.46	2.02	1.66	1.69	1.17	1.97	1.25
Top 20%	3.67	2.24	1.09	3.80	1.99	0.86	1.51	2.43	1.84	2.07	1.96	1.41	2.30	1.33
Q1/Q5	0.65	0.84	0.84	0.69	0.66	0.51	0.69	1.02	0.79	0.44	0.68	0.75	0.70	0.74
Q1-Q5	−1.27	−0.37	−0.17	−1.16	−0.67	−0.42	−0.47	0.06	−0.39	−1.16	−0.62	−0.35	−0.69	−0.34
N	5 578	5 801	4 980	8 485	11 257	7 361	17 428	1 898	9 125	11 574	15 283	6 104	104 875	55 249

Note: EU-12 rates computed as weighted average of country-specific rates.

the bottom and top quintile have been added to ease cross-country comparisons of utilization differences by income level.

It is clear that some countries, notably Germany and Austria, have above-European average rates of utilization for both GP and specialist visits. Some general patterns can be observed. Countries with below-average utilisation rates for both types of visits include Ireland, Netherlands, Denmark, UK, Portugal, Spain and Greece. Belgium and Italy have above-average GP visit rates only and Luxembourg

233

is the only country with above-average specialist visit rates only. Canadian rates of GP and especially specialist use are below the European average. These inter-country differences in mean utilisation levels are probably closely related to GP and specialist availability and remuneration per country.

More interesting for our purposes are the patterns by income. It is striking that in all countries, low income groups are more intensive users of GP care than higher income groups. The discrepancy differs by country but, on average, the bottom decile group reports about 50 per cent more GP visits or about 1.5 extra visit per year. However, after need standardization, the quintile gradients almost disappear in both ratio and difference measures and for almost all countries. In two countries – Austria and Portugal – they even change sign and turn into pro-rich differences. In all other countries, GP utilisation seems to be distributed very much as expected on the basis of reported morbidity.

The picture is quite different for visits to a medical specialist (Tables 6 and 7). The unstandardised use is distributed much more equally across quintiles, with only a slightly higher use for higher income groups in most countries. After standardization, however, all distributions (except the one for Luxembourg) are clearly and significantly in favour of the higher income groups, suggesting that the rich appear to receive a higher share of specialist visits than expected on the basis of their need characteristics. The gradients seem particularly steep in Portugal and Ireland. As in the case of GP visits, the Canadian distribution is quite close to that of the average European country, albeit at a somewhat lower level. Although these differences may appear to be small, their relative magnitude becomes more apparent when expressed in terms of the total populations: even if the richest quintile on average has only 0.5 more visits per adult per year than the poorest quintile, it would require in most countries a redistribution of many millions of visits in order to achieve an equal standardized distribution.

Tables 8 and 9 show the overall picture as the (unstandardized) quintile distributions for all physician visits (*i.e.* the sum of GP and specialist visits) to enable a comparison with the United States. It is worth noting from Table 8 that the average US physician visit rates are much lower than in Europe and somewhat lower than in Canada. In all countries, without any exception, there is a negative difference between the bottom and top quintile rates. However, Table 9 shows that, after standardisation for need differences, the utilisation gradient becomes positive in most countries but the bottom-to-top quintile ratio is substantially below one only in Portugal (0.72), the United States (0.77), in Austria (0.79) and Greece (0.85). This suggests that only in these countries, the standardized doctor use of the poorest quintile is 20-30 per cent lower than that of the richest quintile. In all other European countries and in Canada, this difference is less than 10 per cent suggesting that there is not much of a gradient in utilization left after the standardisation, or a fairly equal treatment for equal need across quintiles.

While quintile distributions are useful for providing insight into the differences in the distributions of physician visits across countries, the methods used to measure inequality differences based on the bottom-versus-top differences and ratios suffer from well-known disadvantages. First, while the use of OLS for the standardisation has the convenient property of preserving the mean in the predictions, its

Table 8. **Mean number of total physician visits by income quintile (unstandardised)**

	Austria	Belgium	Denmark	Germany	Greece	Ireland	Italy	Luxem-bourg	Nether-lands	Portugal	Spain	United Kingdom	EU-12	Canada	United States
Bottom 20%	8.67	8.68	4.39	8.48	4.84	5.28	5.90	6.51	4.78	5.49	5.63	6.22	6.66	5.25	4.56
20-40%	8.91	8.44	4.43	9.14	3.99	5.45	6.51	6.53	5.32	4.79	6.00	5.63	6.87	4.73	3.97
40-60%	7.86	6.54	4.37	8.60	4.05	3.93	5.87	5.37	4.82	4.83	5.81	4.78	6.27	4.23	3.67
60-80%	7.36	5.53	3.94	7.94	3.30	3.56	5.72	5.58	4.46	4.99	4.83	4.20	5.72	3.99	3.89
Top 20%	8.36	6.30	3.33	7.56	3.21	3.33	4.85	4.36	4.16	4.68	4.36	3.88	5.34	3.92	4.14
Mean	8.23	7.10	4.09	8.34	3.88	4.31	5.77	5.67	4.71	4.95	5.33	4.94	6.17	4.42	4.04
Q1/Q5	1.04	1.38	1.32	1.12	1.51	1.59	1.22	1.49	1.15	1.17	1.29	1.60	1.25	1.34	1.10
Q1-Q5	0.31	2.38	1.06	0.92	1.64	1.95	1.05	2.15	0.61	0.81	1.27	2.34	1.32	1.33	0.42
N	5 578	5 801	4 980	8 485	11 257	7 361	17 428	1 898	9 125	11 574	15 283	6 104	104 875	55 249	15 937

Note: EU-12 rates computed as weighted average of country-specific rates.

Table 9.   **Mean number total physician visits by income quintile**

OLS standardised for age, sex and morbidity

	Austria	Belgium	Denmark	Germany	Greece	Ireland	Italy	Luxem-bourg	Nether-lands	Portugal	Spain	United King-dom	EU-12	Canada	United States
Bottom 20%	7.48	7.20	3.83	7.64	3.48	4.56	5.62	5.84	4.28	4.13	5.34	5.08	5.90	4.43	3.59
20-40%	8.24	7.46	3.92	8.44	3.69	4.29	5.92	5.92	4.75	4.41	5.39	4.83	6.20	4.47	3.79
40-60%	8.15	6.82	4.42	8.69	4.22	4.05	5.70	5.68	4.79	4.99	5.35	4.87	6.25	4.35	3.90
60-80%	7.79	6.69	4.36	8.44	3.85	4.27	5.81	5.45	5.03	5.49	5.18	4.96	6.20	4.35	4.26
Top 20%	9.43	7.32	3.93	8.48	4.10	4.37	5.73	5.45	4.66	5.74	5.38	5.00	6.29	4.52	4.67
Q1/Q5	0.79	0.98	0.98	0.90	0.85	1.04	0.98	1.07	0.92	0.72	0.99	1.02	0.94	0.98	0.77
Q1-Q5	−1.95	−0.12	−0.10	−0.84	−0.62	0.18	−0.11	0.39	−0.38	−1.61	−0.04	0.08	−0.39	−0.10	−1.08
N	5 578	5 801	4 980	8 485	11 257	7 361	17 428	1 898	9 125	11 574	15 283	6 104	104 875	55 249	15 937

Note: Results for all non-US countries computed as sums of standardised visit rates for GP and specialist.

use is inappropriate for a non-continuous and non-normally distributed dependent variable with non-negative count data and a lot of zero observations. Second, while quintiles do provide some relevant information on the distribution of the utilization, both of the "range" measures of inequality (*i.e.* the ratio and the difference of the bottom and top quintile) are arbitrary and incomplete in the sense that they are not sensitive to the experience of the middle three quintiles. In the next section we examine whether the general patterns observed are confirmed when we use more appropriate standardisation techniques and inequity measures. We also explore some of the possible determinants of the findings.

4.2. Horizontal inequity indices

The estimated C_M and HI_{WV} indices and their t statistics are presented in Tables 10-12 for all countries[15] for GP visits, specialist visits and the total of the two. In the standardisation procedure, need is proxied by a vector of nine age-sex dummies,[16] four dummy variables for self-assessed health

Table 10.   **HI_{WV} indices for GP visits, 12 EU countries and Canada, 1996**

					HI_{WV} index adjusted for:					
			Need only[1]		Need + region[2]		Need + priv. insurance[3]		Need + both[4]	
	C_M	t[5]	HI_{WV}	t	HI_{WV}	t	HI_{WV}	t	HI_{WV}	t
Austria	−0.0496	−3.45	0.0178	1.34	0.0173	1.31	0.0102	0.78	0.0094	0.71
Belgium	−0.1023	−8.78	−0.0198	−2.25	−0.0194	−2.53	−0.0189	−2.18	−0.0187	−2.46
Denmark	−0.0787	−5.24	−0.0045	−0.32			−0.0053	−0.38		
Germany	−0.0631	−5.04	−0.0188	−1.66						
Greece	−0.1257	−8.06	−0.0109	−0.87	−0.0215	−1.66				
Ireland	−0.1282	−9.39	−0.0430	−2.97	−0.0409	−2.82	−0.0238	−1.64	−0.0226	−1.54
Italy	−0.0642	−3.57	−0.0277	−1.78	−0.0133	−0.89	−0.0271	−1.73	−0.0131	−0.87
Luxembourg	−0.0883	−5.51	−0.0324	−2.14						
Netherlands	−0.0472	−4.59	−0.0034	−0.35						
Portugal	−0.0696	−5.17	0.0146	1.19	0.0087	0.71	0.0188	1.53	0.0128	1.04
Spain	−0.0908	−8.35	−0.0437	−4.12	−0.0402	−3.79	−0.0398	−3.75	−0.0372	−3.51
United Kingdom	−0.1154	−9.7	−0.0145	−1.28	−0.0148	−1.31	−0.0147	−1.29	−0.0144	−1.28
Canada	−0.0795	−11.07	−0.0063	−1.00	−0.0141	−2.27	−0.0149	−2.37	−0.0201	−3.24

Note: Blanks in the table indicate that the relevant standardising variables were missing for the country in question.
1.   Need only = Indirectly standardised for 15 need dummies [age, sex, self-assessed health and (hampered by) chronic condition].
2.   Need + region = ind. stand. includes need plus regional dummies.
3.   Need + private insurance = ind. stand. includes need plus private insurance dummy.
4.   Need + both = ind. stand. includes need, region and private insurance dummies.
5.   t-statistics based on robust standard errors.

235

Table 11. **HI$_{WV}$ indices for specialist visits, 12 EU countries and Canada, 1996**

			HI$_{WV}$ index adjusted for:							
			Need only		Need + region		Need + priv insurance		Need + both	
	C_M	t	HI$_{WV}$	t	HI$_{WV}$	t	HI$_{WV}$	t	HI$_{WV}$	t
Austria	0.0360	1.83	0.0807	3.93	0.0771	3.76	0.0776	3.74	0.0732	3.53
Belgium	−0.0303	−2.46	0.0358	2.93	0.0378	2.56	0.0247	2.07	0.0289	2.05
Denmark	0.0197	0.72	0.0725	2.71			0.0621	2.33		
Germany	0.0150	1.01	0.0587	4.14						
Greece	−0.0360	−2.15	0.0767	5.13	0.0576	3.78				
Ireland	0.0696	3.02	0.1496	6.30	0.1469	6.21	0.0691	2.85	0.0663	2.74
Italy	0.0205	1.26	0.0621	3.95	0.0471	3.17	0.0547	3.52	0.0422	2.88
Luxembourg	−0.0658	−2.51	−0.0041	−0.16						
Netherlands	−0.0206	−1.34	0.0372	2.47						
Portugal	0.0959	3.85	0.1904	7.18	0.1630	6.44	0.1756	6.59	0.1528	5.97
Spain	0.0248	1.65	0.0763	4.86	0.0499	3.26	0.0645	4.13	0.0428	2.79
United Kingdom	−0.0245	−1.12	0.0830	4.12	0.0749	3.78	0.0623	3.10	0.0570	2.88
Canada	0.0009	0.08	0.0631	6.45	0.0608	6.23	0.0514	5.26	0.0500	5.12

Note: See Table 10.

Table 12. **HI$_{WV}$ indices for all physician visits, 12 EU countries, Canada and the United States, 1996**

			HI$_{WV}$ index adjusted for:							
			Need only		Need + region		Need + priv insurance		Need + both	
	C_M	t	HI$_{WV}$	t	HI$_{WV}$	t	HI$_{WV}$	t	HI$_{WV}$	t
Austria	−0.0223	−1.41	0.0403	2.91	0.0389	2.81	0.0340	2.45	0.0320	2.30
Belgium	−0.0866	−9.26	−0.0009	−0.12	−0.0001	−0.02	−0.0030	−0.43	−0.0016	−0.23
Denmark	−0.0564	−3.73	0.0163	1.23			0.0131	0.99		
Germany	−0.0343	−3.21	0.0118	1.32						
Greece	−0.0882	−6.28	0.0273	2.51	0.0127	1.13				
Ireland	−0.1095	−7.56	−0.0112	−0.82	−0.0098	−0.71	−0.0061	−0.44	−0.0053	−0.38
Italy	−0.0492	−2.86	−0.0083	−0.60	−0.0012	−0.09	−0.0095	−0.69	−0.0021	−0.16
Luxembourg	−0.0815	−5.19	−0.0159	−1.11						
Netherlands	−0.0384	−3.64	0.0127	1.38						
Portugal	−0.0274	−1.68	0.0635	4.72	0.0524	3.97	0.0626	4.65	0.0525	3.98
Spain	−0.0602	−5.58	−0.0084	−0.85	−0.0137	−1.39	−0.0091	−0.91	−0.0136	−1.38
United Kingdom	−0.0973	−8.17	0.0094	0.91	0.0074	0.72	0.0043	0.41	0.0034	0.33
Canada	−0.0595	−9.09	0.0107	1.87	0.0044	0.77	0.0013	0.23	−0.0029	−0.51
United States	−0.0209	−2.71	0.0550	5.49	0.0532	5.33	0.0291	2.89	0.0280	2.8

Note: See Table 10.

(SAH) and one or more dummies for the presence of a chronic condition or handicap and the extent to which it hampers the individual in his or her usual activities. These are the same variables as the ones used in the standardised quintile distributions but the regressions are now estimated using the two-part model consisting of a logit and a zero-truncated negative binomial model. The HI$_{WV}$ indices and their robust standard errors were estimated using equation A4 in the appendix. Country indices, ranked by magnitude, along with 95 per cent confidence intervals are also presented in Figures 2-4.

The significantly negative C_M indices in the first column of Table 10 confirm that in all countries, without any exception, lower income groups use GP services significantly more often than higher income groups. However, this unequal distribution largely coincides with the (unequal) distribution of need for such care: both the table and the graph in Figure 2 show that there are few countries with a HI$_{WV}$ index for GP visits that is large (in absolute value) and significantly different from zero. The index

Figure 2. **HI$_{WV}$ indices for GP visits (with 95% confidence intervals), EU countries and Canada**

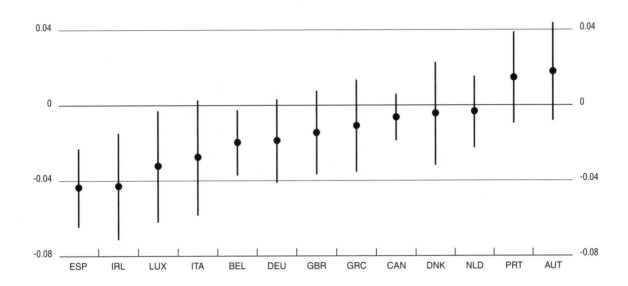

Figure 3. **HI$_{WV}$ indices for specialist visits (with 95% confidence intervals), EU countries and Canada**

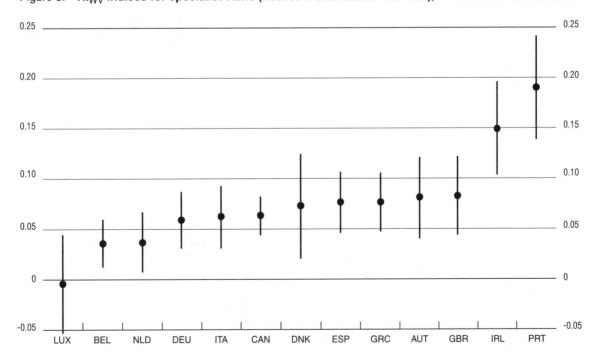

Figure 4. **HI$_{WV}$ indices for all physician visits (with 95% confidence intervals), 12 EU countries, Canada and United States**

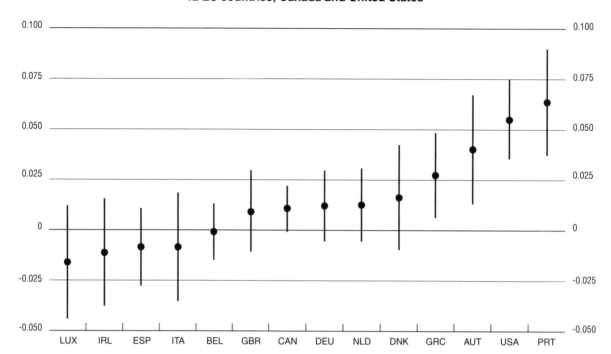

values are negative for Canada and for all European countries except Portugal and Austria, but they are significantly different from zero only in the cases of Spain, Ireland, Luxembourg and Belgium. The latter three countries are all known to have more favourable cost sharing arrangements for certain groups of low-income users of GP care (*cf.* Appendix Table A1). This is not true in Spain where GP visits are free at the point of delivery but there is a 40 per cent copayment rate for prescribed medicines, with cost sharing exemptions for pensioners only. On the other hand, also the Netherlands has free GP care for the sickness fund insured and Germany and Austria also have some copayment exemptions for low income groups but these countries do *not* show significantly negative indices. It appears to matter, therefore, to what extent these copayment exemptions are targeted towards the poorest in society and whether they can be reinsured.

Unfortunately, the ECHP survey does not provide any further detail on the copayment liability per household or individual. Only the variable indicating the presence of some type of private insurance coverage can be used as a proxy for it. We can observe that standardizing for private insurance generally tends to produce only a marginal reduction in the HI$_{WV}$ indices for GP visits. The impact is not negligible in Ireland and it makes the index more negative in the cases of Portugal and in Canada. In Canada it even makes it significant. This means that private insurance in these two countries contributes to a less pro-poor distribution of GP utilisation. But the effect is not very large.

The impact of standardising for regional utilisation differences is similarly small, although it now makes the Ireland and Luxembourg HI$_{WV}$ indices significantly negative. Inclusion of both variables simultaneously only makes the Irish inequity index non-significant and the Canadian inequity index significantly negative. However, all index values are relatively small and, all in all, these findings suggest that there seems to be little to worry about in terms of GP access in most European countries and Canada. There is some slight horizontal inequity in GP use favouring the lower income groups in about a third of these countries only, but the reasons for it seem to have little to do with inequalities in private coverage or regional differences. The only real exception is Ireland, where private insurance coverage does seem to be an important factor contributing to this finding.

Things are quite different with respect to the use of specialist services, as shown in Table 11. Concentration indices for specialist use (C_M) show much less evidence of a concentration of utilization among the less well-off. They are negative and significant only in Belgium, Luxembourg and Greece, while they are not significantly different from zero in any of the other countries except Ireland and Portugal, where they are significantly positive. In all countries except Luxembourg we now find significantly positive HI_{WV} indices, indicating a significant degree of horizontal inequity favouring the rich. Figure 3 shows that this is a general phenomenon but that there are also some important differences between countries. Especially in Portugal and Ireland, the degree of "excess" use of specialist visits by higher income groups (as compared to their needs) is much larger than in the other European countries, which generally show index values between 0.04 and 0.08.

The other columns in Table 11 also shed some light on the sensitivity of these positive index values to insurance and region. Inclusion of private insurance in the standardisation reduces the HI_{WV} index values in all countries where it is available, but most of all in Ireland. The Irish index is more than halved when private insurance is standardised for, indicating that the lack of such cover does seem to act as some access barrier to specialist care for lower income groups, in spite of their entitlement to free specialist care (cf. Harmon and Nolan, 2001). After controlling for private cover, the remaining degree of horizontal inequity is of the same magnitude as that in other countries. In Portugal, on the other hand, the influence of private insurance coverage seems much smaller than the influence of regional utilization differences. This is mainly because private insurance is much less widespread in Portugal. Moreover, even after standardising for region and insurance effects, the Portuguese HI_{WV} index remains very large.

Adjusting for region reduces the degree of inequity in the other southern European countries (Spain, Greece and Italy) and – to a lesser extent – in the UK and Canada. This highlights the fact that in these countries the income-related inequities in specialist use are – at least in part – associated with regional differences in access to such care. Not surprisingly, adjusting for private insurance coverage also reduces the degree of inequity in the UK (where quicker or more convenient access to specialist care is precisely what such cover buys) and to a lesser extent also in Spain, Belgium, Denmark, Austria, Canada and Italy. It is important to note that in none of the countries studied, adjusting for insurance and region makes the inequity index non-significant. This suggests that although region and insurance cover do play some role, they cannot account entirely for the observed inequity in specialist use.

Finally we turn to the results for *all* physician visits in Table 12 and Figure 4, defined as the sum of GP and specialist visits. The main reasons are *i)* to take into account that substitution of GP visits by specialist visits may occur to a different degree among the rich and the poor and *ii)* to enable a comparison with the US 1996 MEPS data which do not allow to distinguish between GP and specialist visits. It is worth noting that this distinction is not always clear in some European countries either. Apparently, also in Luxembourg both GPs and specialists provide primary care services and it is well known that certain specialists, like pediatricians and gynaecologists to a large extent provide primary care services in some countries with direct access to specialist care like Belgium, Italy and Spain. As a result, the separate analysis is not always entirely feasible. On the other hand, of course, the aggregation of GP and specialist visits compounds the problem of quality differences. It is most improbable that GP and specialist visits represent on average the same level of quality. As a result, any equity patterns detected in volume are very likely to underestimate any true treatment inequities taking account of quality differences. Table 12 shows that the use of the aggregate of all doctor visits is unequally distributed in favour of the lower income groups (all C_M indices negative) in all countries, but most of all in Ireland, and least of all in the United States. Further disaggregation of the US visits rate shows that this is mainly due to the major component, *i.e.* office visits, being only slightly pro-poor ($C_M = -0.0044$, $t = -0.55$). The other two types of physician visits, *i.e.* outpatient visits ($C_M = -0.1463$, $t = -3.68$) and especially emergency room visits ($C_M = -0.1865$, $t = -11.12$), show very negative and significant inequality indices. This highlights the fact that the average mix of visits is not the same at every income level.

In all countries, the distribution of all physician visits is also fairly closely related to need since most HI_{WV} indices are not significantly different from zero. There are only four exceptions: Greece,

239

Austria, and especially the United States and Portugal *do* show a significant degree of horizontal inequity favouring the rich. In these countries, lower income groups report significantly lower physician use than can be expected on the basis of average usage patterns. In Greece, this seems to have a lot to do with regional disparities in utilization since the index becomes non-significant after adjusting for region. The fact that the US inequity index is reduced by almost 50 per cent when account is taken of private health insurance cover stems from the fact that, unlike in Europe or Canada, such cover is the *primary* source of coverage for the great majority of the population under 65, but it does indicate that a large part of the inequity seems to be due to gaps and inequalities in such cover. In Portugal, on the other hand, neither adjustment for region, nor for insurance affect the degree of inequity a great deal.

5. Conclusion

In this paper we have compared distributions of doctor visit rates in 12 EU member countries to similar distributions for Canada and the United States in 1996. The identical design and questionnaire used in the European Community Household Panel survey provides a very high degree of comparability across the European countries, but also for Canada and the United States a fairly high degree of comparability could be achieved. We have used both simple quintile distributions and concentration indices estimated by means of two-part models to assess the extent to which adults in equal need for physician care appear to have equal rates of doctor visits. We emphasized that the usefulness of the measurement method crucially hinges on the acceptance of the horizontal equity principle as a policy goal. To the extent that equal treatment for equal need is not an explicit policy objective, the measures cannot, of course, be used for equity performance assessment.

The cross-country comparative results suggest the following conclusions. First, while average annual rates of doctor visits vary substantially between countries, the patterns of their relative distribution across income groups show some remarkable similarities. Secondly, there appears to be relatively little reason for concern about the access to – and distribution of – GP services. The higher use of GP care among lower income individuals that is observed in virtually every country appears to be largely in accordance with the higher needs for such care by these groups, suggesting little or no horizontal inequity. In a few countries only – Spain, Ireland, Belgium and Luxembourg – preferential treatment of lower income groups through copayment reductions or exemptions may explain the (slightly) pro-poor distributions. Third, the fairly equal need-standardised distributions of GP care are hardly affected by regional disparities in GP utilisation or by the presence of private insurance coverage. This is not so surprising given that a good deal of this private cover relates to the use of medicines or buys preferential access to secondary care. Fourth, the distributional patterns are completely different for the use of medical specialist care. In all countries except Luxembourg, significantly positive indices emerge, indicating inequity favouring the higher income users. In two countries, Portugal and Ireland, the degree of such a pro-rich distribution of use is much larger than in all other countries. Fifth, for the use of specialist services, the findings can to some extent be explained by the presence of (additional) private cover and by regional disparities in the availability of such care. Especially in Ireland, but to a lesser degree also in Spain, Belgium, Denmark, Austria, Canada, Portugal and Italy, private insurance seems to be one of the factors contributing to this finding. Similarly, systematic regional differences in utilization play some role in the generation of horizontal inequities in use by income, especially in the Southern European countries. However, neither the adjustment for insurance coverage, nor for the region of residence removes the inequities entirely: even after such correction, a significant degree of horizontal inequity in specialist usage remains in all countries. Sixth, aggregating all physician visits allows for an overall picture which assumes away quality differences between GP and specialist care but enables a comparison with the US results. In most countries, both poor and rich people do get to see a doctor when they appear to need one, but there are important differences in the type of doctor seen. In three European countries – Portugal, Austria and Greece – and in the United States, we find evidence of significant pro-rich inequity in total physician visits. In Greece, this is to a large extent related to regional disparities in doctor visits, while in the United States it is higly related to the presence of private insurance coverage.

The conclusion which emerges, therefore, is that most European countries and Canada appear to have ensured a fair degree of equal access to the GP for people with equal needs but unequal incomes. However, the same horizontal equity goal does not appear to have been attained with respect to the use of specialist services despite the fairly universal coverage of such services for decades now in most European countries and in Canada. Either higher income groups are over-utilising the services of specialists, or some access barriers for those on lower incomes remain. Differences in either insurance coverage or regional disparities appear to be only a small part of the explanation, although we need to point out that both of these variables were measured very crudely in this study. This finding corroborates earlier results for European health care systems and the United States (*e.g.* Van Doorslaer *et al.*, 2000) and for Canada (*e.g.* McIsaac *et al.*, 1997). The fact that it shows up in very different types of health care systems (albeit to differing degrees) suggests that it may have more to do with systematic differences in utilisation behaviour between higher versus lower income (or education) individuals than with the characteristics of health care delivery systems. A crucial question is, of course, whether the remaining systematic differentials in use are largely irrelevant from an equity point of view because they merely reflect differences in "tastes" for specialist services and do not translate into differences in health gains, or whether these use patterns *do* reflect important diagnostic and therapeutic quality differences which translate into the less well-off receiving lower standards of care than the better-off. Only in the latter case, they signal a violation of the equal-treatment-for-equal-need principle.

Disease-specific evidence for certain countries suggests that the differential patterns of utilization are by no means trivial. For example, one Canadian study has looked at differences in access to invasive cardiac procedurs after acute myacardial infarction by neighbourhood income in the province of Ontario (Adler *et al.*, 1999). Whereas the rates of coronary angiography and revascularization were found to be significantly and inversely related to income, waiting times and one year mortality rates were significantly positively related to income. Each \$10 000 increase in the neighborhood median income was associated with a 10 percent reduction in the risk of death within one year. This suggests that differences in diagnostic and therapeutic utilization are not trivial and do appear to translate into differential outcomes by income as well. If such effects on access are so pronounced in a country with universal acces free of charge at the point of use, it is most unlikely that the differences in use of specialized services we find are less worrisome in countries without such universal free access.

Overall, in all countries except the United States, Portugal, Greece and Austria, *total* doctor visits appear to be distributed according to need, although the *type* of doctor seen varies with income. In Europe and Canada, lower income individuals are more likely to consult a GP while higher income individuals are more likely to see a specialist. In the United States, lower income people are more likely to consult a doctor through an emergency room or an outpatient department, while higher income individuals are more likely to consult a doctor in his office. To the extent that the quality of services rendered by these two types of doctors differs, and that the differentials are not merely due to taste differences but to access constraints in terms of either costs or information, this cannot be regarded as "equal treatment" and some concern over horizontal equity remains. This is even more true for the three countries where the use of GP or primary care doctor services does *not* compensate for the pro-rich distribution of specialist visits. In Austria and Portugal this horizontal inequity in overall doctor utilization could not be attributed to differential private coverage or regional disparities. It is worth noting, however, that the utilisation gradient in Austria appears to be of less concern given the very high average utilisation rates. With a (standardised) rate of 7.5 visits to the doctor per year, the bottom quintile can hardly be said to lack access. Perhaps the rate of 9.5 visits per year of the top quintile is more reason for concern!

Comparing our results to findings of others is difficult because of the many differences in approaches. Compared to the results presented in Van Doorslaer *et al.* (2000), there is only one different finding here: no significant inequity in all physician visits in 1996 for the Netherlands whereas we did find such a result for 1992. For Austria, Greece and Portugal we do not have any results of earlier analyses to compare with, but the present study confirms the earlier finding for 1987 for the United States (Van Doorslaer *et al.*, 2000) that access to a doctor is not equal for those in apparently equal need. The pro-rich distribution of office visits is only very partially compensated for by the pro-poor distribution in outpatient and emergency room visits. Indeed the results suggest that, if anything has changed, the distribution has become more pro-rich, since the horizontal inequity index for the United States has gone up from 0.044 in 1987 to 0.055 in 1996.

Our results also compare well to those from a recent Commonwealth Fund study. Schoen *et al.* (2000) have assessed disparities in access to health care by income in five countries using a common telephone survey. Whereas they found those with below average incomes to be in significantly worse self-reported health than average in all countries, these groups were only reporting significantly higher probabilities of a doctor visit in two of the countries studied, the UK and Canada. There were no differential probabilities in two other countries (Australia and New Zealand) and the lower income groups even had a significantly *lower* probability of having seen a doctor in the United States. Although the authors did not statistically standardize for need/morbidity differences across income groups as in our study, the results for the three overlapping countries do seem to point into the same direction: little or no inequity by income in doctor access in Canada and the UK, but substantial inequity in the United States.

All in all, we hope that this paper has helped to demonstrate that even normative concepts like equity in health care access and use can be subjected to positive analysis and measurement using existing data sources if agreement can be reached on what the equity objectives are. The methods used could be adapted to analyze other types of health care use and to address other types of equity concerns (*e.g.* geographical, gender, ethnic or age disparities). The results show that even in the richest group of countries in the world, with fairly universal and comprehensive coverage of their populations some reason for concern about the unequal treatment for equal need remains.

NOTES

1. For various reasons, Finland, France and Sweden could not be included. *Cf.* footnote 8.

2. There is some debate as to whether it is not treatment but access, or rather access costs, which ought to be equalized (Mooney *et al.*, 1991, 1992; Culyer *et al.*, 1992*a*, 1992*b*; Goddard and Smith, 2001). For the present exercise, the difference seems fairly innocuous and mainly related to the interpretation of any remaining differences in utilization after standardising for need differences. To the extent that these are genuinely due to differences in preferences, and *not* due to differences in *e.g.* benefit perceptions resulting from differences in information costs, these would not be regarded as inequitable.

3. Note that this interpretation implies that *"on average, the system gets it right"*. The average relationship between need indicators and utilization, as expressed by the regression coefficients, is the implied norm for assessing equity in this health care system. But this approach to measuring need is not intrinsic to the method of measuring equity. If need estimates could be obtained alternatively (*e.g.* from professional judgement), the equity measures could still be computed in the same way.

4. *Cf.* also footnotes 7 and 8 in Wagstaff and van Doorslaer (2000*a*).

5. One method proceeds by decomposing the total degree of inequality into its various sources and analysing cross-country differennces using a decomposition method proposed by Wagstaff *et al.* (2002). This approach is not pursued here because it requires identical variable definitions across countries.

6. During the first half of 1996, 83 per cent of all Americans were covered by private or public health insurance, leaving 17 per cent of the population, some 44.8 million persons, uninsured (Vistnes and Monheit, 1996).

7. More detailed information on the design and contents of this survey can be found at *www-rcade.dur.ac.uk/echp/*

8. Sweden does not take part in the ECHP. The French questionnaire only includes one question asking for all GP, medical specialist, dentist and optician visits which is not comparable to the other questions. Revised Finnish income data were not released yet at the time of the research.

9. More detailed information on the design and contents of this survey can be found at: *www.stats.gov.nt.ca.*

10. More detailed information on the design and contents of this survey can be found at *www.meps.ahcpr.gov.*

11. The modified OECD scale gives a weight of 1.0 to the first adult, 0.5 to the second and each subsequent person aged 14 and over, and 0.3 to each child aged under 4 in the household.

12. For the ECHP countries, in addition direct standardization for demographic differences was used by imposing the European age-sex distribution on all countries. This ensures that the differences between European countries are not merely a result of demographic differences.

13. Two countries (Luxembourg, Denmark) did not apply cluster sampling while some others (Germany, The Netherlands, Austria and Canada) did not provide the primary sampling unit information for privacy reasons.

14. In other words, the bottom European quintile does *not* contain the 20 per cent Europeans with the lowest incomes but the population-weighted average of the bottom quintile of each of the 12 EU countries.

15. Except for the United States, for which we only have total physician visits.

16. The age intervals used were: 16-29, 30-44, 45-59, 60-69 and 70+.

REFERENCES

ADLER, D.A., NAYLOR, C.D., AUSTIN, P. and TU, J.V. (1999),
"Effects of socioeconomic status on access to invasive cardiac procedures and on mortality after acute myocardial infarction", *New England Journal of Medicine*, No. 341, pp. 1359-1367.

CAMERON, A.C. and TRIVEDI, P.K. (1998),
Regression Analysis of Count Data, Cambridge University Press, Cambridge.

CULYER, A.J., VAN DOORSLAER, E. and WAGSTAFF, A. (1992a),
"Access, Utilisation and Equity: A Further Comment", *Journal of Health Economics*, Vol. 11, No. 2, pp. 207-210.

CULYER, A.J., VAN DOORSLAER, E. and WAGSTAFF, A. (1992b),
"Utilization as a measure of equity by Mooney, Hall, Donaldson and Gerard: Comment", *Journal of Health Economics*, Vol. 11, No. 1, pp. 93-98.

EUROSTAT (1999),
European Community Household Panel (ECHP): selected indicators from the 1995 wave, European Commission, Eurostat, Luxembourg.

GERDTHAM, U.-G. (1997), "Equity in health care utilization: further tests based on hurdle models and Swedish microdata", *Health Economics*, No. 6, pp. 303-319.

GODDARD, M. and SMITH, P. (2001),
"Equity of access to health care services: theory and evidence from the UK", *Social Science and Medicine*, No. 53, pp. 1149-1162.

GREENE, W.H. (1997),
Econometric Analysis, 2nd Edition, Prentice-Hall, London.

HARMON, C. and NOLAN, B. (2001),
"Health insurance and health services utilization in Ireland", *Health Economics*, No. 10, pp. 135-145.

HURST, J. and JEE-HUGHES, M. (2001),
"Performance Measurement and Performance Management in OECD Health Systems", Labour Market and Social Policy Occasional Papers, No 47, OECD, Paris.

JONES, A.M. (2000),
"Health Econometrics", in Culyer, A.J. and Newhouse, J.P., *Handbook of Health Economics*, Elsevier, pp. 265-344.

KAKWANI, N, WAGSTAFF, A. and VAN DOORSLAER, E. (1997),
"Socioeconomic inequality in health: measurement, computation and statistical inference", *Journal of Econometrics*, Vol. 77, No. 1, pp. 87-104.

LERMAN, R.I. and YITZHAKI, S. (1984),
"A Note on the Calculation and Interpretation of the Gini Index", *Economics Letters*, No. 15, pp. 363-368.

McISAAC, W., GOEL, V. and NAYLOR, D. (1997),
"Socio-economic status and visits to physicians by adults in Ontario, Canada", *Journal of Health Services Research and Policy*, Vol. 2, No. 2, pp. 94-102.

MOONEY, G., HALL, J., DONALDSON, C., *et al.* (1991),
"Utilisation as a Measure of Equity: Weighing Heat?", *Journal of Health Economics*, Vol. 10, No. 4, pp. 475-480.

MOONEY, G., HALL, J., DONALDSON, C., *et al.* (1992),
"Reweighing Heat: Response", *Journal of Health Economics*, Vol. 11, No. 2, pp. 199-205.

MOSSIALOS, E. and LE GRAND, J. (1999),
Health care and cost containment in the European Union, Ashgate, Aldershot, pp. 267-302.

MULLAHY, J. (1986),
"Specification and testing of some modified count data models", *Journal of Econometrics*, No. 33, pp. 341-365.

POHLMEIER, W. and ULRICH, V. (1995),
"An econometric model of the two-part decisionmaking process in the demand for health care", *Journal of Human Resources*, Vol. 30, No. 2, pp. 339-361.

SALTMAN, R.B. and FIGUERAS, J. (1997),
European Health Care Reform; Analysis of current strategies, WHO Regional Publications, European Series No. 72, WHO Regional Office for Europe, Copenhagen.

SCHNEIDER, M. (1992),
Complementary Health Schemes in the European Union, Basys, Augsburg, pp. 149-164.

SCHNEIDER, M., BECKMANN, M., BIENE-DIETRICH, P., GABANYI, M., HOFMANN, U., KÖSE, A., MILL, D. and SPÄTH, B. (1997),
Gesundheidssysteme im internationalen Vergleich, Basys, Augsburg.

SCHNEIDER, M., BIENE-DIETRICH, P., GABANYI, M., HOFMANN, U., HUBER, M., KÖSE A. and SOMMER, J. (1994),
Gesundheidssysteme im internationalen Vergleich, Basys, Augsburg.

SCHOEN, C., DAVIS, K.,DESROCHES, C., DONELAN, K. and BLENDON, R. (2000),
"Health insurance markets and income inequality: findings from an international health policy survey", *Health Policy*, No. 51, pp. 67-85.

STEPAN, A. (1997),
Finanzierungssyteme im Gesundheidswesen; Ein internationaler Vergleich, Manzsche Verlags- und Universitätsbuchhandlung, Wien.

VAN DOORSLAER, E., WAGSTAFF, A. and RUTTEN, F. (eds) (1993),
Equity in the Finance and Delivery of Health Care: an international perspective, Oxford University Press, Oxford.

VAN DOORSLAER, E., WAGSTAFF, A. *et al.* (1992),
"Equity in the delivery of health care: some cross-country comparisons", *Journal of Health Economics*, Vol. 11, No. 4, pp. 389-411.

VAN DOORSLAER, E., WAGSTAFF, A. , VAN DER BURG, H., CHRISTIANSEN, T., DE GRAEVE, D., DUCHESNE, I., GERDTHAM, U-G, GERFIN, M., GEURTS, J., GROSS, L., HÄKKINEN, U., JOHN, J., KLAVUS, J., LEU, R.E., NOLAN, B., O'DONNELL, O., PROPPER, C., PUFFER, F., SCHELLHORN, M., SUNDBERG, G., WINKELHAKE, O. (2000),
"Equity in the delivery of health care in Europe and the US", *Journal of Health Economics*, Vol. 19, No. 5, pp. 553-583.

VISTNES, J.P. and MONHEIT, A.C. (1996),
Health Insurance Status of the Civilian Noninstitutionalized Population, Agency for Health Care Policy and Research, Rockville (MD); (1997), MEPS Research Findings No. 1. AHCPR Pub. No. 97-0030.

WAGSTAFF, A. and VAN DOORSLAER, E. (2000*a*),
"Measuring and testing for inequity in the delivery of health care", *Journal of Human Resources*, Vol. 35, No. 4, pp. 716-733.

WAGSTAFF, A. and VAN DOORSLAER, E. (2000*b*),
"Equity in health care financing and delivery", in A.J. Culyer and J.P. Newhouse (eds.), *Handbook of Health Economics*, North Holland, pp. 1803-1862.

WAGSTAFF, A., VAN DOORSLAER, E. and PACI, P. (1991),
"On the Measurement of Horizontal Inequity in the Delivery of Health Care", *Journal of Health Economics*, Vol. 10, No. 2, pp. 169-205.

WAGSTAFF, A., VAN DOORSLAER E. and WATANABE, N. (2002),
"On decomposing the causes of health sector inequalities with an application to malnutrition inequalities in Vietnam", *Journal of Econometrists* (forthcoming).

WHO (1997-99),
Country Highlights, WHO Regional Office for Europe, Copenhagen.

Appendix

COMPUTATION AND TESTING OF INEQUITY INDICES

There are several ways in which these indices can be computed. If m is the sample mean of m_i, C_M can be computed as:

(A1) $$C_M = \frac{2}{N \cdot m} \sum_{i=1}^{N} m_i R_i - 1,$$

where N is the sample size and R_i is the relative rank of the ith person. C_N can be calculated analogously by replacing m_i and m with m_i^* and m^*. Alternatively, C_M and C_N can be computed by means of "convenient" regressions (*cf.* Kakwani *et al.*, 1997). Thus, for example, C_M can be computed using:

(A2) $$2\sigma_R^2 [m_i / m] = \gamma_1 + \delta_1 R_i + u_i$$

where σ_R^2 denotes the variance of the relative rank. The OLS estimator of δ_1 is equal to

(A3) $$\hat{\delta}_1 = \frac{2}{N \cdot m} \sum_{i=1}^{N} (m_i - m)(R_i - \tfrac{1}{2}),$$

which, from equation A1, makes $\hat{\delta}_1$ equal to C_M. For weighted samples, similar results are obtained by using the weighted fractional rank and by applying weighted rather than ordinary least squares (Lerman and Yitzhaki, 1984).

Given that inequity indices are computed from samples, it is important that standard errors be computed to be able to test the statistical significance of indices and of changes over time and differences between countries. Application of OLS to equation A2 automatically provides a standard error for C_M and, when using indirectly standardized values, for C_N. Obtaining a standard error for HI_{WV} is not so straightforward, though, since C_M and C_N are not independently distributed. A standard error for HI_{WV} could be obtained using the following convenient regression:

(A4) $$2\sigma_R^2 \left[\frac{m_i}{m} - \frac{m_i^*}{m^*} \right] = \gamma_2 + \delta_2 R_i + u_i,$$

where m^* is the mean of m_i^*. The OLS estimate of δ_2 will be equal to HI_{WV} and from the regression one obtains a standard error of HI_{WV}. Building on results obtained by Kakwani *et al.* (1997), Wagstaff and Van Doorslaer (2000*a*) also present a slightly more accurate estimator for the standard error of HI_{WV} that takes into account the serial correlation in u_i but it does not correct for heteroskedasticity or clustered sampling. Instead we will estimate robust standard errors for equation A4 using White's and Huber's estimators as implemented in Stata version 7.

Table A1. **Equity-relevant delivery system characteristics and provider incentives**

	GP consultations	GP gatekeeper	Specialist consultations
Austria	Ambulatory care free at the point of delivery, except for farmers and self-employed who pay 20%; mix of capitation and FFS payment; co-payments for drugs, but poor exempt.	Yes.	Ambulatory care is free at the point of delivery, except for farmers and self-employed who pay 20%.
Belgium	Substantial co-payments, reduced rates for widowed, handicapped, pensioners and orphans below income treshold); FFS; co-payments for drugs as well; self-employed not compulsory covered.	No.	Specialists are allowed to overbill ; FFS; self-employed not compulsory covered; direct access.
Canada	GPs paid fee-for-service. No co-payments.	Yes.	Fee-for-service remuneration. Direct access discouraged by lower reimbursement.
Denmark	People can freely choose between group I and group II. GP care free at point of delivery for group I (98% of population) but this group has to accept the same GP for at least 6 months, and she will work as a gatekeeper. Group II has to pay a co-payment for GP care, but can choose their GP freely.	Yes for group I; No for group II.	People in group II have to pay a co-payment for specialist care, but do not need a referral to use it.
Greece	Private sector: primary care physicians (including many doctors working in the public sector) charge on an ATP basis. Hidden payments to doctors (both private and public).	No (in practice).	Public sector: combination of salaried doctors and doctors paid on a FFS basis. Private sector: primary care physicians (including many doctors working in the public sector) charge on an ATP basis. Hidden payments to doctors common (both private and public).
Germany	Free at point of delivery; FFS.	No.	Substantially higher fees for privately insured; some co-payments; FFS.
Ireland	The 35% Irish with the lowest income fall into group I and get free GP care at point of delivery. For this group GP are paid by capitation. Group II has to pay for GP services in full.	Yes for group I, but it can be bypassed by emergency unit of the hospital; No for group II.	All free at point of delivery for group I, and group II only has to pay for routine opthalmological and aural services; specialists receive higher fee for private care patients.
Italy	GPs with special child care training are known as GP paediatricians; free at point of delivery; paid on capitation basis;	Yes, but weakly enforced in practice.	Free at point of delivery; co-payment for diagnostic examinations; ambulatory and day hospital care paid based on diagnosis-related groups.
Luxembourg	Non reimbursable patient's contribution; GP care may also be provided by specialists; FFS.	No.	FFS; unclear distinction between primary and secondary care, many specialists deliver GP services.
Netherlands	Free for public patients, private patients obtain reimbursement of fee if covered; GPs paid capitation for public and FFS for private patients.	Yes.	Most specialists receive a salary from their partnerships, which themselves are paid FFS; other specialists get FFS; academic specialists receive a salary and get FFS for private patients only.
Portugal	Diagnostic test at primary level require co-payments; GPs are salaried.	Yes, but patients often use hospital emergency departments to get referred.	Full time salaried physicians are allowed to have a private practice; co-payments should vary according to a patients (or her family's) income.
Spain	Free at point of delivery; GPs are mainly salaried; private sector patients are paid FFS.	Yes, but emergency departments often used to bypass waiting lists.	Free at point of delivery; Paediatricians deliver primary care to population under 14.
United Kingdom	Free at point of delivery; capitation + fundholding.	Yes.	Free at point of delivery except for opthalmic care, exemptions for the poor.
United States	Cost varies widely depending on nature of insurance plan. Co-payments very common. Uninsured pay full cost of consultation, although charitable care is occasionally provided.	Yes only for 40% of the population with public or private managed care plans.	Depends on the insurance plan. Charges for specialist visits are typically the same as for GPs.

Source: Mossialos and Le Grand (1999); Saltman and Figueras (1997); Schneider *et al.* (1994, 1997); Stepan (1997); WHO (1997-99).

Table A2. **Regional differences and private insurance characteristics**

	Regional differences	Private insurance
Austria	Some variation between regions for nursing homes and hospitals.	1% is uninsured; 38% has supplementary private health insurance which mostly covers sick leave benefits, a more comfortable accommodation in a hospital and free choice of physician.
Belgium	Regional differences in utilisation between Flanders, Wallonia and Brussels.	Many employers offer supplemental insurance to cover public insurance copayments and extra-billing.
Canada	13 different plans, for ten provinces and three territories, but conform to federal Canada Health Act.	Many employers offer supplemental health insurance as benefit to cover services not covered by provincial plans such as prescribed medicines, dental care, etc.
Denmark	Regional organisation of HC; but GPs are evenly distributed across the country.	30% of population; but coverage limited and not very relevant as GP and specialist care are free for 98% of the population.
Greece	Substantial urban-rural variation; primary care by salaried physicians in health centres for rural areas, by FFS physicians in hospital outpatient departments in urban areas.	40% of health expenditure is private.
Germany	Regional negotiations on fees.	< 0.5% uninsured, civil servants different insurance, small percentage private insurance.
Ireland	Planning of health services done by regional health boards.	35% of the population has voluntary health insurance; VHI pays co-payments and for private care; private care available in public hospitals.
Italy	Regional resource allocation to health services; important regional variation in supply of GP care and size of GPs' lists.	20% of total health expenditure is private; private insurance is mostly double coverage; 1.6% has complete double coverage.
Luxembourg	Very small country size.	80% has additional coverage; level of reimbursement is considered high (WHO); there is often an non-reimbursable patient's contribution.
Netherlands	Health care regionally allocated according to need.	> 1% is uninsured; about 1/3 of the population privately insured (no double coverage).
Portugal	1 800 extensions of health centres and health posts seem to ensure a fair distribution of GP-care; large hospitals are unequally distributed; the level of autonomy in the five regions is high.	Private practitioners to be paid by the patients themselves; 10% of the population has some private insurance.
Spain	Regional variations exist as some regions organise most of the health care, whereas others don't. Catalonia and the Basque Country took steps to increase competition among providers.	Private insurance means double cover; most people opt for private insurance in order to bupass waiting list; the private sector has been encouraged as a form of competition.
United Kingdom	Resources are distributed according to formula to ensure equity; geographical variation in private care considerable.	Around 10% of population has (duplicate) private coverage; growth also result of employment benefits packages.
United States	Large variations by state in all types of private health insurance. Some state variation in Medicaid. Less variation in Medicare.	Private insurance provided through an employer plan is the most common form of coverage for those under 65. For those 65 and over, private supplimental insurance for Medicare is extremely common.

Note: see Table A1.

Part IV

BEST PRACTICES IN MEASURING DIFFERENT DIMENSIONS OF HEALTH SYSTEM PERFORMANCE

Chapter 12

MEASURING THE QUALITY OF HOSPITAL CARE: THE STATE OF THE ART

WHAT INFORMATION SHOULD BE MADE AVAILABLE TO THE PUBLIC?

by

Gérard de Pouvourville and Étienne Minvielle[*]

Abstract

The quality of hospital care has become a focal point in the regulation of health systems. This can be put down to several factors: the funding crisis, greater public demands on health care professionals owing in part to the wider availability of health-related information and, finally, the development of new data processing technologies. This combination of factors has caused the medical profession's monopoly to be called into question and has prompted calls for the development of external schemes to monitor, and even control, service provision.

The effect of these demands has been the emergence of a new field of health research focussing on the measurement of health care quality, and in particular outcomes, and initiatives by payers or government agencies aimed at making outcome measurement an integral feature of hospital resource allocation. At the same time, those same players and the popular press have been providing the public with "league tables" comparing hospitals on the basis of selected indicators. The nature and quality of these initiatives vary substantially across OECD countries. The United States, with its competition-led health care system, has been at the forefront in both methodological research and the introduction of external control schemes. In the European and other OECD Member countries, the publication of similar research has taken longer, partly for political reasons but also because of delays in computerisation.

The aim of this paper is to gain insights from experiments conducted in a selection of countries. It addresses two points in greater depth. First, it reviews the state of the art regarding methods of measuring health care quality and outcomes, the main emphasis being on the measurement of hospital care quality in terms of either clinical outcomes or health status. Second, it analyses the use made of these methods by external institutions – payers, government agencies and the popular press – looking at why and how they are used, the problems encountered and, finally, how they are currently assessed and what recommendations can be derived from them.

Introduction

The cost-containing constraints that have been placed on health-care systems in developed countries have led public and private financial sources alike to pay greater attention to unit costs in the delivery of health services. At the same time, however, concern over the quality of care has been growing, with an insistence that efforts to reduce or moderate cost trends should not result in a lower quality of care. On this point, the various stakeholders have adopted different approaches, which may be classified

* Centre for Health Economics and Administration Research, INSERM/CNRS, 80 rue du Général Leclerc, 94276 Le Kremlin Bicêtre Cedex France, *gdepouvo@kb.inserm.fr*

251

into four categories: the professional approach, that of rationalizing practices; the managerial approach, drawing upon experience with managing continuous quality improvement in industry; a competition-based approach, seeking to force health-care providers to publish indicators of the quality of their services; and finally a public policy approach, with the authorities playing a key role in the publication of those indicators either in the name of "accountability" or as an effort to overcome the asymmetry of information between potential users and providers of health services. The latter two approaches lead to the same result – the publication of quality indicators as a basis for evaluating and comparing service performance – but the *modus operandi* is distinct in each case: in one case, it is those who pay for care (most often the insurers) who are taking advantage of competition to demand information from care providers, while in the second case intervention is accomplished through regulation.

These approaches have been implemented at varying paces and in different ways from one country to the next. The United States has had a head start over other OECD countries. For example, the federal Health Care Finance Agency (HCFA), the funding manager for Medicare, has been publishing adjusted mortality rates for Diagnosis-Related Groups since 1986. The Joint Commission on the Accreditation of Health Care Organizations (JCAHO) publishes a guide to the different ways of measuring hospital performance (JCAHO, 2001). In 1991, a number of private businesses and non-profit organisations launched the National Committee for Quality Assurance (NCQA) to provide information on the various health insurance plans available to Americans. This progress can be explained by four characteristics of the United States: the federal and state governments are required to report regularly to their legislatures on their actions; there is a strong belief in competition as the principal regulator of economic activities; consequently , there are many players in the health insurance system; and finally, the health-care system is under constant pressure from the courts in the form of malpractice suits. The United Kingdom has had in place since 1989 a policy of fostering inter-hospital competition, including the publication of regular comparative data on hospital performance. England has limited itself to publishing indicators that reflect the quality of service provided (for example waiting lists) (NHS, 1995) rather than clinical outcomes, and it is only in the last year that the National Health Service has published hospital mortality data. In 2001, however, a private initiative known as "Dr. Foster"[1] has begun posting comparative data on public and private hospitals on an Internet site: these data have sparked lively debate, given the method used to adjust mortality rates. Outcome and process indicators are regularly published in Scotland (Shaw, 1987). Canada publishes an annual survey that compares the quality of services available by geographic zone (Marshall, 2001). It is prepared by the Canadian Institute for Health Information (CIHI, 2001). This annual survey is complementary to an initiative of the Province of Ontario, which has published "Hospital Report Cards" on 95 provincial institutions. In France, it was the media that took the initiative, with publication in 1999 of a hospital quality ranking (*Science et Avenir*, 1999). This list has since been regularly reproduced in other magazines (*Figaro Magazine, Le Point*). Since then, the Ministry of Health has prepared a French model for publishing comparative data on hospital performance (DREES, 1999, 2001), as has the National Health Care Accreditation and Evaluation Agency (ANAES) (Box 1).

This paper attempts to summarize these experiments, focusing on the measurement of hospital performance. The approach excludes the many US studies that evaluate not only health-care providers taken individually but also the health-care plans marketed by "managed care organisations". In the latter case, an evaluation must cover all the services offered by a plan.[2] The paper also limits itself to measuring the clinical outcomes of health care, *i.e.* performance in terms of reduced morbidity, mortality avoided, improved biological and clinical parameters for patients. This excludes the impact of health care on patients' quality of life, which is still at a very experimental stage (Cooper *et al.*, 2001). It also excludes those dimensions of service quality that relate primarily to the patient's physical and psychological comfort, which can be measured either by specific indicators (length of waiting lists) or by patient experience surveys (Coulter and Cleary, 2001).[3] Finally, the paper does not take into account studies on "total quality improvement" management methods, the objective of which is to ensure that an institution maintains permanent control over factors that determine the quality of care.

Box 1. **The Ontario Hospital Report 2001: care indicators**

This comparison of hospital care is based on a selection of ten medical conditions, for which four types of indicators are measured. The conditions are the following:

- Myocardial infarction
- Stroke
- Heart failure
- Community-acquired pneumonia
- Asthma
- Intestinal haemorrhage
- Cholecystectomy
- Hysterectomy
- Prostatectomy
- Carpal tunnel syndrome

The indicators are the following: the number of complications in comparison to the number of cases, readmissions, length of stay, and access to technology or day-hospital care.

The first part of the paper presents what we may call the "technology" of measuring hospital performance. The first segment reviews the principal characteristics of hospital care services, while the second lists their consequences for quality measurement.

The second part of the paper presents the indicators most widely used in various countries, and discusses the limits of some of these indicators.

The third part examines the ways this technology is used and attempts to identify its impacts, on the basis of published information. It looks first at the objectives of those who advocate the production and publication of hospital performance measures, and then examines the impact of these efforts from three points of view: that of the patient, that of the care purchaser (public or private insurers), and that of the authorities.

The final part draws some lessons from the analysis and offers some recommendations for action.

1. Hospital performance measurement technology

1.1. The characteristics of hospital care

A *hospital is, first of all, a multi-service provider*. Using the most common tools for measuring hospital workload, which are systems of the Diagnosis-Related Groups type for classifying hospital stays, a hospital may "produce" between 600 and 1 500 different types of hospitalisation, depending on the degree of refinement of the classification used. This very variety poses a problem, particularly if one is seeking to measure not only workload but also productivity and quality of service. In fact, it requires rigorous measures for each "product". It also means that a hospital can perform well in some activities, and less so in others. At the present time, however, there are no data covering all of a hospital's potential activities.

The first solution is to select a small number of activities, generally those that are most in the media spotlight (heart surgery or obstetrics), those that are frequently performed but are not very serious (treatments that pose no risk to patients), those of an elective nature (where there is a high risk of unnecessary treatment), or those selected on the basis of the target population (hip fractures among the elderly) or the availability of proven databases (resuscitation units). The second solution is to look for indicators that will reflect the overall results of care, such as casemix-adjusted mortality rates. Choosing the first method means that we will have no comprehensive comparison of hospital performance. For patients suffering from a particular condition not covered by the selected indicators, published information will be of

253

---

no interest. To remedy this problem, Eddy (1998) suggests a systematic shift of target pathologies from one year to the next. Mortality rates pose some specific problems, which will be addressed below.

The second characteristic of hospital care is that it represents a complex personal service. The hospital product involves not merely providing a bed but taking charge of an individual, his illness, the dependency induced by that illness, and its treatment. This responsibility involves many inputs: the combination of inputs selected must not only be based on the best available knowledge, but must be delivered efficiently and must be appropriate to each case. This is what Minvielle (1996) calls "managing patient singularity on a large scale". In a service relationship, the patient himself is an input to the process, as a function of his state of health at admission and his genetic inheritance, on one hand, and his degree of cooperativeness under treatment, on the other hand. Finally, the quality of the interpersonal relationship between the patient, his family and the hospital team also contributes to the outcome of the process. For this reason, there is often some confusion about the notion of care quality, *i.e.* between the quality of care considered as an attribute of the outcome of the process (curing a disease, overcoming a handicap, etc.) and the quality of care considered as an attribute of the process itself. It is usual, in the specialized literature on health-care evaluation, to distinguish between two notions of quality: outcome measures and process measures. Among the outcome measures, we may also distinguish between intermediary outcomes, such as controlling high blood pressure or cholesterol levels, and final outcomes, such as cure, remission or death. Finally, the fact that the patient may be both the beneficiary of the process and an input resource to it means that, in comparing different hospitals, their clientele characteristics must be taken into account for their impact on outcomes.

From a theoretical viewpoint, it is best to use outcome indicators: they measure the impact of care on an individual's state of health. These outcome indicators should be specific to each hospital activity. Apart from the complexity of the task, reflecting the variety of hospital activities, there are also some severe methodological limitations in taking accurate and regular measurements of the outcome of care. In the first place, a final improvement in state of health may not appear until well after the period of hospitalisation: this implies long-term patient monitoring. Unfortunately, the data needed for this kind of monitoring are generally not in the control of the hospitals, and collecting them requires cooperation by the patient and by other care providers. In the second place, if the outcome is measured by the non-occurrence of complications, and if these are rare, it will take numerous observations to be sure that measurement is sufficiently precise. Finally, there may be some confounding factors that must be ascertained before imputing outcomes to a given establishment. For these reasons, and provided there is enough convincing evidence on the link between a process characteristic and an outcome, we may replace an outcome measure by a process quality measure. There are however no properly controlled studies of overall hospital care available, and the relationship between process and outcome is not always fully established. This means that respect for a process standard is not a full guarantee of the quality of outcome.

The third characteristic of hospital activity is the stochastic nature of care. There is no determinist relationship between the provision of treatment and its effect on the patient. No treatment is 100 per cent effective, and no treatment is risk-free. In other words, the failure of treatment may be due to random or other factors beyond the control of the hospital team.

The fourth characteristic of hospital care is that it involves medical practice under real conditions. Contrary to what happens in a well-controlled, random clinical task, where patients are carefully selected, and at the end of which we can measure experimental effectiveness, hospitals must adapt their reference treatments to patients who are not part of a clinical test. As a result of ethical concerns (such as over depriving a patient of a therapy of proven effectiveness) and practical reasons (the cost of constantly conducting random tests), hospitals cannot always fully respect decision-making rules based on data for which there is widespread published proof. In this case, again, adhering to good-practice recommendations in the scientific literature is not a complete guarantee that treatment will be effective.

1.2. Consequences for the measurement of health care quality

The first consequence of these characteristics of hospital activity on measuring care quality has already been mentioned: there is no current system that covers all hospital activity, and inter-hospital comparisons are available only for a limited number of pathologies. It can of course be argued that a hospital that does well in several activities is likely to do so in all, but that remains to be demonstrated. There is also debate over the publication of hospital rankings based on combined performance in several dimensions, such as mortality, reputation and other factors (the "league tables"). The aggregation procedure relies necessarily on a relative weighting of various criteria. In general, the choice of these weightings is done empirically, with no scientific basis, by the team publishing the ranking. At best, the relative weights for the different dimensions may reflect the observed preferences for each of these dimensions among the general public. Moreover, aggregation masks performance differentials in each dimension, and can work in favour of hospitals that are merely average on all criteria. In this way, authors recommend the continued publication of non-aggregated results (Eddy, 1998), in order to provide readers with full information.

The second consequence relates to the constraints that statistical method imposes in producing a rigorous demonstration, on one hand, of a hospital's impact on care outcomes (identification of confounding factors) and on the other hand, of significant differences between hospitals. In both cases, these constraints arise, first, from the size of the universe studied, which means that only high-volume activities are selected, or else that data must be gathered over a long period of time in order to achieve a sufficient volume. There is also a further factor of variation – time – during which new technologies or new practices may appear. This means that the publication of comparative results must be significantly hedged, for example by indicating confidence intervals for published indicator values. Uncertainty over the results is the second reason why hospital rankings are criticized: depending on how accurate the measure is, a great number of hospitals may perform equivalently from the statistical viewpoint, and yet may have different rankings. This will make the published results meaningless to a public that is not sufficiently familiar with statistical method, or that does not take the time to examine the results carefully. It can also undermine the ability of insurers to react, if results do not really make it possible to distinguish between various establishments.

The third characteristic relates to the quality of the information systems that are needed to conduct such analysis. Each hospital has to ensure that the data it provides for comparative analysis are accurate and complete. This means controlling the quality of both internal and external data. Data definitions must be strictly the same from one hospital to the next, or the comparison may be distorted. Kritschevsky *et al.* (1999) have shown how different definitions of caesarean section rates can lead to different conclusions in inter-hospital comparisons. Techniques for controlling the impact of confounding factors, for example patient-risk adjustment for mortality rates, can require very detailed clinical data. Such data are often produced for purposes of the care process, but not always systematically (since they are not all required for the medical decision): producing them may therefore require a specific investment by the hospitals being evaluated. In the absence of computerized medical files that are standard from one hospital to the next, there is also a third constraint on the extent of activities covered by a comparative analysis: that of the investment cost in a new computer system for monitoring all hospital activity at a sufficient level of detail. There is debate in the literature over the comparative advantages of specific databases intended to measure care quality for a precise segment of activity (for example, comparing mortality rates for coronary bypass grafts) and databases of the "administrative" kind, *i.e.* consisting of data that are routinely gathered for purposes other than quality evaluation. For example, databases that produce discharge abstracts for measuring the hospital casemix were first used by Medicare, beginning in 1989, to publish casemix-adjusted mortality rates. In the first case, this offers the advantage of data that are specific to a field of pathology, and hence clinically relevant. The results are more convincing, easier to interpret and more acceptable to clinical practitioners. But this comes at the price of an additional investment and a reduced field of analysis. In the second case, in principle, the initial investment cost in the database is low, the field covered is potentially large since it embraces all hospital activity, the data are produced on a regular basis, but the analysis loses its specificity.

2. The main indicators

It should be noted at the outset that this section deals only with indicators that relate to hospitals and that are made available to the general public. Medical practices are also evaluated in many studies that are published in scientific reviews or that are used by hospitals at their own discretion to monitor the quality of the care they provide. We shall adhere to the conventional distinction between outcome indicators and process indicators.

2.1. Mortality rate as an indicator of quality of care

There is *a priori* unanimity on this indicator: death is an event that everyone wishes to avoid, and that can be seen as the ultimate sanction of poor-quality care. It has a strong hold on the public imagination, and when premature or avoidable mortality seems to be linked to dysfunctional procedures, it appears particularly unfair. It is also an indicator about which there is no ambiguity in terms of clinical definition, and it is one that hospitals must measure with the greatest precision, if only because the regulations so demand. Since the first publications from Medicare, and from several American states, a comparative analysis of mortality rates has given rise to many methodological studies, and continues to be used by the media in preparing their "league tables" (Ansari *et al.*, 1999; Chalé and Naiditch, 1999; Iezzoni, 1997; Iezzoni *et al.*, 1995; Landon *et al.*, 1996; Leyland and Boddy, 1998; McKee and Hunter, 1995; Thomas and Hofer, 1999).

In fact, mortality data are not that easy to collect. In the first place, many studies show that the records kept by hospitals are not fully reliable, and that they may show significant and unexplained fluctuations over time. Since hospital deaths are a rare phenomenon, missing data can have an important impact on the outcome. In the second place, in-hospital mortality is not a sufficient basis on which to judge the impact of care on a patient's future prospects. On one hand, the ultimate effect of an intervention may occur well after the first episode of treatment, and the patient may die later at home, or in the course of re-hospitalisation. An acute-care hospital may also have an early-release policy of sending patients to follow-up care facilities, and death that eventually results from the first intervention may occur only in that latter facility. For this reason, it is common to measure not only in-hospital mortality but also mortality within 30 days after discharge (or longer, if relevant), which means that hospitals must monitor their patients after they leave. This requirement can further undermine the accuracy of data if such tracking is not fully reliable.

The remarks above relating to the characteristics of hospital activity also apply with respect to mortality rates. For most pathologies treated in hospital, mortality rates are very low. If we seek to measure them accurately for a given hospital, or to make a useful comparison between hospitals, we must start with a fairly large population. This can be done in two ways: by selecting frequently occurring pathologies, or by selecting data over a period longer than one year. Yet when working with common pathologies, these will often produce a highly favourable prognosis, and hence few deaths.

Moreover, the literature on the measurement of mortality rates stresses the need to take into account confounding factors, and in particular the risk factors that patients present at the time of their admission. Hospitals may differ widely in terms of the profile of the patients they admit. The first adjustment factors to be considered are age and sex. The natural probability of death increases with age, of course, and there is also a difference in mortality at the same age between the two sexes. But other factors must also be taken into account. For any given treatment, patients will present different risk profiles depending on their state of health. The nature of these risks will vary depending on the treatments and the pathologies involved, which means that we must develop specific models and collect specific data for each one.

The models are built on the following principle. An initial medical examination will identify potential risk factors, the impact of which on mortality will then be tested. A multi-centric database is then constructed for hospitals, either on a geographical basis (all hospitals providing treatment in a given state, for example) or on a voluntary basis, or, more rarely, using a predefined stratification. These data can be used to identify significant risk factors and to estimate their relative impact on mortality or on morbidity. This model is then applied to patient characteristics for any given hospital, so as to calculate the expected mortality rates. Next, this expected rate is compared against the rate observed in the hospital, to produce a ratio between the two values. If the observed rate is higher than the expected rate, this may signal a quality problem, while an observed rate lower than the expected rate is a sign of good performance. Generally, it is these observed rate/expected rate ratios that the media use in their published "league tables" for ranking hospitals against each other.

Given the statistical uncertainties surrounding the results, these rankings are unreliable. Observed rates, after all, are derived from a sampling method that will determine the accuracy of the measurement. The coefficients of the statistical models used for calculating the expected rates are themselves estimated, and their accuracy is only relative. It will depend as well on the size of the database and its composition: calibration errors can be suspected if testing the same model on a different basis produces different results, *i.e.* if the risk factors and the coefficients are not the same.

For these reasons, experts have replaced ranking by identifying hospitals that are significantly different from others, the "outliers". This term reflects the notion that the discrepancy between the observed rate and the expected rate for some hospitals is too great to be due solely to chance. An outstanding study of this kind was conducted in New York State hospitals to measure mortality associated with coronary bypass operations (Hannan *et al.*, 1990, 1994, 1995; Naiditch, 1999).

Despite these precautions, the confidence that experts have in the mortality rate (unadjusted and adjusted) for identifying care quality problems is limited (Ansari *et al.*, 1999; Chalé and Naiditch, 1999; Iezzoni, 1997; Iezzoni *et al.*, 1995; Landon *et al.*, 1996; Leyland and Boddy, 1998; McKee and Hunter, 1995; Thomas and Hofer, 1999). There are several reasons for this. In the first place, there are many alternative systems for adjusting risk factors. Iezzoni (1997), Iezzoni *et al.* (1995) and Landon *et al.*, 1996) compared the performance of 12 of these systems for four pathologies or treatments: coronary bypass, myocardial infarction, pneumonia and unoperated cerebral stroke. While the systems' statistical performances are fairly comparable overall, comparing them in pairs produces significant discrepancies, particularly for establishments ranked in the best and worst deciles. In other words, the placement of the "outliers" is unstable from one ranking to the next, even if the rankings are relatively consistent overall. Thomas et Hofer (1999) arrived at identical results, but using a different method. They showed that even if there were a perfect method for adjusting the case mix and the risk factors, systematic errors in the statistical identification of the outliers are such that their positive predictive value is low: in other words, a significant percentage of good-quality hospitals will be found amongst the worst outliers, and *vice versa*. This predictive value increases, nevertheless, with the size of the data samples used for each hospital, but even with samples of 900 patients per hospital the error remains sizeable. Silber et Rosenaum (1997) provided a conceptual critique of the link between mortality rates and quality of care, arguing that not all deaths can be blamed on the quality of care. The general condition of certain patients is such that death is inevitable, and care will merely delay it. On the other hand, the care team must be careful to prevent complications of a condition that could worsen the patient's chances of survival. The rate of complications during hospitalisation is therefore the preferred indicator for measuring quality of care, and it offers two additional advantages. Complications are more frequent than death, and hence the sample size required is smaller. Data are normally gathered systematically from the discharge abstracts, although here the authors call for great caution in using data of this kind.

The mortality rate, then, is a simple and obvious indicator of the quality of care, but it is complicated to calculate with sufficient rigor to be usable and has only weak powers of discrimination between hospitals, once measurement biases are taken into account. Measuring the adjusted mortality rate for one or several pathologies is not sufficient grounds for an overall judgment of the hospital (Rosenthal *et al.*, 1997, Iezzoni *et al.*, 1995). It is not very useful in producing ordinal rankings of the "league tables" type. Finally, it is not clear that it is a good predictive factor for the quality of care, since a high (low) mortality rate is not always synonymous with a poor (good) quality of care. Yet the cumulative and rigorous work that has been done to measure the mortality rate has produced useful lessons: the effort invested in examining patient files so as to ensure the quality of the data and to interpret the results in terms of identifying risk factors has led to progress in reducing mortality rates for certain pathologies, as can be seen from experience with coronary bypasses in New York State (Box 2).

257

Box 2. **The most frequently studied mortality rates**

- Overall case-mix-adjusted mortality
- Mortality following a coronary bypass
- Mortality following a myocardial infarction
- Mortality following severe heart failure
- Mortality following a stroke
- Mortality of patients suffering from pneumonia
- Mortality of patients suffering from an obstructive respiratory illness
- Mortality following intestinal haemorrhage
- Mortality following a total hip replacement
- Mortality of resuscitation patients
- Mortality at birth of underweight infants

2.2. Intermediate outcome indicators

This notion covers several phenomena. The result of any portion of the care process is an intermediate outcome. We also speak of intermediate outcome when we do not know how to cure an illness, but can only stabilize certain of its manifestations. In the area of cancer pathologies, a reduction in the size of a tumour is an intermediate outcome. We also measure an intermediate outcome when the final outcome is observed only after a period of time much longer than the stay in hospital. An example is the time it takes for elderly hip-fracture patients to walk again: the final outcome will be observable, not upon discharge from the hospital that performed the acute treatment, but only after a period of rehabilitation. Finally, the frequency of avoidable, undesirable events is also an intermediate outcome: this is the case with nosocomial infection rates, *i.e.* hospital-acquired infections, the complications rate from specific surgical operations, or the importance of iatrogenicity linked to medication prescriptions. Measuring the frequency of avoidable morbidities represents a large part of the work on intermediary outcomes.

The measurement of intermediate outcomes has been the subject of many studies in recent years, under the heading of "outcome research". In the United States, the Joint Commission for Accreditation of Healthcare Organizations publishes a document listing available tools and methods (the ORYX Initiative). Yet these are little used in inter-hospital comparative studies, even though they provide users with more specific information by identifying hospitals' performance for different pathologies. There are several reasons for this.

As in the study of mortality rates, a comparative analysis of intermediate outcomes between hospitals requires some significant methodological precautions, the main ones of which were discussed earlier: sample size, adjustment for patients' characteristics, data quality, need to use specific clinical or biological data surveys. This complicates the use of comparative data. Secondly, the very variety of the hospital workload is an obstacle to generalizing the studies to a large number of establishments.

This has led to an emphasis on performance indicators that are generic and that can be applied to the entire structure. The rate of nosocomial infections has the advantage of being an intermediate outcome indicator that is not specific to a given pathology. It measures the incidence of hospital-acquired infections in comparison to the volume of hospitalisations, and without any direct relation to the originating illness. This rate is complex to measure, since it requires very rigorously documented medical files. Nosocomial infections may be due to staff negligence or failure to respect hygiene regulations, but there is in fact an irreducible risk that infectious agents will be transmitted in any place as open as a hospital. Finally, a nosocomial infection may be due to technical infrastructure shortcomings that are not readily apparent, as in the case of "legionnaires' disease". Hospital staff may see detailed documentation of cases as a kind of self-incrimination, and they may resist keeping records if the episode ends without major harm to the patient. This suggests that the results of incidence surveys should not lead to direct individual sanctions (or rewards), but rather to efforts to improve the functioning of the service. Otherwise, the data may be falsified. This is particularly a problem if the indicator is to be given wide publication, in which case there will be fears of user complaints and lawsuits.

Nosocomial infections are in fact a good example of the way hospitals should account for the quality of their risk management. Effective surveillance of nosocomial infections requires proper observance of very strict hygiene rules, of course, but it also implies a costly mechanism for tracing sources of infection. Yet the enforcement of rules requires a high degree of confidence among the different people involved in hospital care, so that the controls necessary for surveillance are seen not as a threat of sanctions but as a contribution to improving the overall effort and securing the best outcomes for patients. Only under such circumstances will infections be property documented. In other words, a mediocre hospital could well report low rates of nosocomial infections (because few are reported), while an efficient and transparent establishment could find that the data published on it are much less flattering. If infection rates are to be compared among hospitals, then, we must also ensure that each hospital is organized to monitor this risk effectively (Humphreys et Emmerson, 1993; DREES, 2001).

The number of therapeutic accidents resulting from medication prescription errors is an intermediate outcome indicator with characteristics similar to those of the nosocomial infection rate. Personal responsibility is more important here than in the case of infections, however, where it is impossible to control all the infectious agents present in a hospital. For this reason, observation of these accidents is even more difficult. They are regarded as one of the major sources of medical error, and their cost is considerable. Yet to date they have been the object of no published inter-hospital comparisons.

2.3. *Process indicators*

Process indicators are intended to describe and evaluate the process of providing care. They may refer to a practical rule – "measures to prevent thromboembolism should be taken during orthopaedic surgery" – and the indicator will then show the rate of adherence for the rule. In the best of cases, the rule will have been established as a result of experience demonstrating that a given practice is superior. In many cases, there may be no comprehensive experimental evidence, but rather a collection of elements. Finally, sound practice can be dictated by experts. Thus we may use process indicators as a substitute for measuring the intermediate or final outcomes on which they have an impact. In this way we get around the fact that certain undesirable events occur only rarely.

The care process involves a number of phases, and many different players. We need then to identify the stages of the process that have the most significant impact on care outcomes. This analysis can be used to define sentinel events that will signal that a critical event is imminent, one that will pose a high risk to the quality of care. Identifying these signals is important for day-to-day care management, yet given their number it is impossible to make them public in a systematic way. Attempting such effort would be equivalent, for example, to continuously posting the temperature of molten steel in a foundry, and it would have no meaning for users. This is why, once again, research is directed towards finding simple process markers that are generic and easy to collect. Some of these are clinical in nature, and others are not.

The rate of caesarean sections, and the rate of vaginal births after a first caesarean section, are clinical process indicators. We may also consider them as intermediate outcome indicators, where the final outcomes are the state of health of infant and mother. It has in fact been regarded as a characteristic indicator of the care process, since it involves one method of childbirth. The caesarean rate is an indicator of the quality of care, for this reason: a caesarean section is a surgical procedure that requires an anaesthetic, thereby posing a greater risk to mother and child than does natural childbirth. There are medical indications for the caesarean approach, but with the number of these procedures in developed countries growing (admittedly at different rates) experts have come to question the justification in terms of surgical and anaesthetic risk. Studies have shown that, beyond medically justified indications, caesareans may be used as a birth programming technique; that the abuse of artificial labour inducement can also result in the need for a caesarean section; and finally, in certain countries, that caesareans are used as a very indirect form of contraception, based on the belief that a second pregnancy following a caesarean delivery will be dangerous for the mother, because of the weaknesses caused by scarring of the uterus. In all developed countries, reducing the rate of caesarean sections has been accepted as a public health objective. Moreover, the belief that post-caesarean natural childbirth is dangerous is being countered through training and information for professionals and users alike.

We may say, then, that there is a true consensus on this performance indicator. Nevertheless, methodological precautions are needed if we are to draw valid comparisons between institutions. On one hand, maternity ward admission patterns may differ in terms of the maternal risk profile, and hence the probability of resort to caesarean section for valid medical reasons. Comparisons must therefore be adjusted for these risk factors (Aron *et al.*, 1998). On the other hand, Kritschesky *et al.* (1999) showed that caesarean rate calculation was dependent on conventions relating to the information-keeping systems of each hospital, and that no absolute inter-hospital comparison was possible.

The most frequently used nonclinical process indicators are length of hospitalisation, rates of unplanned readmission, and volumes of activity by type of intervention. Certain magazines that publish "league tables" make the assumption that a short stay in hospital is a sign of good-quality care. On one hand, this is what patients want. On the other hand, a short stay reduces a patient's risk of exposure to prescription errors and to nosocomial infections. This pressure towards shortening the length of hospitalisation also has an economic rationale, in terms of reducing the number of hospital beds. But care must be used in interpreting it. A comparison of length of stay requires adjustment for different factors: the case mix, the severity of cases, and sometimes the socioeconomic status of the patients. On the other hand, we must be careful not to invert the causal relationship. It is true that new treatments have appeared that reduce the need for long hospitalisation, such as endoscopic exploratory and surgical techniques, while at the same time enhancing the quality of care. In this case, it is the improved techniques themselves that have reduced the length of hospitalisation and increased the quality of care. Yet reducing the length of hospitalisation is a parameter that can be manipulated by the hospital. If the hospital has surplus beds downstream in its convalescence or rehabilitation wards, early discharge from acute hospitalisation may lead in the end to a longer convalescence and a less satisfactory quality of care. For this reason, the length-of-hospitalisation measurement must be accompanied by a measurement of the number of premature discharges, and the number of readmissions following on the heels of such discharges (generally within 30 days). In fact, a high number of early readmissions may indicate inadequate patient rehabilitation. This measure is not in itself completely satisfactory: some hospitals may refer their patients to another hospital if they suffer post-operative problems.

Using the workload by type of intervention is based on a simple idea that originated in industrial economics: cumulative experience in executing a task improves the performance of the operator. Several studies have attempted to discover this "experience effect" in the health system, particularly for surgery or diagnostic tests (Hillner *et al.*, 2000; Nathens *et al.*, 2001; Phillips *et al.*, 1995; Ritchie *et al.*, 1999). Since the intent is to show the effect of experience not only on the time spent in surgery, or the cost of the procedure (primary productivity), but also on the quality of the outcome, measured for example by the number of peri- and post-operative complications or deaths attributable to surgery, it is important in these studies to observe the same methodological precautions as in other performance measurement research. In particular, patients cared for by different surgeons must have identical risk factors, and the surgical technique employed must be the same. Some studies look at cumulative experience over time, and this raises the problem of the appearance of new techniques. In the end, the relevant level of analysis is not solely the intervention of the surgeon, but the overall volume of a team's activity. A team that does few operations of any one type but that has a high overall level of activity will have more experience than a team that does few operations of any kind because its overall workload is low. Finally, the analysis must apply to the entire operating team and not only the surgeon.

This experience effect has been applied (with due regard for the above factors) to certain surgical procedures, such as total hip replacement, peritoneoscopic surgery and open-heart surgery, to mention only a few. The volume of activity by type of operation is often used as a process criterion in inter-hospital comparisons, and particularly in the preparation of rankings. Yet these rankings should not be interpreted too literally. In the first place, studies show a significant statistical link between volume and outcome, but this link is not enough to move directly to a ranking. Suppose, for example, that 30 per cent of inter-hospital performance discrepancies can be explained by the volume effect. The fact remains that 70 per cent of the differential must be explained by other factors. To jump directly to a ranking will give rise both to positive errors (where hospitals may be highly ranked on the basis of their high volume, without deserving it) and negative errors (where hospitals are poorly ranked, and improperly so, because of low volumes). Consider for example a surgical team that performs a high volume of operations, but at the price of overworked support personnel and long days in the operating room for the surgeon. Studies have shown that when surgical teams approach the saturation point there is a high risk to the quality of their work, because of fatigue and inattentiveness. Another reason for avoiding ordinal rankings is that volume effects are not continuous: a hospital that does 152 operations a year is not necessarily performing better than one that does only 151. It is important therefore to establish workload thresholds.

In terms of the information that should be given to users, an indication of volume is not sufficient. We must also indicate whether the operating team follows the rules in terms of the pace of work and recovery time. We must also know if other, more specific process criteria are being respected: for example, the systematic use of prophylactic precautions during intestinal surgery to avoid post-operative infections. These process indicators are generally studied in the course of accreditation. This opens the question of the publicity given to these reports, which contain the most extensive available information on a hospital 's working methods.

2.4. Lessons

Several lessons can be drawn from the experience described above in terms of a comparative evaluation of hospitals. In the first place, all authors insist on the issue of the quality of information systems and the degree of standardization required to ensure that studies are conducted rigorously.

Investment in the establishment and maintenance of databases is thus a cost that must not be underestimated. Nor should we underestimate the skills that may be required to manage them and to analyse the data. We have already pointed to the methodological precautions that must be taken in order to reflect confounding factors in inter-hospital comparisons. Consequently, any organisation, public or private, that seeks to develop an analysis of this kind will have to recruit high-level statisticians and enlist the cooperation of expert clinicians in interpreting the results.

The last point concerns the publication of hospital rankings in the form of "league tables". The media are fond of presenting results in this way, because it is simple and attention-grabbing and good for circulation. But there are sound reasons for thinking that these rankings are spurious, in the sense that they do not really reflect inter-hospital differences in the quality of care. We have discussed these reasons: the results are tainted with uncertainty and the indicators are not direct and unequivocal measurements of quality. A further reason is that these publications attempt in the end to impose a weighting on the different dimensions of quality, for example by giving more weight to mortality than to length of hospitalisation. Yet this weighting function has no justification in science, in politics (the results of a vote) or in economics (marketing surveys that might determine consumer preferences). The final ranking is thus sensitive to the choice of weightings.

Such information is supposed to help users to become enlightened consumers, so they can choose the hospital where they will go for treatment. If the information is erroneous, then the media are providing poor guidance for these decisions and could, in theory, be responsible for severe patient disappointment. They might even find themselves liable to lawsuit for providing false information occasioning personal injury. Low-ranked hospitals might also consider themselves libelled. At the very least, it would be wise to publish, not ordinal rankings, but comparisons between groups of hospitals with statistically comparable levels of performance.

3. The impact of comparative evaluations

We shall analyse this impact from three viewpoints, that of the providers of health care, those who use them, and those who pay for them. There has in fact been little effort to evaluate the impact of these inter-hospital comparisons.

3.1. Impact on care providers

The publishers of these data expect that the impact will be to improve the performance of each care provider. This improvement will itself depend on the structure of incentives contained in the original program. In a conventional competition model, the provision of information on product quality does not necessarily produce an incentive to low-quality producers to improve their performance. In fact, they may conclude that some consumers are price-sensitive and willing to settle for lower quality. These producers will be able to find their own market niche. At the very most, there may be regulations establishing a minimum quality threshold below which no one may operate. Why does any producer seek to improve his quality? He will do so if he thinks he can earn a return on his investment, through a larger market share and higher profits.

In the health care sector, we must anticipate, then, that the publication of comparative data on quality of care will have a quality-improvement impact only on those providers seeking to expand their market share and hence their revenues or profits.

The health-care industry has a number of specific features. One of these is the high price/quality elasticity of users, *i.e.* users accord great value to quality and are ready to pay much more in order to guarantee that quality.[4] In other words, publishing comparative results could provoke significant shifts of clientele between establishments (or, in the case of systems where there is heavy litigation pressure, such as in the United States, the fear of malpractice suits could induce the poorest-ranking hospitals to improve their performance). If hospitals feel that this threat is high, they will have an incentive to invest in quality. Yet the perception of this risk is tempered, in the case of hospital care, by the issue of geographic accessibility (how far people are willing to travel in order to obtain a higher quality of care) and the degree of competition within the local catchment area (a hospital with a local monopoly will have no incentive to change). Finally, for any given hospital, we may assume that the decision to take action is a function of perceived cost in comparison to expected returns, and this is also a function of the gap separating the hospital from the average of the hospitals with which it is being compared. If this gap is narrow, the incentive to take action is likely to be weak, and the hospital can ascribe the discrepancy to statistical error. For hospitals ranked above the mean, we may also assume that they will have little incentive to try to catch up with the leaders if the perceived cost of such an effort is high.

A second specific feature of the health-care industry is the involvement of a third-party purchaser, the insurer (public or private). The price/quality relationship is negotiated between the insurer and the care provider. In the case of private insurers in a competitive market there are two possibilities. The insurers may deem the price/quality relationship to be satisfactory (for example quality and price are both low), in which case there will be no incentive to change, in the absence of evidence that the insured clients are unhappy with the situation. If an insurer feels that that the price/quality relationship is inadequate, it may threaten to withdraw its accreditation of the hospital, or reduce the price it will pay. This threat will be all the more credible if the insurer is a dominant source of financing for the hospital, or if all insurers adopt the same strategy. In this case, the hospital will be forced to take steps to improve the quality of the care it offers.

In the case of a public insurer, we may assume that it is in a monopoly situation. In this case, it is politically difficult not to take action when quality discrepancies between the various hospitals under its control become too great. Here we may identify four possible situations:

Price/Quality	Low	High
Low	1	2
High	3	4

The public insurer may find that there are hospitals 1) of low quality and low unit cost, 2) of high quality and low unit cost, 3) of low quality and high unit cost, and 4) of high quality and high unit cost. In 1), it should in principle condition its financing of the hospital on steps to improve quality. Those establishments that fall under 2) will constitute a reference group. Hospitals in 3) should ultimately face financial penalties, with demands that they improve their quality. Those in 4) should be asked to reduce their unit costs while maintaining their current quality levels. There is no incentive, then, for a hospital to make an effort unless the purchaser has the technical means to perform a unit cost/quality analysis, and the political clout to enforce it. In fact, this means a redeployment of resources among hospitals, which may mobilize their local political resources to influence the decisions taken.

In short, for a hospital with a mediocre record, the incentive to act arises from a) the fear of acquiring a negative reputation that will over time result in fewer patients; b) the quality gap by which it falls short of the average hospital; c) this fear may be tempered in the short term by the hospital's relative positioning in its local competitive environment; d) it also depends on the pressure exerted by the insurers; e) this depends on the insurers' perception of the price-quality relationship.

This means, in effect, that the reaction to published results is likely to depend on the particular circumstances of each hospital, and that it is difficult to predict any general tendency. Yet this reasoning holds only at a given point in time. If the results are published repeatedly, showing that certain hospitals are making no effort, then they will sooner or later find themselves obliged to take corrective action. In terms of measuring the impact of comparative evaluations, this means that the effort must be maintained over the long term. In the case of a public purchaser, however, it must ultimately accept responsibility for correcting discrepancies, especially in the case of hospitals where quality is low and unit costs are low.

Does the literature back up these predictions? The evidence is too fragmentary to permit definitive conclusions, but we may discern some indications. The experiments cited as having had their impact on the behaviour of care providers evaluated are based primarily on voluntary participation by hospitals, which in fact pay for a portion of the studies. This means that those hospitals consider *a priori* that gaining recognition of their relative performance is sufficient benefit to offset the risk of a negative image, assuming that consumers and insurers will give them credit for having taken the risk of being shown to be underperforming. They are thus in a position where they must make every effort possible: if their results are mediocre, they will have to take action so as not to lose the confidence of their respective clientele.

One of the first large-scale experiments conducted in the United States involved the regular publication of casemix-adjusted mortality rates by the Pennsylvania State Department of Health. This experiment went quite far, and involved the publication of physician-specific data. Launched in 1989, it was suspended in 1993 after a series of disputes over the quality of the adjustments made and the appropriateness of using mortality as a performance indicator.

The most famous example in many respects is the coronary bypass mortality study in New York State (Hannan *et al.*, 1990, 1994, 1995; Chassin *et al.*, 1996; Naiditch, 1999). This was an exemplary study on several scores. It involved all the New York State hospitals performing coronary bypasses. It was financed by the state Department of Health, which committed itself to long-term funding. The study lasted from 1990 to 1997. It gathered specific clinical data involving long-term patient tracking, and data quality was monitored regularly. Results could thus be properly adjusted for risks. The teams met frequently to analyse the results. Results were presented, not as rankings, but as a three-tiered grouping of hospitals: those with better-than-average scores, those with scores around the average, and those below average. Initially, to encourage surgeons to sign on to the project, it was agreed that the results would not be published until the entire study was completed. Partway through the study, however, a journalist, claiming freedom of information, challenged this understanding in court. Following the first publication of results, mortality declined by 41 per cent, while it went down by only 18 per cent in the rest of the country, and patient severity rose. Part of this improvement was due to the fact that the less successful teams, in general those with the lowest workload, abandoned the market, but the systematic study of the most successful working methods also helped other teams to progress, and to understand the factors for success with the treatment.

Another large-scale experiment that gave rise to a number of published studies was conducted in Ohio, under the name Cleveland Health Quality Choice (CHQC) (Rosenthal *et al.*, 1998). This project dates from 1988 and represents a joint effort by several groups of stakeholders: the hospital association, the physicians' association, employers and the chamber of commerce. It assembles data from 30 hospitals, covering the following areas: mortality associated with eight pathologies, length of hospitalisation for 13 pathologies, mortality and length of hospitalisation for resuscitation patients, rate of caesarean sections and rate of vaginal births after caesarean section, indicators of hospital iatrogenicity, and a survey of patient satisfaction. The published studies on the impact of this program show a decline in the caesarean section rate, an increase in the rate of vaginal births after caesarean section (Caron and Neuhauser, 1994), a reduction in post-resuscitation mortality rates together with a reduction in the length of stay, and this despite a heavier patient load (Sirio *et al.*,1994). Rosenthal *et al.* (1998) cite four case studies of hospitals participating in the experiment that took steps to improve their results in three areas: length of hospitalisation for coronary bypass, pneumonia-associated mortality, and the caesarean section rate and the rate of vaginal births after caesarean section. An external evaluation of the Cleveland experiment was published by Rosenthal *et al.* (1997), who examined the mortality rates for the eight pathologies selected at the outset of the experiment and performed a statistical analysis comparing these rates with those before and after the CHQC. They concluded that there was a significant reduction in risk-adjusted mortality for the eight pathologies, totalling 13 per cent over two years, with a 20 per cent improvement for heart failure, intestinal haemorrhage, colectomy and coronary bypass. Given the nature of these data, the analysis does not permit a solid inference that this trend is attributable to the project. A very similar experiment was undertaken in California, known as the California Hospital Outcomes Project (Romano *et al.*, 1995). This project was limited to three problems: mortality after myocardial infarction and after vertebral disk surgery, and the caesarean section rate. Finally, Epstein and Kurtzig reported in 1994 that 38 American states had established databases to assess hospital performance (Epstein and Kurtzig, 1994).

The Cleveland experiment is instructive on several points. Initially based on voluntary participation through a steering group that included all partners in collective decision-making, it experienced a number of tensions over the release and use of results. One partner used published results to renegotiate its contracts with the hospitals, but without notifying the other members, and the hospitals threatened to withdraw from the project unless there was proper consultation before any of the data were used for taking decisions. Secondly, the program was limited to producing comparative information, but it was left to the initiative of individual hospitals to take improvement measures. The project group never provided hospitals with any assistance in these actions. Thirdly, the hospitals shouldered 75 per cent of the overall cost of the project, amounting in 1998 to some $3 million for the 30 hospitals, or about $100 000 each.

In the United Kingdom, Bucknall *et al.* (2000) showed that introducing a simple system for auditing the care accorded to asthma patients resulted in closer observance of good-practice recommendations.

In conclusion, the published data suggest that the establishment of comparative databases on hospital performance, if they are constructed with rigorous methodological principles and based on cooperation with the participating hospitals, can provide highly useful knowledge for improving performance. Publishing the results is an essential step, but the potential threat that this represents for participating hospitals must be tempered by predetermined rules governing use of the resulting information, as well as the publication format. The authors, here again, stress the difficulty of producing high-quality data. We can identify efforts that hospitals have made to improve their performance in the wake of published evaluations, but these are not systematic to all institutions. It would seem, in the end, that there is an overall effect, but it is difficult to attribute this to the comparative analysis alone. It is likely that these improvements are also the result of a more demanding external environment for hospitals.

3.2. Impact on users

The publication of hospital performance data will have an impact if users use this information in selecting their care provider. From an economic theory viewpoint, such publicity is justified because it reduces the asymmetry of information between service providers and beneficiaries. From a public policy viewpoint, this publicity is desirable as a means of bringing the needed transparency to public services. These principles are hard to contest. In practice, patients suffering from certain chronic diseases (such as renal failure or HIV/AIDS) have demonstrated that they are able to acquire some real practical knowledge about their disease and the treatments they need. They are in a position to truly express an autonomous demand for health services. But these expert patients are not the rule, and in most cases demands for health care are not planned carefully ahead of time. The question that arises then is this: what is the best way to publicize this information so that it will be truly useful to beneficiaries of the services, and will not lead to mistaken judgments? From this viewpoint, debate over the publication of "league tables" takes on a new perspective. These rankings offer a highly simplified account of relative hospital performance. As we have seen, ranking hospitals in terms of mortality rates, for example, has no scientific value and transmits spurious information. "Sound" information is that which groups hospitals with similar performances (within a single confidence interval), yet even this kind of grouping is not error-free. In other words, selecting a hospital from a list simply because it is in first place is no guarantee that it will give a better quality of care than the second or third-placed hospital. It may even present a risk of poor-quality care. This "true" information may be too complicated to be acceptable, however, and may even undermine a lay reader's confidence in the researchers' work.

This information should be useful for the following kinds of decisions:

- In the case of a sick person, what is the treatment best suited to his condition?
- Which service providers offer these treatments, and at what level of quality?

We have discovered little research on this issue. We do not know the initial public impact of publishing comparative data: how many people read them, with what degree of attention, and what credibility they may accord the data provided. Voelker (1995) notes that data from the accreditation surveys conducted by the JCAHO are available to the press and to the general public, but they are seldom consulted. Even when this information is accessed, we do not know what role it may eventually play in individual decision-making. For example, we have little evidence on the impact that a published hospital ranking may have on admissions in a given hospital. On the other hand, Hibbard et al. (1996) conducted studies in order to 1) evaluate people's understanding of quality indicators and 2) describe the most effective means of communicating results. Their work attempted to assess the impact of comparative information in terms of facilitating the choice of a health insurer. Their findings can be summarized as follows.

In the first place, these authors point out that published studies are not the only source of comparative information available to beneficiaries. Competing or supplementary sources include past experience with a hospital, word-of-mouth, the personal physician's opinion, surveys published by patients' or consumers' associations, and other sources of information offered by the media. Measuring the impact of published data requires complex research tools for observing the decision-making behaviour of individuals in a "realistic" situation, either through experimentation or through interviews. No such studies have yet been performed.

Jewett and Hibbard (1996) highlighted the complexity of information on the quality of hospital care. Using the focus group method, where a limited number of individuals are asked to pass judgment on assertions or to respond to questions, and where group dynamics encourage people to speak out more freely and to be more explicit in their responses than they would in a questionnaire-based survey, they found that a significant percentage of people had a poor grasp of what the indicators mean, and that they either misinterpreted them or did not understand them at all. This was particularly true for indicators relating to undesirable events. Under these conditions, we must ask how we can present data so that people will accept them as reliable, i.e. how to indicate their degree of accuracy. Hibbard et al.

(1997) suggest the need for efforts to explain the data and place them in context. People at whom the information is targeted should be told why a certain indicator has been selected, how it actually measures the quality of care, and what questions it can answer. This exercise can become very difficult, however, especially if the indicators selected are published with the statistical notes demanded by sound methodology. Finally, the authors note that the relative sophistication of published information makes it inaccessible to people with a low level of education.

Aggregating the different dimensions of performance poses another problem. In the studies published by the mass media, this issue is resolved through an arbitrary "in-house" weighting of these different dimensions. Yet without such aggregation, the reader himself will have to impose his own trade-offs between the various dimensions of quality. According to Hibbard *et al.* (1997), empirical studies on decision-making show that individuals find it very difficult to make trade-offs between conflicting dimensions. In this case, they will try to construct an analytical framework that will favour one dimension over the other, at the risk of underestimating or ignoring significant pieces of information.

For all these reasons, and in an effort to improve the decisional utility of the information provided to patients, Hibbard *et al.* (1997) and Sisk (1998) propose assigning an important interpretive role to mediators, who should ideally have three types of skills. First, an understanding of the questions that patients ask before deciding on hospitalisation for a given pathology: these questions are likely to concern the procedures involved in the treatment as much as the risks associated with it. Secondly, an understanding of the way in which hospitals actually deal with these problems: this will require further and more refined studies of process, hospital by hospital. Finally, an understanding of the use and limitations of available outcome indicators that make it possible to explain a situation and place it in context. Patients' associations might play this role, as well as people's personal physicians, provided they have access to all this supplementary information. Publishing comparative data would therefore mean not only printing tables of results in the press, but also giving people access to a network of accredited intermediaries for advice.

Finally, there is much stress on the credibility of the information produced. This credibility has three dimensions: the independence of the producers of comparative information, the reliability of the data (which is linked to the degree of standardization in calculating the indicators) and their accuracy (the quality of the information systems). In an effort to certify this credibility, given the profusion of initiatives for publishing comparative results among care providers and health insurance plans in the United States, an evaluation and accreditation body, the Consumer Assessment of Health Plans Study, was created in 1996.

3.3. Impact on the purchasers

This point was already addressed in part during our discussion of care providers. In principle, awareness of hospitals' relative performance in terms of care quality should have an impact on their financing, as a function of the cost-quality relationship sought by the purchaser. We can imagine three decisions that might be related to the relative performance of the care provider: the decision whether or not to send insured patients to this provider, the decision to sign a selective contract with a provider (where the insurer selects a set of treatments from among the full range offered), and finally the negotiation of the price-quality relationship. In this last case, a provider offering higher-than-average quality could also demand a higher price. On the other hand, the purchaser might refuse the price demanded by a provider whose level of care is not up to the purchaser's expectations. Such a trade-off requires the ability to make simultaneous price-quality comparisons among care providers.

Generally speaking, the first decision is taken on the basis of an accreditation process entrusted to an independent agency. Accreditation is in principle the cornerstone of systems for measuring the quality of care. Detailed information on a given hospital will be made available to potential purchasers and, to a partial extent, to the public. Information of this kind will attract less public attention than the league tables, no doubt because the reports containing it are so lengthy and so technical. The care provider's accreditation level is thus an essential parameter of its relationship with a provider. But in a country where accreditation has been in force for a long time (as in the United States), nearly all hospitals are accredited at a satisfactory level, and it is no longer possible to discriminate among them on that basis. There are many examples of selective contracting between purchasers and hospitals: if the level of performance for a segment of activity is not satisfactory, the purchaser will refuse to refer patients needing such treatment to that hospital. In health care systems where there is a strong public sector presence, this is done through selective accreditation procedures: only those hospitals that meet a certain number of criteria (generally process criteria) will be allowed to practice that segment of activity. The segments most often cited are heart surgery, cardiology institutes, organ transplant centres, and maternity hospitals. Outside the United States, these accreditation procedures are based primarily on process criteria, and not on outcome indicators.

Cost remains a dominant criterion of the relationship between purchaser and provider, particularly in competitive health insurance systems. In the United States, where such competition is sharp, the quality of the health plans offered to insurers has become an important business consideration with insurees and their employers, who generally pay for these programs. In systems where the public sector plays a major role, the quality and safety of health care have become a significant political issue. In other words, it would seem inevitable that negotiations between purchasers and providers are going to become an increasingly important part of this dimension of the qualitative performance of health care. The studies published on this topic are intended primarily to evaluate whether pressure on costs leads to deterioration in the quality of care provided to the insured. On the other hand, since these negotiations are conducted in private, there are no published studies for determining how economic agents make their trade-offs between quality and cost.

We may suggest the following hypotheses. First, we may suppose that the unit cost of service rises with its quality: this is the dominant assumption, that quality is expensive. In a system where purchasers are in competition, and where service providers are also in competition, the purchasers have only partial information available on the relative quality of the providers. They have the basic guarantee offered by accreditation. They may also resort to selective contracting. But the published indicators cover only a portion of providers' activities. The purchaser must therefore make the assumption that if a hospital is doing well in one part of its activity, there is a good probability that it will do so in all activities. On the other hand, the indicators make it difficult to discriminate between providers: the league tables are misleading, by any rigorous standard, and can at best classify providers into three or maybe five groups: high-quality, average/acceptable, low-quality. The economic calculation whereby the purchaser will determine the trade-offs between a marginal unit of additional quality and the unit cost of the service is not easy to perform without a specific examination of each provider. Moreover, it can take two or three years of data collection to confirm an initial ranking. Finally, purchasers are subject to geographic constraints: in any given zone, there are only a finite number of providers. It is generally impossible to select a provider from beyond the residential zone of the insured. Under these conditions, purchasers are likely to avoid the lower-ranked hospitals as far as possible, and to make competition work for them (in terms of costs and prices) among those ranked in the middle. On the other hand, they are not likely to have much bargaining strength with the small number of high-quality establishments. There will always be a degree of heterogeneity, therefore, in the quality of care.

In a system of universal health insurance with a single purchaser, that purchaser will face the same difficulties in making fine distinctions between providers on the basis of their performance and their price-quality ratio. Yet the purchaser has to operate under the constraint of treating all providers equally in terms of their quality of care. Assuming that cost increases with quality, then it is the purchaser's responsibility to make more resources available to the lower-quality providers so that they can catch up with the others. If the results are published, the purchaser may be subjected to heavy pressure from voters (*i.e.* the insured) to upgrade the quality of service and hence to provide more resources across the board.

In both cases, average quality will increase along with costs. In the first case, the poorer providers will be forced out of the market if they cannot shape up, while in the second case the public authorities will guarantee to all providers the means to achieve the best level of performance. We may have some doubts about this scenario, however. In fact, the notion that "quality is expensive" may be true once all providers have reached the same level of performance, but that is far from being the case today. In other words, it is quite possible for providers to enhance their performance while reducing their unit costs. For example, many studies have shown that there is a positive correlation between workload and clinical outcomes. In the hospital business, where fixed costs are high, unit costs will decline as a function of volume. Sending patients to high-volume hospitals, then, can serve both to improve clinical outcomes and to reduce costs. The purchaser can make a quality-cost trade-off only if it is in a position to know the relationship between those two factors, activity by activity. We have already pointed out that only a small part of hospital activity is covered at this time by performance indicators, which means that we are surely far from having exhausted the potential for improving outcomes without increasing costs. There is a further difficulty: the people insured by a given purchaser will not necessarily have the same profile as the average for patients of a given hospital. Since performance indicators cover all of these patients, there may be a performance estimation bias in one direction or the other, depending on whether the purchaser's clients present a greater or lesser risk.

We are faced, then, with a sharp asymmetry of information between insurers and providers, to the detriment of the former, in terms of the quality of care, despite the development of comparative indicators. The purchaser must find incentives that will induce the care provider to make visible efforts to improve its results and to share any productivity gains with the purchaser. For these efforts to be monitored, the provider will have to develop an information system that goes beyond producing the indicators most widely used today. Consequently, transaction costs between the two players will have to rise.

We can now see why studies that attempt to measure the impact of competition on the quality of care tend to produce contradictory results, quite apart from the methodological difficulties of measuring this competition (McLaughlin and Ginsburg, 1998). On one hand, it is by no means certain that the purchaser can really observe the provider's effort to improve its performance. In this case, costs may decline and performance may deteriorate without the purchaser's being aware, or the costs of quality may be shifted to another purchaser or another segment of activity where performance is not measured; or there may be cost-reduction gains resulting from improved performance that are not shared with the purchaser. On the other hand, the intensity of competition may vary depending on the segment of activity of each provider.

3.4. *Summary*

The lessons available about the impact of publicizing hospital performance indicators come mainly from United States, where publicity of this kind is a feature of the competition among purchasers to win insurance clients, and among providers to win purchasers. US experiments have been based on the principle of the "informed consumer", to the point where one initiative, the Consumer Assessment of Health Plans Study, guarantees the quality of information provided by the various open health insurance plans. The weight of consumerism in the United States makes itself felt as well, in the role played by patients' or consumers' associations in publishing comparative health-care studies. The climate is not the same in England, where "league tables" have existed since 1993, but where publication of mortality data began only in 2000. Nor is it the same in France, where publication of comparative performance data began in 1999, and remains the preserve of the mass media. Public purchasers in these two countries have not really introduced any mechanisms for care providers to compete on the basis of their clinical performance. The impacts observed in the United States are thus greater than we should expect to find in a country where the public purchaser is in a monopsonistic position.

We find, then, that the publicity given to comparative studies has had an impact on a portion of the providers concerned, but not on all of them. Some hospitals have undertaken corrective actions and have succeeded in improving their performance significantly in particular treatments. These actions have been most systematic when the study was clearly targeted at improving performance in a particular treatment. In other experiments, such as that in Cleveland, the initial objective was rather to make comparative data available to all players as a basis for making enlightened choices, but the initiative to take corrective action was left to each provider. That initiative is no doubt itself dependent on the provider's competitive position, its negotiating strength with purchasers, and the political clout exerted by local consumers' groups. Despite this limitation, these experiments provide important and useful knowledge to all players on the critical factors in clinical performance. Finally, the impact on patients is ambiguous. The published articles show that information of the clinical type is complex and often misunderstood, and the uninitiated are likely to prefer patient satisfaction indicators to clinical indicators. The publicity given in the press to the ratings awards apparently have a short-term impact, but not a lasting one. There are no studies to reveal how the general public has used this information in choosing a treatment or a hospital. This does not mean that such efforts should be abandoned, but rather that more effective and better-targeted means of communication are required.

4. Recommendations

Publicizing comparative results between hospitals, health services and insurance plans would appear to be an irreversible trend, for several reasons. Rationalizing resource use in health systems implies reducing informational asymmetry between the players, to the benefit of patients and the public or private insurers that speak for them. This publicity is equally justified whether in an American-style competitive system or in public systems that are accountable to their citizens for the quality of tax-funded service. The irreversible nature of the trend is reinforced by the growing ease of access to general information on diseases and their treatments, even if such access is still highly unequal. Yet if publicity is to be of real benefit to the community, it must meet requirements in terms of 1) information systems, 2) partnership with providers, 3) communication with the beneficiaries of health services, and 4) formalizing the price-quality relationship with purchasers.

4.1. Information systems

All the authors stress that a great deal of work will be needed to ensure a) a standardized definition of the data to be collected, b) the regular collection of data, c) the accuracy of information, and d) the quality of statistical manipulation. Such work must be accepted as a responsibility by each provider, of course, but also by the organisation seeking to constitute a comparative database. At the outset, the experiment will require a long training and breaking-in period. During the course of the experiment there will have to be regular audits, with frequent resort to medical files and discussion with the care team to ensure that the information is valid. Each new participant will add to the value of the database, but there will be few benefits of scale when this happens, since while the organisation managing the data may have acquired a degree of expertise, any new participant will still have much to learn. The slightest slippage in terms of quality will throw into question the value of the conclusions and credibility of the database itself.

There is debate over the best way to constitute these databases. In order to reduce the costs of constituting and managing them, some experts recommend making maximum use of existing databases, either administrative or regulatory. The best-known tool is the discharge abstract, which serves among other things to identify a hospital's output in homogeneous patient groupings (the Diagnosis-Related Groups or any other hospitalisation classification system). Yet these data have a drawback in that they are produced for rate-setting purposes, and their coding thus follows precise criteria that may fall far short of a rigorous description of the care process. Moreover, the medical data available are not always sufficiently detailed to measure the outcome of the care process. This is why other experts recommend constituting specific databases, drawing upon detailed clinical data collected during the patient 's period of hospitalisation. In this case, data production is more expensive and data quality is more difficult to maintain. In fact, the health teams must routinely gather data that they will use only briefly in the care process, but that they have no need to memorize. The utility of such an effort is apparent only after the analysis has been done, long after the data are gathered. It is difficult to decide between these two approaches. We do not really know their consequences in terms of costs, compared to the expected benefits of more specific information in the second case. For countries with a shorter history than the

269|

United States has in gathering discharge abstracts, it would be a mistake to think that they can produce prompt results with existing data: American-style discharge abstracts already contain more detailed information then those used in European countries. Some authors place great store in the spreading use of computerized medical files. Yet here again, we must not underestimate the difficulty of developing a common structure of medical files for any country, or a standard definition of all the items involved.

4.2. *Partnership with the medical profession*

These databases serve to compare the performance of medical teams. Physicians are of course ready to participate in efforts to improve their results, but they will be suspicious about the penalties, whether economic or legal, that may be entailed. They are particularly sensitive to the image that a hospital may acquire after publication of negative results in the media. Yet they are a critical and indispensable resource for conducting any such studies. It is they who produce the basic data on the system. They are thus in a position to undermine databases by simply relaxing their vigilance over the quality of information produced. Indeed, such behaviour may be justified if the published data are going to be used to bring malpractice suits against practitioners (Liang, 2000). They are also the principal players in interpreting the results and in translating these into their practice. Finally, their cooperation is likely to be required over the medium term in order to produce significant results. The rules of the game in terms of communicating results, and the decisions that flow from them, should therefore be negotiated in advance and respected for as long as the database is in use. In the Cleveland experiment, for example, cooperation nearly collapsed when one of the partners, the purchaser, reversed its initial commitment and decided to make use of the study results for selecting between hospitals, without submitting the issue to the whole group in advance. It was not the decision itself that was criticized, but the failure to respect the group's written rules. This warning should be understood as a plea to accord medical personnel a degree of immunity: it reflects the clear finding that, even if it is easier today to monitor their behaviour and hold them accountable, they still have considerable discretionary power to justify their decisions *a posteriori*. Informational asymmetry may be reduced, but it does not disappear.

4.3. *Communication with patients*

We know little about the impact of rankings published in the press (or by other means) comparing clinical outcomes for hospitals. It is time to examine this question in greater depth. The most plausible hypothesis is that the attention effect will be short-lived, and will fade over time. This is logical enough: the information produced will be useful mainly to someone who is sick or undergoing treatment, if the ranking provides specific information on that disease and its treatment. Yet this is clearly not the most important point. The fact is that information on clinical outcomes is very complex, particularly if it is given with the kind of methodological reservations favoured by statisticians. It may be misunderstood or its meaning may be completely inverted. It often does not meet the real expectations of the general public, who tend to be more interested in indicators that look at the interpersonal relationship dimension in the caring process and patient satisfaction. People with less education might find clinical outcomes data even more incomprehensible. And these data do not cover all pathologies.

What is needed, then, is to find efficient ways of communicating this information. This can be done by improving the form of the published documentation, which should include several levels of communication and explanation ("layered information") so that everyone can delve further into topics of interest. The information also needs to be contextualised, *i.e.* the cognitive space in which it has meaning should be explained. It is not enough to report outcomes: the treatment process must also be explained. The use of mediators – patients' associations, for example – can be effective in responding to people's questions. Finally, the means of communication must be adapted to the target audience. This in effect might mean launching a process of acculturating the general public to information on the clinical outcomes of hospitals.

We took a critical look at "league tables" earlier in this paper. Rankings of this kind reflect only very roughly the real differences in performance between institutions, and many institutions could well be entitled to demand amends for attacks on their reputation. It is tempting to reproach the media for sensationalism in publishing data in the form of unvalidated rankings. Yet since we do not really know the impact of such publications on the reputation and attractiveness of hospitals, it is difficult to measure their negative effects. There is evidently an effect on hospitals that feel unfairly treated in the rankings: exercising their right of response will not command the same audience as the initial publication. Three solutions suggest themselves for insuring that publications are more rigorous. First, a competing publication might seek to produce a counter-assessment relying on a more rigorous approach, or demonstrating the progress that may have been made since the previous ranking. Second, dialogue could be encouraged between experts and journalists, leading gradually to the publication of more rigorous data with due regard to statistical limitations (Chassin *et al.*, 1996; Rosenthal *et al.*, 1998). Third, the organisations producing the studies could arrange to disseminate them themselves, with the help of communication experts.

4.4. Quality-cost trade-offs

Whether we are speaking of a competitive system or one dominated by the public sector, the link between performance and financing remains largely informal. There are two reasons why this should not surprise us. On one hand, despite the progress in performance measurement studies, hospital activity is so varied that it is difficult to summarize with a few indicators. The relationship between the level of these indicators and the cost of care has yet to be thoroughly examined. Study of this relationship is called for, using benchmarking methods among others. If such benchmarking is to be effective, hospital cooperation is indispensable. Incentives must therefore be found to encourage such cooperation, by sharing the risks and benefits of efforts to provide a better understanding of hospital performance. On the other hand, formalizing this price-quality relationship will require purchasers to be explicit about the price they are ready to pay for an additional unit of quality. A purchaser operating in a competitive environment should in theory obtain this information from the market, while a public purchaser should in principle rely on democratic debate in setting its price. Yet revealing popular preferences is a very difficult task for any government, whether in the health field or in other areas of public policy.

NOTES

1. The sole clinical outcome indicator in Dr. Foster is mortality. The Web site also publishes a descriptive fact sheet for each hospital, comparative outcomes focused primarily on waiting times for each specialty, the number of complaints and the number of complaints processed.

2. In order to compare the performance of health plans, the NCQA has developed a comparative database known as HEDIS (Health Plan Employer Data and Information Set) to which NCQA-accredited plans contribute on a voluntary basis.

3. For the sake of style, we shall use here the terms performance and quality of care interchangeably, to designate, on one hand, indicators that focus on outcomes measured on a biological or clinical basis, and on the other hand the level achieved by a hospital against these indicators. We are not speaking here of efficiency measurement, which would also take into account patient need satisfaction in other dimensions, compared to the costs involved.

4. It may also be that quality preferences are relatively insensitive to the client-perceived level of risk. In France, for example, a significant obstacle to introducing a maternity system ranked in terms of its ability to treat high-risk pregnancies is that low-risk women, who could comfortably give birth in "level 1" facilities, nevertheless prefer the security offered by the high-tech "level 3" maternity hospitals, even when they do not need such care.

REFERENCES

ANSARI, M.Z., ACKLAND, M.J., JOLLEY, D.J., CARSON, N. and MCDONALD, I.G. (1999),
"Inter-hospital comparison of mortality rates", *International Journal of Quality in Health Care*, Vol. 2, No. 1, pp. 29-35.

ARON, D.C., HARMER, D.L., SHEPARDSON, L.B. and ROSENTHAL, G.E. (1998),
"Impact of risk-adjusting Cesarean delivery rates when reporting hospital performance", JAMA, Vol. 279, No. 24, pp. 1968-1972.

BUCKNALL, C.E., RYLAND, I., COOPER, A., COUTTS, H., CONNOLLY, C.K. and PEARSON, M.G. (2000),
"National benchmarking as a support system for clinical governance", *Journal of the Royal College of Physicians of London*, Vol. 34, No. 1, pp. 52-56.

CARON, A. and NEUHAUSER, D. (1999),
"The effect of public accountability on hospital performance: trends in rates for Cesarean section rates and vaginal births after Cesarean section in Cleveland, Ohio", *Quality Management in Health Care*, Vol. 7, No. 2, pp. 1-10.

CHALÉ, J.J. and NAIDITCH, M. (1999),
"Retour sur une enquête controversée", *La Recherche*, No. 324, pp. 71-74.

CHASSIN, M.R., HANNAN, E.L. and DE BUONO, B.A. (1996),
"Benefits and hazards of reporting medical outcomes publicly", NEJM, Vol. 334, No. 6, pp. 394-398.

CIHI (2001),
Hospital Report 2001. www.cihi.ca/HospitalReport/

COMAROW, A. (2000a),
"Higher volumes, fewer deaths", USNews, July 17.

COMAROW, A. (2000b),
"Picking the top centers. Reputation, outcomes and technology all count", USNews, July 17.

COOPER, J.K., KOHLMANN, T., MICHAEL, J.A., HAFFER, S.C. and STEVIC, M. (2001),
"Health outcomes. New quality measure for Medicare", *International Journal for Quality in Health Care*, Vol. 13, No. 1, pp. 9-16.

COULTER, A. and CLEARY, P. (2001),
"Patients' experience with hospital care in five countries", *Health Affairs*, Vol. 20, No. 3, pp. 244-252.

DREES (1999),
"Les éléments de la 'performance' hospitalière", *Études et Résultats*, No. 42, Paris.

DREES (2001),
"Eléments pour évaluer la performance des établissements hospitaliers", *Dossiers solidarité et santé*, No. 2, Paris.

EDDY, D.M. (1998),
"Performance measurement: problems and solutions", *Health Affairs*, Vol. 17, No. 4, pp. 7-25.

EPSTEIN, M. and KURTZIG, B. (1994),
"Statewide health information: a tool for improving hospital accountability", *The Joint Commission Journal of Quality Improvement*, Vol. 20, No. 7, pp. 370-375.

HANNAN, E.L., KILBURN, J.F., O'DONNEL, J.F. *et al.* (1990),
"Adult open heart surgery in New York State. An analysis of risk factors and hospital mortality rates", JAMA, pp. 2768-2774.

HANNAN, E.L., KILBURN, J.F., RACZ, M. *et al.* (1994),
"Improving the outcomes of Coronary Bypass Surgery in New York State", JAMA, No. 271, pp. 761-766.

HANNAN, E.L., SIU, A.L., KUMAR, D. *et al.* (1995),
"The decline in Coronary Bypass Graft Surgery Mortality in New York State. The role of surgeon volume", JAMA, No. 273, pp. 209-213.

HIBBARD, J.H., SLOVIC, P. and JEWETT, J.J. (1997),
"Informing consumer decisions in health care: implications from decision-making research", *The Milbank Quarterly*, Vol. 75, No. 3, pp. 395-414.

HIBBARD, J.H., SOFAER, S. and JEWETT, J.J. (1996),
"Condition-specific performance information: assessing salience, comprehension, and approaches for communicating quality", *Healthcare Financing Review*, Vol. 18, No. 1, pp. 95-111.

HILLNER, B.E., SMITH, T.J. and DESCH, C.E. (2000),
"Hospital and physician volume or specialization and outcomes in cancer treatment: importance in quality of cancer care", *J Clin Oncol*, Vol. 18, No. 11, pp. 2327-2340.

HUMPHREYS, H. and EMMERSON, A.M. (1993),
"Control of hospital acquired infection: accurate data and more resources, not league tables", *Journal of Hospital Infection*, No. 25, pp. 75-78.

IEZZONI, L. (1997),
"The risks of risk adjustment", JAMA, Vol. 278, No. 19, pp. 1600-1607.

IEZZONI, L., SCHWARTZ, M., ASH, A.S., HUGHES, J.S., DALEY, J. and MACKIERNAN, Y.D. (1995),
"Using severity-adjusted stroke mortality rates to judge hospitals", *International Journal for Quality in Health Care*, Vol. 7, No. 2, pp. 81-94.

JEWETT, J.J. and HIBBARD, J.H. (1996),
"Comprehension of quality indicators: differences among privately insured, publicly insured and uninsured", *Healthcare Financing Review*, Vol. 18, No. 1, pp. 75-94.

Joint Commission on Accreditation of Health Care Organizations (2001),
The Self-assessment Checklist: Hospitals, Oakbrook terrace, Illinois, United States.

KRITSCHESKY, S.B., BRAUN, B.I., GROSS, P.A., NEWCOMB, C.S., KELLEHER, C.A. and SIMMONS, B.P. (1999),
"Definition and adjustment of Cesarean section rates and assessments of hospital performance", *International Journal for Quality in Health Care*, Vol. 2, No. 4, pp. 283-291.

LANDON, B., IEZZONI, L., ASH, A., SHWARTZ, M., DALEY, J., HUGUES, J.S. and MACKIERNAN, Y.D. (1996),
"Judging hospitals by severity adjusted mortality rates: the case of CABG surgery", *Inquiry*, No. 33, pp. 155-166.

LEYLAND, A.H. and BODDY, F.A. (1998),
"League tables and acute myocardial infarction", *The Lancet*, No. 351, pp. 555-558.

LIANG, B.A. (2000),
"Risks of reporting sentinel events", *Health Affairs*, Vol. 19, No. 5, pp. 113-120.

LOMBRAIL, P. and NAIDITCH, M. (1999),
"Comment partager l'information ?", *La Recherche*, No. 324, pp. 75-78.

MARSHALL, R. (2001),
"Where We Get the Best Health Care", *Macleans*, No. 114, pp.31-36.

MCCORMACK, L.A., GARFINKEL, S.A., SCHNAIER, J.A., LEE, A.J. and SANGL, J.A. (1996),
"Consumer information development and use", *Healthcare Financing Review*, Vol. 18, No. 1, pp. 15-31.

MCKEE, M. and HUNTER, D. (1995),
"Hospital league tables: do they inform or mislead?", *Quality in Health Care*, No. 4, pp. 5-12.

MCLAUGHLIN, C.G. and GINSBURG, P.B. (1998),
"Competition, quality of care and the role of the consumer", *The Milbank Quarterly*, Vol. 76, No. 4, pp. 737-743.

MC MULLAN, M. (1996),
"HCFA's consumer information commitment", *Healthcare Financing Review*, Vol. 18, No. 1, pp. 9-15.

MINVIELLE, E. (1996),
"Gérer la singularité à grande échelle", *Revue Française de Gestion*, No. 109, pp. 119-124.

NHS (1995),
The NHS Performance Guide 1994-1995, London.

NAIDITCH, M. (1999),
"L'exemple de la chirurgie cardiaque new-yorkaise", *La Recherche*, No. 324, pp. 66-70.

NATHENS, A.B., JURKOVICH, G.J., GROSSMAN, D.C., MACKENZIE, E.J. and RIVARA, F.P. (2001),
"Relationship between trauma center volume and outcomes", JAMA, Vol. 285, No. 9, pp. 1164-1171.

PHILLIPS, K.A., LUFT, H.S. and Ritchie, J.L. (1995),
"The association of hospital volumes of percutaneous transluminal coronary angioplasty with adverse outcomes, length of stay, and charges in California", *Medical Care*, Vol. 33, No. 5, pp. 502-514.

LE POINT (2001),
"Hôpitaux. Le Palmarès 2001", No. 1151, August 31.

RITCHIE, J.L., MAYNARD, C., CHAPKO, M.K., EVERY, N.R. and MARTIN, D.C. (1999),
"Association between percutaneous transluminal coronary angioplasty volumes and outcomes in the Health Care Cost and Utilization Project 1993-1994", AM J *Cardiol*, Vol. 83, No. 4, pp. 493-497.

ROMANO, P.S., ZACH, A., LUFT, H.S., RAINWATER, J., RELY, L.L. and CAMPA, D. (1995),
"The California Hospital Outcomes Project: using administrative data to compare hospital performance", *The Joint Commission Journal on Quality Improvement*, Vol. 21, No. 12, pp. 668-685.

ROSENTHAL, G. (1997),
"Weak association between hospital mortality for individual diagnoses: implications for profiling hospital quality", *American Journal of Public Health*, Vol. 87, No. 3, pp. 429-433.

ROSENTHAL, G.E., QUINN, L. and HARPER, D.L. (1997),
"Declines in Hospital Mortality associated with a regional initiative to measure hospital performance", *American Journal of Medical Quality*, Vol. 12, No. 2, pp. 103-112.

ROSENTHAL, G.E., HAMMAR, P.J., WAY, L.E., SHIPLEY, S.A., DONER, D., WOJTALA, B., MILLER, J. and HARMER, D.L. (1998),
"Using hospital performance data in quality improvement: the Cleveland Health Quality Choice Experience", *The Joint Commission Journal on Quality Improvement*, Vol. 24, No. 7, pp. 347-360.

SHAW, C.D. (1997),
"Health-care league tables in the United Kingdom", J. Qual. Clin. Practice, No. 17, pp. 215-219.

SILBER, J.H. and ROSENBAUM, P.R. (1997),
"A spurious correlation between hospital mortality and complication rates: the importance of severity adjustment", *Medical Care*, No. 35(suppl.), pp. OS77-OS92.

SIRIO, C.A., ANGUS, D.C. and ROSENTHAL, G.E. (1994),
"Cleveland Health Quality Choice (CHQC) – An ongoing collaborative, community based outcomes assessment program", *New Horizons*, Vol. 2, No. 3, pp. 321-325.

SISK, J. (1998),
"Increased competition and the quality of health care", *The Milbank Quarterly*, Vol. 76, No. 4, pp. 687-707.

THOMAS, J.W. and HOFER, T.P. (1999),
"Accuracy of risk-adjusted mortality rate as a measure of hospital quality of care", *Medical Care*, Vol. 37, No. 1, pp. 83-92.

VOELKER, R. (1995),
"Why has historic' diclosure of hospital performance data attracted so little attention?", JAMA, Vol. 273, No. 9, pp. 689-690.

Chapter 13

MEASURING THE QUALITY OF LONG-TERM CARE IN INSTITUTIONAL AND COMMUNITY SETTINGS

by

Naoki Ikegami[*], John P. Hirdes[**] and Iain Carpenter[***]

Abstract

Our objective lies in clarifying the basic issues in long-term care (LTC) policy, describing instruments for the comprehensive assessment of those receiving LTC in institutional and community settings, and demonstrating how the assessment database could be used to measure quality.

A clearly defined LTC policy is needed to avoid distortions and fiscal strains in programmes designed for health, social welfare and housing. Since the need for LTC services can be broadly interpreted, policy-makers should first focus on developing entitlement standards to ensure equitable access. Next, the focus should be on measuring quality by collecting data on the process of care and how it impacts on the functional, cognitive and emotional status of the recipients.

The development of the MDS (Minimum Data Set) in the United States was a break through towards obtaining accurate data for this purpose. The MDS has been mandated in virtually every nursing home in the United States since 1991, and also in Iceland and two provinces in Canada. It has been translated and validated in over 20 countries. A home care version of the MDS, the MDS-HC, has been developed by interRAI, an international non-profit organisation of researchers and clinicians. This development shares core assessment items so that seamless care can be provided regardless of site, while also having specific items tailored to meet the unique needs in home care.

Using the databases of the MDS and MDS-HC, quality indicators have been developed to compare quality among providers within and across countries. In Canada, data for hospitals providing complex continuing care in the province of Ontario showed that a third of patients were restrained on a daily basis, which might lead to pressure ulcers. This finding contributed to the recent adoption of more restrictive policies on restraint use in Ontario. Otherwise, the pilot implementation of quality indicators in single point entry agencies to community and institutional services still in Ontario showed that a high proportion of clients who would potentially have benefited from rehabilitation did not receive such services.

---

[*]   Professor, Department of Health Policy & Management, School of Medicine, Keio University, Tokyo, Japan.
[**] Associate Professor, Department of Health Studies and Gerontology, University of Waterloo, Ontario, Canada.
[***] Reader, Centre for Health Service Studies, University of Kent, UK.

Acknowledgements: The authors would like to gratefully acknowledge an earlier paper commissioned by the OECD entitled "The potential for micro-data in assessing performance, needs and outcomes for long-term care at the international level" by G.I. Carpenter, J.P. Hirdes, B.E. Fries, D. Frijters, and R. Bernabei; and also for the support from interRAI.

1.   Basic issues in long-term care

1.1. *The rationale for establishing a long-term care social policy*

Since there is some confusion on what exactly is "long-term care" (LTC), the definition given by the Institute of Medicine (1986) is a useful start. This states that LTC is "a variety of ongoing health and social services provided for individuals who need assistance on a continuing basis because of physical or mental disability. Services can be provided in an institution, the home, or community, and include informal services provided by family or friends as well as formal services provided by professionals or agencies". A careful reading of this brief explanation provides us with some hints as to why it has been difficult to establish LTC as an integral part of social security (Ikegami and Campbell, 2001).

The first lies in the difficulty of defining the proper line between public and private responsibility. It is easy to agree that care for an elderly woman who is alone, impoverished, and frail should be a public responsibility. But what if her husband is alive and fairly healthy? Or what if there is money in the bank, or an asset like a house or car? Should she still be eligible for publicly funded services? If so, should her children inherit those assets? If the children are well-off, should they contribute? Or if nearby children could provide hands-on care? In fact, most hands-on care for frail older people in the community is provided by family members (OECD, 1996). If formal services were provided, would families withdraw? Conflicting views on these issues make it difficult to achieve a consensus on LTC policy.

A second problem is that LTC requires "a variety of ongoing health and social services". Health and social service professionals have very different goals and working styles (Kane, 1999). In general, health professionals may try to focus on objective measures of change in health status, and they may become disinterested if improvement is unlikely. On the other hand, social service professionals may be more empathetic and may pay insufficient attention to the possibilities of improvement with medical treatment. These differences in education and training may make it difficult for members of the two professions to collaborate in teams. Differences in how medical and social services are organised and financed may make cooperation even harder to develop and sustain at the institutional level.

The third and perhaps most crucial reason for the reluctance to think seriously about expanding LTC is simply cost. The governments of all the industrialized nations are worried about the increasing burdens of population ageing on their pension and health care systems. In that context, taking on long-term care as a new, costly entitlement programme may seem foolhardy.

However, despite these formidable obstacles, no one can deny that there will be an increasing demand for formal LTC services because of the ageing of society and the decline in family support.[1] If this demand could not be met appropriately, it would cause distortions and fiscal strains in programmes designed for other purposes, such as health insurance, social welfare, and housing. The strains fall particularly on the hospital services that are usually available on a universal basis, in contrast to the restricted means-testing in social welfare. This would not only be inefficient, but would also be inequitable because, under strained systems, the limited resources are likely to be allocated in a way that would be perceived as unfair by the public. These concerns led the OECD nations in 1998 to agree on trying "to co-ordinate the roles of health and social care systems so they provide appropriate and integrated care for those with long-term needs".[2] Thus, the policy objective is to design, implement and monitor a LTC programme that is both equitable and efficient. For that purpose, the measuring of quality plays a crucial role.

1.2. *Equitable access as the first criterion for quality*

Since the need for LTC services can be so broadly interpreted, governments should first focus on developing entitlement standards that determine access to services partly or totally publicly funded. As in health care, fair access should be regarded as the first criterion for measuring quality in LTC. However, unlike health care, the task of allocating resources cannot be left simply to the professional judgement of individual physicians. There is no one profession that has the required expertise in all the various aspects of LTC who would be trusted by the public. Thus, the standards must be clear, objective and be regarded as fair by both the public and providers. In order to achieve this objective, the following must be developed.

- An assessment instrument that objectively evaluates the individual's (and where deemed appropriate, the family's) status;
- Explicit guidelines or an algorithm that allocates the amount of entitled benefits according to the assessed information;
- Training staff to appropriately use the assessment instrument;
- Establish formal mechanisms for monitoring the eligibility process by the government and for accepting appeals of adverse decisions from beneficiaries.

Of particular importance is the development of an assessment instrument to evaluate the individual's physical abilities (*e.g.*, degree of assistance needed in performing daily tasks such as eating or bathing) and mental status (*e.g.*, memory, ability to make decisions). The accurate measurement of these attributes is essential for developing the criteria for allocating benefits. Once the programme is established, these same measures can be used for evaluating the quality of care or for on-going monitoring of service delivery. Each item should have high reliability and validity because the rating on any one of the items could become the key aspect for deciding their eligibility status. This status would be directly reflected in the amount of services that would be made available to individuals and, ultimately, the financial burden that would be ultimately placed on society.

If such eligibility standards could be established, containing costs in LTC should be an easier task compared with acute health care for the following reasons. First, LTC has different norms with respect to what is "equitable". In acute health care, the public expects that whatever is medically necessary should be provided – even at high cost – and treatment should not be related to the ability to pay. In contrast, it may be more acceptable to argue that everyone is entitled to some minimum standard of LTC, but those with more money can live more comfortably for what is at stake is more a matter of degrees of comfort and unpleasantness than life versus death. Thus, compared with health care, LTC expenditures should be relatively predictable and controllable at both the individual and the system levels because levels of need do not change as rapidly, life-or-death interventions and high-cost technology are not as important, and organisational routines rather than independent professionals can control more of the decision-making.

Second, not all elderly individuals would want to consume the full amount of services they may be entitled to if these services were explicitly categorized as "LTC".[3] Some may prefer the care given by their family or friends, and not welcome care workers coming into their homes. In acute care, patients are much more likely to take full advantage of whatever benefits they may be entitled to. The fact that the use of LTC services may be discretionary has been borne out in Japan's first year's experience of implementing its public LTC insurance programme: expenditures have been more than 10 per cent less than projected and about the same level as before the implementation (Ikegami, 2001).

In addition, savings may also be realized through more appropriate placement in LTC of individuals who might otherwise occupy acute care beds. Thus, formally establishing LTC as an independent social security programme may not be as costly as some may fear. The issue hinges on whether fair, transparent and sustainable eligibility standards can be developed. Policy-makers must decide the criteria which best reflect the prevailing societal values. What the research community can contribute is to provide a scientific basis for evaluating each option and the development of measurement instruments.

1.3. Measuring the quality of LTC services

Once there is equitable access to publicly funded LTC services, the next question is what can governments do to ensure their quality? As noted earlier, most LTC will continue to be provided informally by family or friends even when formal services become readily accessible. One might argue that the goal of formal services is to deliver the kind of devoted care that families provide to their members. However, although this may well be the first aspect of quality in LTC, the amount of love and devotion that professionals and care-workers may provide is difficult to measure.

The second aspect of quality is the same as in any service industry: the friendliness of the staff and, in institutional care, the comfort and cleanliness of the rooms, the tastiness of the food etc. At a more basic level, there are standards for preventing fire hazards, maintaining sanitation and monitoring staff negligence. However, these features are not unique to LTC and can be readily adapted from what has been developed in other sectors.

The third aspect of quality is through the licensing and certification of institutional facilities and home care agencies by the government. This will be based on the facility requirements that have already been dealt by the second aspect, and on the hiring of appropriately trained staff. Quality will be measured by whether they have professional qualifications or licensures for having undergone some formal training. However, this may be a necessary, but not a sufficient condition for quality.

The last aspect of quality is how the services impact on the status of the recipients. Although most LTC may continue to be provided by families or friends, instructions may be needed on how they should do so. Providing information and training to informal caregivers are the responsibility of the formal services. In addition, in institutional settings, and in the care that requires more technical expertise (such as treating pressure ulcers), professionals and care workers are directly responsible for the quality of care they provide. Those receiving LTC are not in a state of steady and irreversible decline: the quality of life of individuals and their informal caregivers can be improved, accidents (such as falls) avoided and the rate of decline slowed down. For example, appropriate handling of problem behaviour of those with Alzheimer's disease could alleviate some of its devastating consequences. Adequate nutrition could prevent hospitalisation for dehydration. Periodic turning over of the body would prevent pressure ulcers.

Monitoring the quality of LTC could be an easier process than in acute care, because those receiving LTC tend to be more homogenous in their attributes and the service options are more limited. Moreover, those receiving LTC are, by definition, doing so on a continuous basis. Thus, any lapse in the care provided could have immediate impact on the individual. For example, failing to periodically turn over someone who is completely immobile may lead to the development of pressure ulcers the next day. In contrast, we need to wait for the results of the five years' survival rate for the treatment of cancer. However, in order to measure quality, accurate assessments of the individual's status must be made in order to provide a base-line, and to compare quality among providers. This will be the subject of the next section.

2. The RAI (Resident Assessment Instrument) and the RAI-HC (Home Care)

2.1. *The development and use of the RAI*

The RAI (Resident Assessment Instrument) was originally developed in the United States in response to an Institute of Medicine (IoM) study calling for the creation of a uniform, comprehensive resident assessment system to improve the quality of care in nursing homes (Institute of Medicine, 1986). It has three components. The first is a comprehensive set of standardised items, the MDS (Minimum Data Set), for assessing the strengths and weaknesses of residents, and the care provided in institutional settings (see Table 1). The second component consists of the Resident Assessment Protocols (RAPs) that provide guidance for best practice in care planning for problems, risks and potential for improvement in 18 domains identified by the assessment items (see Table 2). Each RAP has a unique set of items called "triggers", that if checked, prompt the assessor to explore issues that are relevant for the problem, risk or potential for improvement triggered by the item (Table 3). For example, if the resident is checked for the item "dizziness", that resident needs to be examined in the RAP area of "Falls". In this way, the RAPs provide clinicians with a systematic method that promotes best practice in identifying and planning care for the wide range of complex problems faced by older people admitted to long term care (Morris *et al.*, 1996). The third component is the utilisation guidelines that are instructions on when and how to use the RAI.

Table 1. **Sections of the Resident Assessment Instrument (RAI)**

• Identification and background information	• Physical functioning and structural problems
• Communication/hearing patterns	• Vision patterns
• Mood and behaviour patterns	• Psychosocial well-being
• Activity pursuit patterns	• Medication use
• Medications	• Continence in last 14 days
• Special treatments, devices, procedures, and supplies	• Disease diagnoses/health conditions
• Skin condition and foot care	• Oral/dental status
• Oral/nutritional status	• Participation in assessments
• Cognitive patterns	

Source: Morris *et al.* (1996).

Table 2. **Domains of the Resident Assessment Protocols (RAPs)**

• Delirium	• Cognitive loss/dementia
• Visual function	• Communication
• ADL Functional/rehabilitation	• Urinary continence/catheter
• Psychosocial well-being	• Mood state
• Behaviour problems	• Activities
• Falls	• Nutritional status
• Feeding tubes	• Dehydration/fluid maintenance
• Dental care	• Pressure ulcers
• Psychotropic drug use	• Physical restraints

Source: Morris *et al.* (1996).

The RAI was implemented in the United States in 1991 and is required for all nursing home residents (regardless of whether they are paid for by government funding or not) in virtually all nursing homes in the nation. The federally mandated nursing home survey system also audits the assessments and their use by facilities in care planning as part of assuring compliance with acceptable standards of care. All facilities nation-wide must implement computerised reporting and a national archive for research and monitoring purposes is being developed.

In a national evaluation of its implementation, there were the following major findings.[4]

• An increase in the comprehensiveness and accuracy of the information available in residents' medical records.

Table 3. **Structure of the Resident Assesment
Instrument (RAI)**

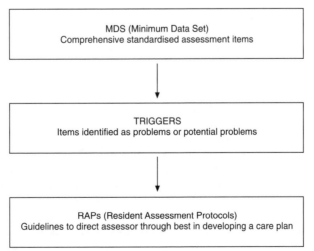

Source: Morris *et al.* (1996).

- An increase in the comprehensiveness of care planning, with care plans in the post implementation period addressing a greater percentage of residents' health problems, risk factors, and their potential for improved function.

- Improvements in a wide array of other care processes that affect residents' quality of care and quality of life, including increased involvement of families and residents in care planning, increased use of advance directives, increased use of behaviour management programs, increased involvement in activities, and decreased use of problematic interventions, such as indwelling urinary catheters and physical restraints.

- Significant reductions in decline among residents in such areas as physical functioning in ADLs, cognitive status, and urinary continence.

- A significant reduction in the number of nursing home residents who were hospitalised, with no increase in mortality.

Outside of the United States, the RAI has been translated and validated in over 20 countries. At present, its use is mandated in Iceland and two provinces of Canada. In Japan, the government-sponsored translation of the manual sold over 300 000 copies and virtually introduced the concept of comprehensive care planning. The inter-observer reliability of the assessment items undertaken in eight countries shows that the values are of the same high level as the original (Hawes *et al.*, 1995; Sgadari *et al.*, 1997). Its use in other countries has illustrated important lessons about making comparisons from one country to another. These include wide variation in the characteristics of residents of institutions that may be referred to as "nursing homes" (Fries *et al.*, 1997). Furthermore, by examining resident level information one can begin to understand how expenditures in LTC result in providing care to different sections of the population (Carpenter *et al.*, 1999).

2.2. *The development and use of the* RAI-HC

The home care version of the RAI, the RAI-HC, was developed in 1996 by an international consortium of researchers in LTC, the interRAI, and tested in multiple countries before its completion. Its assessment form, the MDS-HC (Minimum Data Set – Home Care), is broader in scope in order to be able to assess the unique aspects of home care such as the role of informal support, indicators of elder abuse, IADL performance (Instrumental Activities of Daily Living, such as preparing meals), adherence to care programmes, environmental situation and a variety of health conditions including preventative health measures. At the same time it is shorter in length than the nursing home version in order to accommodate the more limited time available for assessment in a home care situation. This was made possible by relying more extensively on the second level detailed assessment in the Client Assessment Protocols (CAPs) for the areas that are triggered for further investigation. There are 30 CAPs, including new domains such as "Institutional Risk", "Health Promotion", "Elder Abuse" and "Adherence", while retaining the same domains such as "Depression and Anxiety", "Behaviour" and "Psychotropic Drugs" of the original nursing home version. In addition, they include background information and detailed care planning guidelines to serve as a training manual and reference. Cross-training and self-education to possess adequate knowledge of both the health and social service sectors become particularly important in home care because, unlike in institutional settings, they are usually working alone.

Where an assessment concept makes sense in both the nursing home and community settings, identical items are used. These items compose about half of the about 200 items in the home care version. In the key areas of cognition, communication, vision, mood, behaviour, ADL and continence, 30 of the 32 home care items are identical with the nursing home version. Thus, it is possible to track individuals as they move back and forth between community and institutional care, while at the same time, being sensitive to the unique aspects that need to be assessed in each. Moreover, since they will both be using essentially the same care planning methodology, dialogue between professionals in the two sectors will be greatly facilitated. These assessment instruments therefore comprise an integrated health information system (Hirdes *et al.*, 1999).

The inter-observer reliability results of the home care version were equally high in all the five countries tested in the developmental stage and equivalent to levels achieved in the original (Morris *et al.*, 1997). It has subsequently been translated and validated in over ten countries. Governments have implemented, or are about to do so, in nine US states, five Canadian provinces and several regions in Italy. It is the most widely used assessment instrument in Japan and is being used for an EU Vth Framework study that compares recipients of home care and the structural and organisational characteristics of service agencies in 11 European Countries (interRAI 2000). Preliminary cross-national comparisons of home care clients show that there are wide differences in their characteristics.

3. The use of MDS for measuring quality

3.1. Using quality indicators (QIs) in institutional settings

Quality of care assessment has traditionally been a survey of a facilities' capability to perform care (staffing levels, physical facility standards etc.) or reliance on patient ratings given in satisfaction surveys. Facility inspections are often not informative because they do not deal directly with the quality of care received by individual residents and facility attributes may not be the primary determinant of the individual's quality of life in the facility. Patient satisfaction surveys are plagued by numerous serious limitations including inadequate response rates, response bias (*e.g.*, due to fear of reprisal), and exclusion of individuals with cognitive impairment. The MDS permits a more sensitive and meaningful measure of service quality by focussing on standardised measures of the process and outcomes of care (Hirdes *et al.*, 1998; Mor *et al.*, 1998; Phillips *et al.*, 1997; Zimmerman *et al.*, 1995).

The most recent version of the Quality Indicators (QIs) is shown on Table 4 (Center for Health Care Systems Research and Analysis, 1999). There are 24 indicators that directly examine care processes (*e.g.*, polypharmacy, restraint use) and clinical outcomes (*e.g.*, appearance of cognitive impairment, decline in range of motion). The former focuses on the prevalence on a cross-sectional basis, while the latter focuses on incidence for the changes in conditions between two assessments. All data are abstracted from the assessment form, so that there is no need to collect additional data for the purposes of evaluating quality. In the United States, the QIs are being used by state surveyors for

Table 4. **Quality indicators (QIs) for evaluating institutional care**

QI 1 Incidence of new fractures
QI 2 Prevalence of falls
QI 3 Prevalence of behavioral symptoms*
QI 4 Prevalence of symptoms of depression
QI 5 Prevalence of symptoms of depression without antidepressant therapy
QI 6 Use of nine or more different medications
QI 7 Incidence of cognitive impairment
QI 8 Prevalence bladder or bowel incontinence*
QI 9 Prevalence of occasional or frequent bladder or bowel incontinence without a toileting plan
QI 10 Prevalence of indwelling catheters
QI 11 Prevalence of fecal impaction
QI 12 Prevalence of urinary tract infections
QI 13 Prevalence of weight loss
QI 14 Prevalence of tube feeding
QI 15 Prevalence of dehydration
QI 16 Prevalence of bedfast residents
QI 17 Incidence of decline in late-loss ADLs
QI 18 Incidence of decline in ROM (Range of Motion)
QI 19 Prevalence of antipsychotic use in the absence of psychotic or related conditions*
QI 20 Prevalence of any antianxiety/hypnotic use
QI 21 Prevalence of hypnotic use more than two times in the last week
QI 22 Prevalence of daily physical restraints
QI 23 Prevalence of little or no activity
QI 24 Prevalence of Stage 1-4 pressure ulcers*

* Different rates calculated for those at "high risk" and "low risk" for these conditions.
Source: Center for Health Care Systems Research and Analysis (1999).

283

evaluating the quality of care in nursing homes. In Canada, the Canadian Institute for Health Information (CIHI) has for the last three years released provincial status reports on the quality of complex continuing care in Ontario (Teare *et al.*, 2000). The 1999 CIHI report helped to bring the issue of physical restraint use to the public forefront by showing that about one third of complex continuing care patients are restrained on a daily basis. In the following year's report, a special feature on restraints provided a comprehensive analysis of predictors and outcomes associated with their use. In 2001, a private members bill in the provincial legislature received a rare unanimous vote in favour of more restrictive policies on restraint use in Ontario. While these reports were by no means the sole influence in this debate, this new legislation provided a compelling example of the value of evidence in supporting decision-making. The Ontario Hospital Association also now makes extensive use of QIs as part of a new public report card on the quality of complex continuing care hospitals/units. The Canadian Council of Health Services Accreditation (CCHSA) has also recently included QIs in the list of indicators employed in its Achieving Improved Measurement (AIM) standards for accreditation.

Tables 5 to 7 provide the results for three QIs for Ontario Complex Continuing Care hospitals/units, by region (see Teare *et al.*, 2000 for a detailed report on these findings). These QI results are based on 33 071 assessments (based on 16 042 individuals) and 32 437 (based on 16 107 individuals) in 1997-98 and 1998-99, respectively.

Table 5 provides the results for pressure ulcers of various levels of severity ranging from areas of persistent redness (Stage 1) to breaks in the skin exposing muscle or bone (Stage 4). The pain associated with pressure ulcers has serious negative quality of life consequences for the institutionalised elderly, and they are costly to treat and prevent from the facility's perspective. Regions 1 and 4 tended to have the highest rates of pressure ulcers among high-risk patients in both years, whereas the other regions were reasonably comparable to each other for that group. However, in both years the rate of pressure ulcers in the low risk group was lowest in Region 3, the Greater Toronto area. Region 1 tended to have high rates for both groups, but it did show some improvement in pressure ulcer rates for the low risk group in 1998-99.

Table 6 shows the prevalence of use of anti-psychotic medications in the absence of psychotic and related conditions. Anti-psychotic medications can be appropriate for use with some populations (*e.g.*, persons with schizophrenia), but they may be associated with adverse outcomes such as falls or changes in cognitive function. For both the high risk and the low risk groups the rates of this quality indicator were lowest in Region 3 and highest in Region 5, Southwest Ontario. In both years, the rate of

Table 5. **Prevalence of stage 1-4 pressure ulcers by risk status,
Ontario complex continuing care hospitals/units, 1997-1999**

Ontario regions		1997-98	1998-99
Region 1	High risk*	23.2	25.5
	Low risk	14.2	10.9
Region 2	High risk	18.3	18.7
	Low risk	10.4	9.4
Region 3	High risk	20.0	18.6
	Low risk	6.3	7.0
Region 4	High risk	25.4	26.3
	Low risk	9.4	9.4
Region 5	High risk	19.0	18.8
	Low risk	9.7	7.5
All regions	High risk	21.2	21.0
	Low risk	9.0	8.5

* High risk is defined based on the presence of one or more of the following conditions: comatose; impaired bed mobility; impaired transferring; end stage disease with life expectancy of less than six months; left 25% of food uneaten at most meals in the last seven days.
Source: Teare *et al.* (2000).

Table 6. **Prevalence of anti-psychotic drug use in the absence of psychotic and related conditions by risk status, Ontario complex continuing care hospitals, 1997-1999**

Ontario regions		1997-98	1998-99
Region 1	High risk*	37.8	43.0
	Low risk	10.8	9.6
Region 2	High risk	34.4	36.2
	Low risk	10.8	11.5
Region 3	High risk	29.5	30.9
	Low risk	8.2	7.2
Region 4	High risk	33.4	34.5
	Low risk	9.0	9.1
Region 5	High risk	45.8	46.8
	Low risk	17.5	18.7
All regions	High risk	34.2	35.7
	Low risk	10.2	9.9

* High risk is defined based on the presence of one or more of the following conditions: cognitive impairment, verbal abuse, physical abuse and socially inappropriate/disruptive behaviour.
Source: Teare et al. (2000).

anti-psychotic use in the low risk group in Region 5 is more than double the rate in Region 3 and the rate in the high-risk group is about 50 per cent greater (in relative terms).

Table 7 shows the QI for the prevalence of tube feeding that is not adjusted for risk. Unlike the other two indicators, Region 3 has a substantially higher rate of tube feeding compared with other jurisdictions and is more than double that of Regions 1 and 5. The reasons for this difference are not clear at this time, but they reflect important differences in practice patterns requiring additional investigation. It is possible, for example, that physicians in large metropolitan areas may have a different view on the utility of tube feeding compared with their colleagues in other jurisdictions. On the other hand, cultural differences in Toronto-based patients and their families may make them more likely to select aggressive interventions at the end of life than in other parts of the province. A second point of particular interest for this table is that tube feeding rates are going up in all regions of the province. Again, the reason for this is not yet known, but one possible explanation is generalized reductions in staffing levels across the province.

For administrative purposes, the quality results can be compared and evaluated in a variety of ways. Simple comparisons of the absolute values of incidence and prevalence rates for specific indicators can be used to compare different facilities or for internal comparisons within facilities over time. One may also place facilities in rank order based on their rates with the aim of computing a percentile rank. In the United States, state surveyors tend to focus their follow-up inquiries on those facilities with rates that exceed the 90th percentile for the industry. However, from a normative perspective, this must be done

Table 7. **Prevalence of tube feeding, Ontario complex continuing care hospitals, 1997-1999**

	1997-98		1998-99	
	Prevalence	N	Prevalence	N
Region 1	9.8	2 222	11.5	2 028
Region 2	13.0	3 064	15.2	3 581
Region 3	21.0	8 075	23.5	7 913
Region 4	12.5	4 838	15.2	4 702
Region 5	10.5	2 570	12.5	2 276
All regions	15.3	20 769	17.7	20 500

Source: Teare et al. (2000).

Figure 1. **Radar plot of percentile ranks by quality indicator, anonymous Ontario facility, 1995**

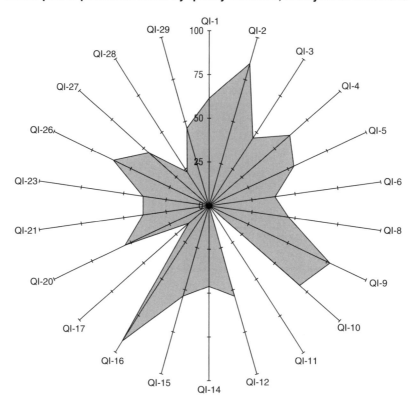

Source: Hirdes *et al.* (1998).

with some caution because the industry as a whole may perform poorly (*e.g.*, uniformly high rates in one indicator) and this would not be detected using only comparisons of ranks.

In addition to their use in monitoring performance and focusing quality improvement efforts, QIs have a number of other uses. They may be incorporated into consumer report cards so that the lay public can gain information on the performance of specific facilities based on scientifically sound measures. The objective performance data for each facility can be helpful to external assessors for accreditation purposes. A facility can also use the indicators to demonstrate a track record of previous performance, as well as the effects of remedial interventions aimed at improving previous quality concerns.

It should be noted that the indicators measure discrete areas for quality: there is no composite score for evaluating overall quality. In practice, a facility may perform well in several areas but usually not in all. This provides opportunities for improving care in the problem areas and for ensuring the staff that they are doing well in others. No health facility, no matter how excellent, performs well in all areas of quality. Figure 1 plots the QIs for a facility as it ranks in percentiles among the Ontario chronic-care hospitals: the further out each indicator is plotted from the centre of each radar axis (the shaded area), the greater the proportion of facilities which have better quality (the indicators shown are the old version so they do not correspond to those listed in Table 4). So for example, QI16, which measures those with dehydration, this particular hospital performs well, but for QI17, measuring those who are bedfast, the hospital performs poorly.

3.2. An alternative method for measuring quality across countries

Unfortunately for the purposes of international comparisons, there are caveats in the QIs that are now currently used in the United States and Canada. These indicators have been developed for the purposes of comparing the quality of facilities that provide care for residents having relatively similar medical and functional characteristics. Although this may be the case for nursing homes within each state of the United States and for the Ontario Complex Continuing Care hospitals/units, it would not be so across countries where LTC facilities have different functions. In order to solve this problem, more sophisticated risk-adjustments must be made. First, the indicators must be adjusted according to the conditions of the residents newly admitted to that nursing home. For example, if a nursing home admits a high proportion of residents with pressure ulcers or restraints from hospitals, it can be expected that their prevalence would be high at any given point of time. The second is adjusting for the difference in the subsequent decline in the residents already admitted. For example, if current residents have a relatively high proportion of faecal incontinence or pressure ulcers, it is expected that a higher ratio of indwelling catheters would be placed. For the first condition, adjustments must be made according to the admission assessment data. For the second condition, multiple assessments of the same resident are needed. The statistical methodology for making sophisticated risk-adjustments at these two levels, the second generation Mega QI Project, has just been completed by a team headed by John Morris. However, the databases needed for making these adjustments have yet to be built in jurisdictions other than the United States and Ontario.

Given these circumstances, to illustrate the potentials of using the assessment data for international comparisons on quality, we have used the following cruder methods for risk-adjustment by respectively dichotomising residents according to physical (using a six-category ADL self-performance index for six ADL items, Morris *et al.*, 1999) and cognitive (using the MDS cognitive performance scale, Morris *et al.*, 1994) disabilities. Thus, the quality is compared for each of the following four groups:

- Good physical/good cognitive (*i.e.*, less physically dependent, less cognitively impaired).
- Poor physical/good cognitive (*i.e.*, more physically dependent, less cognitively impaired).
- Good physical/poor cognitive (*i.e.*, less physically dependent, more cognitively impaired).
- Poor physical/poor cognitive (*i.e.*, more physically dependent, more cognitively impaired).

The data came from Denmark, Iceland, Italy, Japan and the United States. In Iceland and six states in the United States, the data were gathered administratively and representative of the population. In the other countries, it was obtained from research and development projects. The clinical indicators used for evaluating quality were the following:

- *Falls* (*i.e.*, fell in the previous month).
- *Pressure ulcers* (*i.e.*, presence of any pressure ulcers stage 2 or above, with pressure ulcer stage 2 meaning a partial loss of skin layers that presents clinically as an abrasion, blister, or shallow crater).
- *Faecal incontinence* (*i.e.*, once a week or more frequently).
- *Restraint use* (*i.e.*, daily use of any physical restraint, such as limb restraint, trunk restraint or chair that prevents rising).
- *Social engagement* (*i.e.*, a social engagement scale score of less than 3). This scale, calculated from how resident scored in six assessment items and ranging from zero to six, indicates the extent to which residents interact with others, are involved with establishing their own goals and take part in activities within the nursing home (Mor *et al.*, 1995). A score of six is given if the resident is active in all items, and zero if active in none.

Table 8 shows prevalence of these indicators. In this table, cells marked with an asterisk indicate where the prevalence is significantly different (chi-sq. $p < 0.01$) from that expected if there were no association between country and clinical indicators. Within each country, the prevalence of problems tends to be higher as expected for people with physical disability, particularly when associated with cognitive impairment. Between countries, there are large differences in prevalence within the subgroups with no one country "outperforming" the others in all the indicators. The United States ranks first or second in prevalence of falls and restraint use in all sub-groups. In contrast, the percentage of residents with little to no social engagement is the lowest in all sub-groups when compared with

Table 8. **Prevalence of selected clinical indicators stratified by physical and cognitive functioning**

	Number of residents	Fell in last 30 days (%)	Pressure ulcers (%)	Faecal inc. Min. 1/wk (%)	Restraints Any daily (%)	Low Social engagement < 3 (max 6) (%)
Good physical function/good cognition		*	*	*	*	*
Italy	292	7.5	1.7	14.4	4.1	61.3
Denmark	1 454	11.0	0.5	9.4	0	..
USA	8 083	9.3	0.4		0.6	42.9
Japan	665	3.3	0	3.9	0.6	51.1
Iceland	667	4.5	0.3	3.1	0	55.0
Poor physical function/good cognition		*			*	*	*
Italy	207	7.8	2.9	77.3	20.8	72.9
Denmark	924	14.1	2.9	32.8	2.4	..
USA	10 602	16.9	2.1	34.5	12.6	56.4
Japan	208	6.3	1.0	54.8	4.3	87.0
Iceland	224	8.5	0	17.0	6.3	60.7
Good physical function/poor cognition		*			*	*	*
Italy	63	3.2	1.6	27.0	9.5	85.7
Denmark	349	7.7	0.3	17.5	0	
USA	907	14.1	0.3	23.9	3.5	70.1
Japan	43	4.7	0	30.2	0	86.0
Iceland	81	8.6	0	8.6	2.5	85.2
Poor physical function/poor cognition			*			
Italy		*	7.4	*	*	*
Denmark	229	7.5	2.9	92.6	35.7	90.3
USA	715	14.6	3.0	70.5	7.8	..
Japan	7 652	10.7	0.9	81.6	37.9	89.5
Iceland	324	1.9	0.7	86.7	12.3	96.6
	276	3.6		57.2	33.0	97.1

* Cells where distribution is significantly different (chi sq. p < 0.01) from that expected if there were no association between country and clinical indicators.

Source: Reproduced from Carpenter *et al.* (1999).

the other countries. Italy has a higher prevalence of faecal incontinence and restraint use compared with the other countries. Japan has a higher prevalence of faecal incontinence in all but the least dependent groups. Denmark (for whom social engagement data were incomplete) has a lower prevalence of most of these markers with the exception of falls and faecal incontinence in the most independent residents, and falls in the most dependent. Pressure ulcers were more common in those with greater physical dependency, but Iceland and Japan had virtually no pressure ulcers, even in residents with poor physical and cognitive function.

3.3. Quality Indicators (QIs) for home and community-based care

Quality Indicators for home care (HCQIs), using data from the home care assessment form, are in the process of development. Drawing on the experience gained in developing the sophisticated risk-adjustment methodology for nursing homes, 30 tentative home care QIs have been constructed (Table 9). The domains evaluated include: physical function, cognitive function, nutrition, medication, incontinence, ulcers, pain and environmental factors. The quality of community-based care is more difficult to evaluate because, some, if not most, of the care will continue to be provided by family or friends. Under these circumstances, except in cases of blatant abuse, it is difficult for governments to take direct action. However, if formal services are being provided, it should be possible for professionals to inform the informal caregiver about the appropriate way of providing care and the adverse consequences of not following such advice. Also, it would be their responsibility to notify the physician if there appears to be problems in the medical treatment. Thus, for home care agencies showing poor scores, detailed evaluation of individual records to confirm whether appropriate actions by professionals had been taken should be made.

Table 10 shows selected HCQI results from a study of Ontario Community Care Access Centres (CCACs), which act as single point entry agencies providing access to community and institutional

Table 9. **Home Care Quality Indicators (HCQI)**

Prevalence indicators	Incidence indicators

Nutrition
  – Inadequate meals
  – Weight Loss
  – Dehydration
	Incontinence
	  – Failure to improve/incidence of bladder
	  continence

Medication
  – No medication review
	Ulcers
	  – Failure to improve/incidence of skin ulcers

Physical function
  – No assistive device among clients with
  difficulty in Locomotion
  – ADL/rehabilitation potential and no therapies
	Physical function
	  – Failure to improve/incidence of decline on ADL
	  long form
	  – Failure to improve/incidence of impaired
	  locomotion in the home

Psychosocial function
  – Social isolation w/distress
  – Delirium
  – Negative mood
	Psychosocial function
	  – Failure to improve/incidence of cognitive
	  decline
	  – Failure to improve/incidence of difficulty in
	  communication

Pain
  – Disruptive/intense pain
  – Unmanaged pain	

Safety/environment
  – Falls
  – Any injuries
  – Neglect/abuse	

Other
  – Not receiving influenza vaccination
  – Hospitalisation	

Draft indicators for home care developed by interRAI (2001).

services. Case managers in ten different cities implemented the home care assessment form on a pilot basis, and a task force has recently forwarded a recommendation to the Ontario Ministry of Health and Long Term Care to implement the instrument on a provincial basis. There is a 2.6 fold difference in the rates of inadequate pain control among existing CCAC clients, with prevalence rates reaching a high of almost 47 per cent of clients. There is somewhat less variability among all CCACs in the failure to receive flu shots in the previous two years, but there remains an absolute difference in excess of 20 per cent between the CCACs with the highest and lowest rates of flu shot uptake among their clients. A

Table 10. **Prevalence of selected quality indicators among existing clients of ten Ontario Community Care Access Centres (CCACs)**

Home Care Agency	Percentage of clients with Home Care Quality Indicator (HCQI)		
	Pain without adequate control by medication	No flu vaccine in last 2 years	Capacity to improve function but not receiving therapies
CCAC 1	26.1	42.6	74.7
CCAC 2	18.2	21.2	63.8
CCAC 3	38.1	20.4	70.8
CCAC 4	29.2	20.2	63.2
CCAC 5	24.1	16.8	85.1
CCAC 6	32.0	43.2	70.5
CCAC 7	32.5	25.9	72.8
CCAC 8	46.8	20.4	77.1
CCAC 9	42.2	32.8	87.9
CCAC 10	19.5	28.8	75.6

Source: Hirdes, J.P. (2001), *The RAI-Health Informatics Project* (RAI-HIP), Final Report to the Health Transition Fund, University of Waterloo, Waterloo.

somewhat different pattern is noted in the indicators dealing with receipt of rehabilitation therapies among clients with the potential for functional improvement. While there is again an absolute difference of more than 20 per cent in extreme values for this indicator, the most striking aspect of this column is the high overall rate of no access to rehabilitation among Ontario home care clients in need. That is, in each CCAC, a clear majority of clients who had the potential to benefit from rehabilitation were not receiving those services.

Some adjustments in the indicators may need to be considered as they have been developed in the United States and Canada where the services are heavily targeted on health care. In European countries and Japan, the emphasis of home care may be more on social services such as the national performance standards that are being developed in the United Kingdom (Department of Health, 1998).

4. Concluding remarks

In order to evaluate quality in LTC, the following are needed:

1. Reliable and valid assessment instruments
2. Methodology for interpreting the data
3. Databases of the assessment information

With the development of the nursing home and the home care versions of the RAI, and their respective Quality Indicators, the first and second conditions have already been met. To fulfil the remaining third condition, governments must commit themselves to establishing databases and taking a proactive role in monitoring the quality of care. For this purpose, the RAI instruments provide an efficient basis for doing so because they were primarily designed for planning care at the clinical level. Thus, the clinical data generated can also be used for administrative purposes at little extra cost.

This process could be made even more efficient if the data were to be used also for payment purposes. For institutional care, it is possible to do so by paying facilities according to the Resource Utilization Groups – Version III (RUG-III). Each patient falls into one of the 44 groups according to how they are assessed by the MDS. A per-diem reimbursement rate is set for each group that is based on the relative use of resources (Fries *et al.*, 1994). Because the same assessment data are used for the purposes of both payment and quality audit, facilities have two counter-balancing incentives that lead to accurate assessments. For example, the presence of pressure ulcers will place the patient in a high resource group because the care will cost more. Thus, the facility would have every incentive to assess even marginal cases as a "pressure ulcer". However, if the facility has too many residents with pressure ulcer, it will be evaluated to be of poor quality. Therefore, in order not to be scrutinised for problems in quality, the facility would have every incentive not to assess the condition as a "pressure ulcer". The RUG-III is used in the United States by Medicare to pay nursing homes and Ontario has also recently begun to use a similar payment system for its complex continuing care hospitals/units. The RUG-III has been validated in Sweden, Japan, the United Kingdom and Spain (Carpenter *et al.*, 1997) and also in Finland (Björkgren *et al.*, 1999).

For the home care data, another potential use is for determining and monitoring the eligibility status. As noted in the first section, equitable access to care is the primary criterion for quality and having accurate assessments is the initial step towards meeting this goal. In the state of Michigan, the MI-Choice algorithm for placing individuals on Medicaid has been developed to meet the equity norms and services available in that state. MI-Choice has taken several items from the MDS and, in some cases simplified them, in order to develop its single sheet assessment form. This methodology could be applied for developing similar algorithm in other countries.

The RAI concept and methodology will continue to expand. For mental health, a RAI-MH for institutional care has been developed in Ontario and is about to be implemented there (Hirdes *et al.*, 2001). A community care version of this mental health version is now being developed. These instruments share core items so that individuals can be monitored across different settings, but also have specific items to meet the unique needs of each system. In the future, it may be possible to construct a comprehensive database for addressing the quality of care and costs across all settings and service configurations.

However, in order to reap these dividends, policy-makers should be aware that investments must initially be made to adequately train the clinicians who will be actually using these instruments, and the administrative staff who will be analysing and monitoring the data. Long-term care has been an area that has not received the attention it deserves and the barrier that divides health and human service professionals has yet to be bridged.

NOTES

1. Some argue that medical and life-style advances will produce a "compression of morbidity" and drastically reduce the demand for long-term care (Jacobzone *et al.*, 1998). Manton and Gu (2001) argue that even absolute numbers of elderly needing institutionalisation are declining in the United States, and that the rate of "compression" is accelerating, but for most countries this effect will probably not be enough to outweigh the simple increase in numbers of frail elderly.

2. "The New Social Policy Agenda for a Caring World", Meeting of the Employment, Labour and Social Affairs Committee at Ministerial Level on Social Policy, OECD, Paris, 23-24 June 1998 (OECD, 1999).

3. If cash benefits are made available, as in Germany, then all who consider themselves eligible might apply for benefits. In Japan, cash benefits are not available, which is one of the reasons why expenditures are lower than estimated.

4. These findings can be found in a final report to HCFA (Phillips *et al.*, 1996) and in a series of papers (Fries *et al.*, 1997*a*; Hawes *et al.*, 1997*a*; Mor *et al.*, 1997; Phillips *et al.*, 1997*a*).

REFERENCES

BJÖRKGREN, M.A., HAKKINEN, U., FINNE-SOVERI, U.M. and FRIES, B.E. (1999),
"Validity and reliability of Resource Utilization Groups (RUG-III) in Finish long-term care facilities", *Scandinavian Journal of Public Health*, Vol. 27, pp. 228-234.

CARPENTER, G. I., IKEGAMI, N., LJUNNGREN, G., CARRILLO, E. and FRIES, B. E. (1997),
"RUG-III and Resource Allocation: comparing the relationship of direct care time with patient characteristics in five countries", *Age and Ageing*, Vol. 26-S2, pp. 61-65.

CARPENTER, G. I., HIRDES, J., RIBBE, M. W., IKEGAMI, N., CHALLIS, D.J., STEEL, K., BERNABEI, R. and FRIES, B. E. (1999),
"Targeting and quality of nursing home care. A five nation study", *Aging Clin. Exp.Res.*, Vol. 11, No. 2, pp. 83-89.

CENTER FOR HEALTH SYSTEMS RESEARCH AND ANALYSIS (1999),
Facility Guide for the Nursing Home Quality Indicators – National Data System, Center for Health Care Systems Research and Analysis, University of Wisconsin, Madison.

DEPARTMENT OF HEALTH (1998),
Modernising Social Services, London.

FRIES, B. E., HAWES, C., MORRIS, J. N., PHILLIPS, C. D., MOR, V. and PARK, P. S. (1997),
"Effect of the National Resident Assessment Instrument on selected health conditions and problems", *Journal of the American Geriatrics Society*, Vol. 45, pp. 994-1001.

FRIES, B. E., SCHNEIDER, D. P., FOLEY, W. J., GAVAZZI, M., BURKE, R. and CORNELIUS, E. (1994),
"Refining a case-mix measure for nursing homes: Resource Utilization Groups (RUG-III)", *Medical Care*, Vol. 32, pp. 668-685.

FRIES, B. E., SCHROLL, M., HAWES, C., GILGEN, R., JONSSON, P. V. and PARK, P. (1997),
"Approaching cross-national comparisons of nursing home residents", *Age and geing*, Vol. 26-S2, pp. 13-18.

HAWES, C., MORRIS, J. N., PHILLIPS, C. D., MOR, V., FRIES, B. E. and NONEMAKER, S. (1995),
"Reliability estimates for the Minimum Data Set for Nursing Home Resident Assessment and Care Screening (MDS)", *The Gerontologist*, Vol. 35, pp. 172-178.

HAWES, C., MOR, V., PHILLIPS, C. D., FRIES, B. E., MORRIS, J. N., STEEL-FRIEDLOB, E., GREENE, A. M. and NENNSTIEL, M. (1997),
"The OBRA-87 nursing home regulations and the implementation of the resident assessment instrument: Effects in process quality", *Journal of the American Geriatrics Society*, Vol. 45, pp. 977-985.

HIRDES, J.P., ZIMMERMAN, D., HALLMAN, K.G. and SOUCIE, P.S. (1998),
"Use of the MDS quality indicators to assess quality of care in institutional settings", *Canadian Journal for Quality in Health Care*, Vol. 14, No. 2, pp. 5-11.

HIRDES, J.P., FRIES, B.E., MORRIS, J.N., STEEL, K., MOR, V., FRIJTERS, D., JONSSON, P., LABINE, S., SCHALM, C., STONES, M.J., TEARE, G. SMITH, T., MARHABA, M. and PEREZ, E. (1999),
"Integrated health information systems based on the RAI/MDS series of assessment instruments", *Healthcare Management Forum*, Vol. 12, No. 4, pp. 30-40.

HIRDES, J.P., MARHABA, M., SMITH, T.F., CLYBURN, L., MITCHELL, L., LEMICK, R.A., CURTIN TELEGDI, N., PÉREZ, E., PRENDERGAST, P., RABINOWITZ, T. and YAMAUCHI, K. (2001),
"Development of the Resident Assessment Instrument – Mental Health (RAI-MH)", *Hospital Quarterly*, Vol. 4, No. 2, pp. 44-51.

IKEGAMI, N. (2001),
"Population ageing and impact on the organisation, delivery and financing of long-term care: An innovative approach from Japan", *www.chera.ca/program.html*.

IKEGAMI, N. and CAMPBELL, J.C. (2001),
"Designing an independent LTC system: In general and in Japan, Discussion paper for 4-Country Conference on 'Aging and Health Policy'", Gananoque, Ontario.

INSTITUTE OF MEDICINE (1986),
Improving Quality of Care in Nursing Homes, National Academy Press, Washington, D.C.

interRAI EUROPEAN COLLABORATION (2000),
   "The Aged in Home Care (ADHOC) project", 2000, EU Vth Framework project No. QLRT-2000-00002.

JACOBZONE, S., E. *et al.* (1998),
   "Long Term Care Services to Older People, A Perspective on Future Needs: The Impact of An Improving Health
   of Older Persons", Working Paper AWP 4.2, "Maintaining Prosperity In An Ageing Society: The OECD Study on
   the Policy Implications of Ageing", OECD, Paris.

KANE, R.A. (1999),
   "Commentary: Preparing health and social clinicians for holistic care", in J.C. Campbell and N. Ikegami (eds.),
   Long-Term Care for Frail Older People – Reaching for the Ideal System, Springer-Verlag, Tokyo.

MANTON, K.G. and GU, X.L. (2001),
   "Changes in the prevalence of chronic disability in the United States black and nonblack population above
   65 from 1982 to 1999", PNAS Early Edition, *www.pnas.orgycgiydoiy10.1073ypnas.111152298.*

MOR, V., MORRIS, J.N., LIPSITZ, L. and FOGEL, B. (1998),
   "Benchmarking quality in nursing homes: The Q-Metrics System", *Canadian Journal of Quality in Health Care*, Vol. 14,
   pp. 12-17.

MOR, V., K. BRANCO, FLEISHMAN, J., HAWES, C., PHILLIPS, C., MORRIS, J.N., and FRIES, B.E. (1995),
   "The structure of social engagement among nursing home residents", *Journal of Gerontology: Psychological Sciences*,
   Vol. 50, No. 1, pp. 1-8.

MOR, V., INTRATOR, O., FRIES, B. E., PHILLIPS, C., TENO, J., HIRIS, J., HAWES, C. and MORRIS, J.N. (1997),
   "Changes in hospitalization associated with introducing the Resident Assessment Instrument", *Journal of the
   American Geriatrics Society*, Vol. 45, pp. 1002-1010.

MORRIS, J. N., FRIES, B.E. and MORRIS, S.A. (1999),
   "Scaling ADL's within the MDS", J *Gerontology* , Vol. 4, No. 11, pp. M546-553.

MORRIS, J.N., MURPHY, K., NONEMAKER, S., FRIES, B.E. *et al.* (1996),
   Resident Assessment Instrument Version 2.0, Government Printing Office, Washington DC.

MORRIS, J. N., FRIES, B.E., MEHR, D.R., HAWES, C., PHILLIPS, C., MOR, V. and LIPSITZ, L.A. (1994),
   "The MDS Cognitive Performance Scale", *Journal of Gerontology*, Vol. 49, No. 4, pp. 174-182.

MORRIS, J. N., FRIES, B. E., STEEL, K., IKEGAMI, N., BERNABEI, R., CARPENTER, G. I. GILGEN, R., HIRDES J. P. and
   TOPINKOVA, E. (1997),
   "Comprehensive clinical assessment in community setting – Applicability of the MDS-HC", *Journal of the American
   Geriatrics Society*, Vol. 45, pp. 1017-1024.

MORRIS, J. N., C. HAWES. C., FRIES, B.E., PHILLIPS, C., MOR, V., KATZ, S., MURPHY, K., DRUGOVICH, M.L. and
   FRIEDLOB, A.S. (1990),
   "Designing the National Resident Assessment Instrument", T*he Gerontologist*, Vol. 30, No. 3, pp. 293-307.

OECD (1999),
   A Caring World – The New Social Agenda, Paris.

PHILLIPS, C., HAWES, C., MOR, V., FRIES, B. and MORRIS, J. N. (1996),
   Evaluation of the Nursing Home Resident Assessment Instrument: Executive Summary, Health Care Financing
   Administration, Washington, D.C.

PHILLIPS, C. D., ZIMMERMAN, D., BERNABEI, R. and JONSSON, P. V. (1997),
   "Using the Resident Assessment Instrument for quality enhancement in nursing homes", *Age and Ageing*, Vol. 26-
   S2, pp. 77-81.

SGADARI, A., MORRIS, J., FRIES, B.E., LJUNGGREN, G., JONSSON, P., DUPASQUIER, J.-N. and SCHROLL, M. (1997),
   "Efforts to establish the reliability of the Resident Assessment Instrument", *Age Ageing*, Vol. 26-S2, pp. 27-30.

TEARE, G., HIRDES, J.P., ZIRALDO, M., PROCTOR, W., and NENADOVIC, M. (2000), *Provincial Status Report – The Quality
   of Caring – Ontario April 1998-1999*, Canadian Institute of Health Information, Toronto.

ZIMMERMAN, D., KARON, S., ARLING, G., CLARK, B., COLLINS, E., ROSS, R. and SAINFORT, F., (1995),
   "The development and testing of nursing home quality indicators", *Health Care Financing Review*, Vol. 16, pp. 107-128.

Chapter 14

DEVELOPING COMPOSITE INDICATORS
FOR ASSESSING HEALTH SYSTEM EFFICIENCY

by

Peter Smith[*]

Abstract

There exist several dimensions along which health system performance might be measured, and numerous indicators of performance have been proposed. Many such indicators do indeed capture important aspects of system behaviour, but each is to some extent partial, and as a result potentially misleading. Given the intense policy interest in system performance, the question therefore arises: can some form of aggregation of indicators yield a more satisfactory insight into performance than the partial view offered by individual indicators? This paper examines the extent to which some sort of aggregation is possible and useful. It starts with a discussion of some of the key economic concepts associated with system performance. The paper then examines the rationale for moving from separate to composite indicators. It discusses four important elements of a composite indicator, namely: the separate dimensions of performance to be measured, the selection of operational indicators to be used, the transformation of such indicators into common units, and the weights then to be applied to derive the composite indicator. The paper makes some observations on inferring system efficiency from composite indicators. Four concrete examples of operational composite indicators are discussed, and good (and bad) practice in the development of composite indicators is inferred. The paper concludes with a discussion of the circumstances in which composite indicators are useful, and the extent to which their development yields improvements over presentation of separate indicators.

Introduction

All societies and nations have developed some sort of health system, which can be defined as those purposive activities "whose primary purpose is to promote, restore or maintain health" (World Health Organization, 2000). Of course the nature and extent of a health system depends heavily on the circumstances, means and preferences of the society it is designed to serve. However, all systems have (broadly speaking) similar objectives of improving the length and the quality of citizens' lives. And many systems also seek to address equity issues, in the form of the distribution of health between individuals.

Given the large proportion of the global economy spent on health systems, it seems reasonable to ask the question: is the investment in health systems spent wisely? This question has two components: first, given the technologies currently available to mankind, is the proportion of the global economy

* Centre for Health Economics, University of York, York YO10 5DD, United Kingdom (Phone: +44 1904 433779, Fax: + 44 1904 433759). Email: *pcs1@york.ac.uk*

I should like to thank Geoff Anderson, Jeremy Hurst, Gaetan Lafortune, Andrew Street and Alan Williams for comments on an earlier draft, and for additional material made available by John Appleby and David Andrews. Any errors are of course my responsibility.

devoted to health justified? And – assuming it is justified – do individual health systems in practice deploy the resources at their disposal to best effect? The first question is clearly of central importance, and is a matter of continuing debate. However, this paper focuses on the second question.

If the objectives of health systems were uncontentious in definition and simple to measure, addressing this issue would be reasonably straightforward. However, even though there is likely to be broad agreement that health systems are seeking to enhance both the levels and distribution of individual health, there is little consensus on how these broad principles can be made operational.

In this paper I nevertheless assume objectives can be agreed, and define *health system performance* to be the extent to which those agreed objectives are achieved. This definition is analogous to the WHO definition of health system "attainment" (World Health Organization, 2000). There is a widespread belief that health system performance is multidimensional in nature, embracing objectives that – if they can be measured at all – can be captured only on very different scales of measurement. Many existing performance indicators capture important aspects of health system behaviour. However, each is to some extent partial, and as a result potentially misleading. The phenomenon of multidimensional performance is not unique to health systems. Indeed, one of the central themes of modern management is the complex multidimensional nature of most concepts of organisational performance, and the need to develop a "balanced scorecard" if one is to capture the concept satisfactorily (Kaplan and Norton, 1992).

Multidimensionality has led to the development of composite measures of health system performance. The rationale for developing a composite measure is that no single metric can capture the concept of system performance. Instead, one must first measure each of the component dimensions of performance, and then in some way combine the various components into a single measure of whole system performance.

In order to address the efficiency with which health systems use the resources at their disposal, one must examine performance in relation to some measure of resource use, usually summarized in the form of costs. Economists would often define the ratio of performance to costs as a measure of cost-effectiveness. However, for the purposes of this paper I refer to it as *health system efficiency*.

The purpose of this paper is to examine the rationale underlying the development of composite measures of health system performance and the associated concept of health system efficiency. It starts with a discussion of the purpose of developing indicators of health system performance, and the rationale for moving from separate to composite indicators. The paper presents four concrete examples of publicly available composite indicators, and good (and bad) practice in their development is inferred. In the light of these examples, four important elements of a composite indicator are discussed, namely: the separate dimensions to be measured, the selection of operational indicators to be used, the transformation of such indicators into common units, and the weights then to be applied to derive the composite indicator. The paper concludes with a discussion of the circumstances in which composite indicators are useful, and the extent to which their development yields improvements over presentation of separate indicators.

In the interests of space, I avoid discussion of certain important principles underlying the development of composite indicators. For example, discussion of what is meant by the health system is side-stepped. Although this can be loosely defined as the set of institutional arrangements put in place to further the population's health, making this concept operational is difficult. Clearly the health system extends well beyond health care. But should it embrace, for example, income redistribution, often cited as a powerful influence on population health? I also assume system objectives can be agreed, and that the ultimate purpose of developing the composite is to assess the efficiency with which system resources are deployed. These important issues of principle deserve extensive discussion, but this paper concentrates principally on the technical issues underlying the development of composite indicators.

1. Why composite indicators?

Table 1 summarizes two aspects of health system performance in OECD countries. The first indicator is life expectancy for females at age 65. This indicator captures what most people would

Table 1. **Two indicators of health system performance in OECD countries**

	Life expectancy 1995: females at age 65		Infant mortality 1996: deaths per 1 000 live births	
	Years	Rank	Rate	Rank
Australia	19.5	8	5.8	16
Austria	18.7	15	5.1	10
Belgium	19.6	7	6.0	17
Canada	20.1	4	5.6	13
Czech Republic	16.1	27	6.0	17
Denmark	17.6	23	5.6	13
Finland	18.6	17	3.9	3
France	20.6	2	4.8	7
Germany	18.5	18	5.0	9
Greece	18.4	19	7.3	22
Hungary	15.8	28	10.9	26
Iceland	19.4	9	3.7	1
Ireland	17.4	24	5.5	11
Italy	19.4	9	6.2	20
Japan	20.9	1	3.8	2
Korea	17.0	25	7.7	24
Luxembourg	19.2	11	4.9	8
Mexico	18.3	20	17.0	28
Netherlands	18.7	15	5.7	15
New Zealand	19.0	13	7.3	22
Norway	19.1	12	4.1	5
Poland	16.6	26	12.2	27
Portugal	17.8	22	6.9	21
Spain	19.9	5	5.5	11
Sweden	19.7	6	4.0	4
Switzerland	20.2	3	4.7	6
Turkey	14.2	29	42.2	29
United Kingdom	18.3	20	6.1	19
United States	18.9	14	7.8	25

Source: OECD (2000).

consider to be an important aspect of health system performance. Other things being equal, a higher life expectancy indicates better performance. However, life expectancy is a profoundly inadequate and incomplete as a summary of overall system attainment.

For example, we might wish to consider the life expectancy indicator in conjunction with a second measure of system outcome, such as the infant mortality rate, also presented in Table 1. Other things being equal, lower scores indicate better system performance. When viewed in conjunction with the life expectancy indicator, inferences about system performance are far from clear-cut. For example, Finland secures a very low infant mortality rate of 3.9, but manages only mediocre life expectancy of 18.6 years for females at age 65.

Almost any examination of overall system performance therefore runs into a difficulty. How are important dimensions of performance measured on different scales to be combined meaningfully? The advocates of composite indicators would argue that the answer is to apply a system of weights to the individual performance indicators. In its simplest manifestation, therefore, the composite indicator takes a linear form, such as:

$$C_i = \alpha_1 P_{i1} + \alpha_2 P_{i2} + ... + \alpha_n P_{in} = \sum_j \alpha_j P_{ij}$$

where C_i is the composite score for system i, P_{ij} is the individual measure for attribute j in system i, and α_j is the weight attached to attribute j. Other methods of combining performance measures into a composite score can of course be envisaged, but I shall assume this simplest of forms throughout.

Central to the construction of the index is the need to specify a set of weights $\alpha_1, \alpha_2, ... \alpha_n$ to attach to the component indicators. The intention of the weights is to indicate the relative importance of the

297

indicators. Specifically, the ratio α_1/α_2 should indicate the sacrifice in objective 2 that the user is prepared to make in order to gain an extra unit of objective 1. Note that the weights are analogous to prices for the outputs. For a fuller treatment of the economic implications of seeking to develop a composite indicator, see the technical appendix.

The broad arguments for developing a composite indicator of performance are that it offers a more rounded assessment of system performance than piecemeal inspection of individual performance indicators, and that it facilitates judgements on overall system efficiency. Under my chosen definition, securing a measure of system efficiency based on this composite score is in principle a trivial matter. All that is needed is to calculate the ratio of the performance score to the costs of the health system, although this simple concept is often complicated in practice by the difficulty of securing reliable estimates of costs and the need to adjust for external influences on performance that the health system cannot control.

2. Four examples

In order to motivate the following discussion, in this section I outline four published examples of composite measures of system performance, and offer a brief commentary on each. The examples are taken from US Medicare, Canadian regional health care, UK health authorities, and the WHO ranking of national health systems.

2.1. *United States Medicare*

Jencks *et al.* (2000) report a multivariate assessment of the quality of care delivered to fee-for-service Medicare beneficiaries at the state level. The objective is to provide a performance monitoring system to support continuous quality improvement. The emphasis is on the process of care, rather than outcomes. Clinical topics were selected according to five criteria:

- The disease is a major source of morbidity or mortality;

- Certain processes of care are known to improve outcomes;

- Measurement of these processes is feasible;

- There is substantial scope for improvement in performance;

- Managerial intervention can potentially improve performance.

Twenty-two process measures were developed for six clinical areas: acute myocardial infarction (6 indicators), heart failure (2), stroke (3), pneumonia (7), breast cancer (1) and diabetes (3).[1] Each of the indicators reports the percentage of relevant patients receiving a specified intervention relevant to the condition (Table 2).

Each of the 50 states (plus District of Columbia and Puerto Rico) is ranked on each of the measures. That is, each percentage score is transformed to an ordinal scale ranging from 1 to 52. A composite performance measure is produced by computing each state's average rank. Standard deviations are also reported. Northern and less populous states are found to perform better than southern and more populous states.

The Medicare analysis was picked up by the popular media, in the form of Harpers magazine, which published a map of the composite quality scores for states (Holmes and Pennington, 2001). The Harpers item also gave an indication of *per capita* spending levels, suggesting an interest in efficiency that the original analysis did not pursue.

The authors acknowledge that – although the choice of process measures is based on strong science and professional consensus – there are circumstances in which delivery of the chosen process of care is inappropriate. Furthermore, for some measures, the denominator in the indicator is small, leading to rather large standard errors in some states. There are some more general concerns about data reliability for a few indicators.

Table 2. **Quality indicators for care of Medicare beneficiaries**

Inpatient setting

Acute myocardial infarction
1. Administration of aspirin within 24 h of admission (Aspirin 24 h)
2. Aspirin prescribed at discharge (Aspirin disch)
3. Administration of b-blocker within 24 h of admission (BB 24 h)
4. B-blocker prescribed at discharge (BB disch)
5. ACE Inhibitor prescribed at discharge for patients with left ventricular ejection fraction, 40% (ACEI in AMI)
6. Smoking cessation counseling given during hospitalisation (Smoking)
7. Time to angioplasty, min (PTCA min)*
8. Time to thrombolytic therapy, min (Lytic min)*

Heart failure
9. Evaluation of left ventricular ejection fraction (LVEF)
10. ACE Inhibitor prescribed at discharge for patients with left ventricular ejection fraction, 40% (ACEI in HF)

Stroke
11. Warfarin prescribed for patients with atrial fibrillation (Afibrillation)
12. Antithrombotic prescribed at discharge for patients with acute stroke or transient ischemic attack (Antithrombotic)
13. Avoidance of sublingual nifedipine for patients with acute stroke (Nifedipine)

Pneumonia
14. Antibiotic within 8 h of arrival at hospital (Antibiotic time)
15. Antibiotic consistent with current recommendations (Antibiotic Rx)
16. Blood culture drawn (if done) before antibiotic given (Blood culture)
17. Patient screened for or given influenza vaccine (Flu screen)
18. Patient screened for or given pneumococcal vaccine (Pneu screen)

Any setting

Pneumonia
19. Influenza immunization every year (Flu immun)
20. Pneumococcal immunization at least once ever (Pneu immun)

Breast cancer
21. Mammogram at least every 2 years (Mammography)

Diabetes
22. Hemoglobin A1c at least every year (HbA1c)
23. Eye examination at least every 2 years (Eye exam)
24. Lipid profile at least every 2 years (Lipid profile)

* Not used in the composite.
Source: Jencks *et al.* (2000).

The choice of measures is clearly constrained by data availability and gives an unbalanced picture of health services, with inpatient and preventative services over-represented. Furthermore, because each indicator is given equal weight, the use of eight indicators for AMI care means that that clinical area contributes much more heavily to the composite than (say) breast cancer, for which there is only one indicator.

Also, the use of league table ranking as the basis for the composite implicitly assumes that identical differences in ranking are equally important, regardless of the intervention to which they refer, or where in the league table they occur. So, for example, the small difference between (say) Puerto Rico (59 per cent) and New Jersey (61 per cent) on ACE inhibitor prescribed at discharge makes the same contribution to Puerto Rico's composite score as the massive difference between Puerto Rico (38 per cent) and next worse Florida (76 per cent) on antibiotic administered to pneumonia patients within 8 hours of hospital arrival. If Puerto Rico wishes to improve its composite score, the incentive is to concentrate on activities such as ACE inhibitor prescription for which movement up the league table may be readily secured, rather than those that offer most potential health gain.

Even if absolute scores had been used (rather than rankings) the impact on health outcomes of a one percentage point variation in performance might vary considerably between indicators. For example, a one per cent improvement in (say) aspirin prescribed at discharge may have a very different impact on health outcome for AMI patients than would a one per cent improvement in smoking cessation counselling. However, the incentive is for states to concentrate on areas where the costs associated with securing an improved ranking are least.

2.2. Canadian regional health care

The Canadian Institute for Health Information has instituted a series of annual reports that survey the state of the Canadian health care system (Canadian Institute for Health Information, 2001a). Associated with the report, a series of health indicators for the 63 largest regions (covering 90 per cent of the population) is published separately (Canadian Institute for Health Information, 2001b). The Institute avoids any attempt at aggregating the indicators. However, the weekly magazine *Macleans* publishes an annual "Health Report" that seeks to rank regions on the basis of the data. The intention is to present information on health care that "truly matters to Canadians" in a digestible format (Marshall, 1999).

The third *Macleans* report uses what it refers to as the "15 best nationally recognized indicators" of health care performance grouped into six categories, as shown in Table 3: outcomes; prenatal care; community health; elderly services; efficiencies; resources (Marshall, 2001). All 54 regions with populations over 125 000 are covered. Where data are missing, scores are inferred from performance on non-missing data. Each of the 15 indicators is rescaled to have a mean of 80 and a standard deviation of 10 (with a higher score implying better performance).

Within each of the six categories, the constituent scores are then combined using weights "based on expert judgement" to produce six category scores. The six categories are then in turn combined with weights: outcomes 0.2; prenatal care 0.2; community health 0.2; elderly services 0.1; efficiencies 0.2;

Table 3. **Indicators for Canadian regions**

Outcomes
  1. Life expectancy at birth, based on average mortality rates between 1995 and 1997.
  2. Heart attack survival: probability that heart attack patients will die in hospital within 30 days of admission.

Prenatal care
  3. Low birth weight: the proportion of live births weighing less than 2 500 g.
  4. Caesarean sections: the percentage of women who have babies by c-section.
  5. Births after c-section percentage of women who previously gave birth by c-section who have a vaginal birth in hospital.

Community health
  6. Hip fractures: age standardised hospitalisation rates for those aged over 64.
  7. Pneumonia and flu: age standardised hospitalisation rates for those aged over 64.

Elderly services
  8. Hip replacements: age standardised rate of total hip-replacements per 100 000 population up to a cut-off of 80 per cent of communities.
  9. Knee replacements: age standardised rate of total knee-replacement surgeries per 100 000 population – scores do not increase for rates above the national average.

Efficiencies
  10. Possible outpatients: percentage of acute care hospialisations for conditions not requiring admission.
  11. Early discharge: variation from the expected length of stay, standardised for age and diagnosis.
  12. Preventable admissions: age standardised hospital admissions per 100 000 people for conditions (such as diabetes or asthma) where appropriate ambulatory care reduces the need for hospitalisation.

Resources
  13. Physicians: active GPs and family practitioners per 100 000 people up to a cut-off of the highest mark in the bottom 80 per cent of communities.
  14. Specialists: active medical specialists per 100 000 people up to a cut-off of the highest mark in the bottom 80 per cent of communities.
  15. Local services: ratio of total hospitalisations taking place in region to total hospitalisations generated by residents in the region.

Source: Marshall (2001).

resources 0.1. The composite performance scores range from 89.5 (North/West Vancouver, British Columbia) to 73.4 (North Bay/Huntsville, Ontario).

The *Macleans* approach seeks to secure a more rounded assessment of system performance than the Medicare example, incorporating issues such as health outcome and efficiency. Furthermore, the sequential approach to assigning weights (first to indicators within categories, and then to categories) allows a more careful treatment of priorities. However it nevertheless suffers from the same weaknesses related to incompleteness of coverage, and in practice the weighting scheme is very rudimentary.

Moreover, the combination of outcome measures, process measures and efficiency measures leads to some confusion about the concept of performance that the composite measure is capturing. Efficiency is treated not as the extent to which objectives are secured in relation to expenditure, but rather as just another objective that contributes to the chosen concept of performance.

2.3. British health authorities

English Health Authorities and their Scottish and Welsh equivalents are responsible for planning health care for and promoting the health of their populations, which average 500 000 people. The UK television broadcaster Channel 4 commissioned a study from researchers at the King's Fund that sought to rank the overall success of health authorities in pursuing these objectives. The intention was to "measure the standard of healthcare against public expectations", and the results were broadcast on 20 February 2000 (Channel Four, 2000).

Six indicators of health authority performance were selected from readily available data produced by the national NHS Executive:

- Deaths from cancer (per 100 000 people),
- Deaths from heart disease (per 100 000),
- Total number of people on hospital waiting lists (per 1 000),
- Percentage of people on waiting lists who had been waiting over 12 months,
- Number of hip operations (per 100 000),
- Deaths from "avoidable" diseases (per 100 000).

A central focus of this study was to attach weights to these indicators based on public preferences. To this end, the polling organisation MORI undertook a survey of 2 000 members of the public to seek out public priorities. Respondents were asked to allocate a "budget" of 60 chips between the six performance indicators. This gave rise to the average distribution shown in Table 4, which was found to be very little changed amongst different population groups.

The weights shown in the last column of the table were computed by simple rescaling (the negative sign on hip operations merely indicates the "more is better" nature of that indicator). A crude composite performance indicator was then calculated by multiplying the individual performance scores by the associated weight and summing.

Table 4. **Average allocation of 60 chips between six performance indicators for UK health care**

Indicator	Chips	Weight
Reducing deaths from cancer	16	1.00
Reducing deaths from heart disease	12	0.75
Reducing total number of people on hospital waiting lists	10	0.63
Reducing number of people waiting over 12 months	9	0.56
Increasing number of hip operations	5	−0.31
Reducing deaths from "avoidable" diseases	8	0.50

Source: Appleby and Mulligan (2000).

The researchers were concerned that some of the raw performance indicators had skewed distributions, and that they were not all measured on the same scale. They therefore undertook a further analysis in which some of the indicators were transformed in order to approximate more closely to a normal distribution. The data were then rescaled to have a mean of zero and standard deviation of one (a z-score). The revised composite indicator did not result in major changes in health authority rankings.

A final refinement was to adjust the scores for the level of deprivation found in each health authority, considered an important uncontrollable influence on performance. The composite indicator was regressed against a widely used measure of local deprivation (the under-privileged area score). This explained 43 per cent of the variance in the composite indicator. The residuals from this analysis form the basis of a revised composite measure, and suggest substantial changes in rankings (Appleby and Mulligan, 2000).

This study suffers from the same problems of limited scope of data as the first two examples, but has made a more concerted effort to assign meaningful weights to the composite. Furthermore, the researchers recognized that relative weights are implicit in the scales used to measure success. However, it is not at all clear that the survey methodology used in the study has necessarily succeeded in inferring the weights needed for computing a composite indicator, namely the relative *marginal* valuation of an extra unit of performance. Respondents may instead, for example, have concatenated the required valuations of lives saved with irrelevant considerations, such as perceptions of the size of the problem (absolute numbers of deaths) or the effectiveness of health systems in saving lives.

2.4. *The World Health Report* 2000

The *World Health Report* 2000 published by the World Health Organization reported for the first time an attempt to rank the performance of the health systems in individual nations. The intention was to examine "whether a health system is performing as well as it could" (World Health Organization, 2000). The WHO composite index of health system achievement was based on five dimensions of health system performance:

- Overall health outcomes (measured by disability-adjusted life expectancy),

- Inequality in health (measured by an index based on child mortality),

- Overall health system responsiveness, reflecting respect for persons and client orientation (as assessed by a panel of key informants),

- Inequality in health system responsiveness (as assessed by the key informants),

- Fairness of financing (measured by an index based on the proportion of non-food expenditure spent on health care).

For most countries direct estimates of all of these variables were not available, so values were inferred using econometric techniques.

In order to construct a composite measure of overall attainment, the relative importance of the five objectives was assessed on the basis of a survey of about 1 000 "informed" respondents, of which over half were WHO staff. The set of weights shown in Table 5 was inferred from the survey. Before the weights were applied, each of the five raw performance measures was transformed according to the formula in the last column of Table 5. The intention was to place each score on an interval from 0 to 100, with 100 being the highest possible level of attainment (Murray *et al.*, 2000). The consequent composite scores ranged from 35.7 (Sierra Leone) to 93.4 (Japan). Confidence intervals were reported for all estimates.

Unlike the previous three examples, the WHO composite measure of attainment was then used as the basis for estimating overall health system efficiency.[2] This stage entailed econometric modelling of system attainment as a function of a) health expenditure and b) exogenous influences (years of schooling) using frontier statistical models. The distance from the estimated production frontier was the basis for the estimate of overall health system efficiency. Although this method of analysing efficiency

Table 5. **Weights and transformations used for five objectives in the *World Health Report* 2000**

Objective	Weight	Transformation
H: Overall health outcome	0.250	(H-20)/(80-20)*100
HI: Distribution of health outcome	0.250	(1-HI)*100
R: Overall responsiveness	0.125	(R/10)*100
RI: Distribution of responsiveness	0.125	(1-RI)*100
FF: Fairness of financing	0.250	FF*100

Source: World Health Organization (2000).

may be unfamiliar to some, it yields an estimate of the familiar ratio of health system performance to expenditure, after adjusting for presumed uncontrollable influences on performance.

The WHO ranking has unleashed a remarkable flurry of commentary and debate that cannot be rehearsed here (Navarro, 2000; Murray and Frenk, 2001; Navarro, 2001; Williams, 2001*a* and 2001*b*; Murray *et al.*, 2001; Almeida *et al.*, 2001; Appleby and Sheet, forthcoming). In particular, the chosen methodology has attracted fierce criticism, most especially in its methods of measuring performance, its treatment of missing or poor quality data, and its econometric methods. These important issues are beyond the scope of this paper, although they do indicate the sorts of difficulties that arise when seeking to develop a universal measure that seeks to embrace all aspects of health system performance. Data and measurement metrics may be in short supply, so contentious methods may be needed to fill the gaps. I do not dwell here on these issues, and instead focus on the construction of the composite index.

Fundamental to the composite is the set of weights applied to the constituent indicators. The chosen weights were based on responses from an internet survey of WHO staff and other interested parties (Gakidou *et al.*, 2000). This approach was justified on the basis of its high speed, low costs and the difficulty of securing meaningful responses on such a complex topic from members of the general public. Clearly the representativeness of the sample is a major issue that deserves careful scrutiny.

However, the approach adopted is also questionable from a technical perspective. Respondents were asked to supply weights on the basis of pie charts and rankings. It is not at all clear what the responses indicate. For example, it may the case that the weights allocated by some respondents will reflect judgements about the appropriate *effort* to be expended on each objective. However, the discussion above has indicated that the weights used should reflect respondents' *valuations* of achievement against the objectives. In principle, this requires them to offer valuations of a one year improvement in disability adjusted life years against (say) a one unit improvement in the WHO compound index of fairness of financing. It is difficult to see how the responses secured that objective. In short, given the rubric attached to the questionnaire, it is highly unlikely that respondents provided the marginal valuations required to derive the composite weights. The method of deriving the WHO index of system attainment is therefore highly questionable.

The frontier statistical methods used to secure estimates of system efficiency are the subject of intense econometric debate that has yet to be resolved satisfactorily. Amongst the model specification issues to which results are likely to be sensitive are: the choice of functional form, the choice of error structure, the choice of covariates, and the treatment of exogenous influences on performance. Research elsewhere on far more extensive datasets has highlighted the high sensitivity of stochastic frontier results to model specification (Li and Rosenman, 2001; Jacobs, 2001).

Furthermore, a highly contentious transformation of the dependent variable (health system attainment) is made to reflect the level of attainment that would exist "even in the absence of any health system inputs".This adjustment appears to be analogous to the more conventional approach of entering an exogenous environmental influence on performance on the right hand side of the regression, albeit with a fixed coefficient. In the light of the large number of technical judgements required, it seems premature to base high profile national rankings on such exploratory techniques and specifications.

The extensive publicity attracted by the WHO rankings has nevertheless undoubtedly pushed system performance to the topic of the agenda of many health policy makers. Indeed Williams (Williams, 2001a) characterizes the exercise is a marketing ploy rather than a serious scientific contribution. It can be argued that early exposure of data and techniques – however unsatisfactory – to public scrutiny will lead to faster improvements in data and methodology than more traditional research endeavour. The key question is whether the increased urgency of debate and research the WHO exercise has undoubtedly secured outweighs any dysfunctional consequences of premature publication based on poor quality analysis, such as inappropriate policy responses in some countries.

3. Practical approaches to developing composite indicators

The examples outlined above and the technical appendix hint at the numerous practical problems that arise when seeking to develop composite indicators of health system performance. This section summarizes six of the more important issues that must be addressed: what should be measured, collinearity of component measures, identifying the composite weights, transforming the component measures, environmental influences on performance, and analytic approaches to inferring efficiency.

3.1. *What should be measured?*

The development of a composite indicator suggests an interest in moving towards a comprehensive measure of system performance. This implies that important aspects of performance that are difficult to measure should nevertheless appear in the composite. Considerable ingenuity may therefore be required to develop a satisfactory proxy for the problematic dimension of performance. In practice, as shown above, many existing composites are either opportunistic and incomplete (measuring only aspects that are readily captured in existing data) or based on highly questionable sources of data. Either weakness can seriously damage the credibility of the composite.

One of the most problematic aspects of assessing health system performance is that observed health status is often the result of years if not decades of population exposure to the health system. Therefore, although contribution to health status (in the form of length and quality of life) should in principle be the ultimate touchstone of system performance, they are in practice often difficult to interpret. In short, one can rarely be confident that current health status is an accurate indicator of current health system performance. For this reason, some commentators advocate the use of measures of health system *process* in preference to health status measures as the basis for indicators of system performance (Crombie and Davies, 1998). Providing the chosen measures of process are known to be unambiguously associated with future health outcomes, they are often likely to offer a more satisfactory measure of contemporary system performance than contemporary health status measures.

A further disadvantage of health status measures, relative to process measures, is that it may in many circumstances be difficult to attribute the observed outcome to the health system. For example, to what extent is the good health status observed in Japan, Italy and France attributable to the health system? If the definition of system is very broadly defined to include concepts such as diet and lifestyle, this may not matter. If however the interest is in a more circumscribed definition of system, confined to purposive actions on the part of certain agencies, then the influence of such external factors may be profoundly misleading.

On the other hand, a countervailing advantage of health status measures is that they are good summary measures of a system's historical success in combating ill-health from whatever source. Mortality is a good indication of failure across all serious conditions, and does not need to be tailored to specific circumstances. Process measures, on the other hand, are usually far more specific than outcome measures and need to be tailored to the details of a particular condition. Furthermore, what is an appropriate high technology process in (say) a high expenditure system may be wildly inappropriate in a low expenditure health system. Any set of process measures chosen to indicate system performance is therefore likely to appear lengthy yet incomplete. See for example the US Medicare example discussed above (Jencks *et al.*, 2000). Any attempt to measure system performance based on process measures therefore tends to lead to a proliferation of indicators.

3.2. Collinearity of components

There will almost always be some positive correlation between different measures of system performance because many programmes implemented by the health system tend to yield benefits in several aspects of performance. This gives rise to a degree of collinearity (or correlation) between constituent performance indicators, which has often troubled designers of composite indices. The fear is that – by combining variables with high degrees of correlation – one may introduce an element of double counting into the index. The response has therefore often been to seek to seek to choose only indicators exhibiting a low degree of collinearity.

Of course, minimizing the number of variables in the index may be highly desirable on other grounds such as transparency and parsimony, and can be guided by multivariate techniques such as factor analysis. However, it is not strictly necessary from a technical point of view. For the purposes of illustration, consider two *identical* indicators. If these are both included in the index with weights α_1 and α_2, then the associated dimension of performance is represented in the index with weight $(\alpha_1 + \alpha_2)$. This is not problematic, providing the weights have been chosen correctly.

This argument is readily extended to the case when variables are highly but not perfectly correlated. If statistical techniques are used to develop the index, variables for inclusion might be chosen on the basis of statistical significance. In this case it is likely that there will not be a great deal of collinearity between the chosen variables. However, if there are high levels of collinearity between *potential* candidates for inclusion in the index, the precise variables indicated for inclusion in the index may be highly dependent on the model selection procedures used, and therefore somewhat arbitrary. In these circumstances, the choice of one variable at the expense of another collinear variable should not alter the rankings greatly, but may be subject to dispute and challenge, and may materially affect the judgements made on a small number of observed systems.

3.3. Identifying the composite weights

As noted above, the weights $\alpha_1, \alpha_2, \ldots \alpha_n$ attached to the component indicators should indicate the relative importance of the indicators. The ratio α_1/α_2 indicates the sacrifice in objective 2 that the user is prepared to make in order to gain an extra unit of objective 1. Under this definition, the weights are dependent on the scale of measurement for each indicator. For this reason, many analysts seek to rescale the constituent indicators in order that the weights have more intuitive meaning. For example, one possibility would be to transform each indicator P_{ij} so that the it captures performance as a percentage of the sample mean. Mathematically, this takes the form:

$$P_{ij}^* = \frac{P_{ij}}{\mu_j} * 100$$

where μ_j is the associated population mean. Using this transformation means that the ratio of revised weights α_1/α_2 should now indicates the percentage points improvement in indicator 1 that will compensate for a one percentage point worsening of indicator 2. Thus the transformation does not alter the structure of the index in any way, but it may assist in the specification and comprehension of weights.

Although a great deal of appropriate economic methodology exists for inferring weights, the examples cited above suggest that its principles have not yet filtered through to the development of composite indicators of health system performance (Dolan *et al.*, 1996). Merely asking respondents how much importance they attach to an objective is unlikely to yield the marginal trade-off valuations required. Methodologies do exist for inferring what are effectively willingness to pay valuations. For example, with a suitably large sample, techniques such as conjoint analysis could infer weights from respondents' ranking of alternative scenarios (Ryan and Farrar, 2000). And direct interview techniques have been found to elicit meaningful responses on the extent to which the public is prepared to sacrifice health gain in order to reduce health inequalities (Shaw *et al.*, 2001). There are particular challenges in applying these methods to composite indicators of health system performance. For example, many of the measures used to construct a composite – such as the WHO inequality indices – may be difficult to explain to respondents. But, if meaningful preference weights are to be developed, that may suggest a need to simplify the measures rather than to resort to more arbitrary weighting schemes.

3.4. *Transforming the constituent indicators*

An associated question is whether any of the constituent indicators should be subject to some sort of mathematical transformation before entering in the index. For example, two of the four variables comprising the the Townsend Index of local deprivation (long used in UK sociological studies) were transformed on the grounds that they were not symmetric (Townsend, 1987). This is a spurious rationale, as the statistical distribution of the underlying variables is immaterial to the specification of the composite index.

Rather, assuming a linear composite of the sort we are using, the principal theoretical justification for transforming indicators is to ensure that the weights used in the composite remain valid throughout the range of observed performance. Recall that the ratio α_1/α_2 is intended to indicate the sacrifice in objective 2 that the user is prepared to make in order to gain an extra unit of objective 1. This price should remain constant whatever the observed values of the indicators. The purpose of transformation is in principle to ensure that such invariance is secured (a very tall order in practice!).

One commonly used transformation is to take the logarithm of all variables. Under this transformation, the weight ratio α_1/α_2 now indicates the *percentage* improvement in variable 1 that would compensate for a 1 per cent reduction in variable 2. It is particularly useful when (as is often the case) the marginal utility of improving an indicator is known to decrease as performance improves. That is, the transformation will lead to a higher weighting for a unit improvement from a low level of performance than an identical unit improvement from an already high level of performance.

3.5. *Environmental influences on performance*

There are numerous potential influences on composite measures of health system performance:

1. variations due to *differences in health status* of the citizens being served;
2. variations due to the *external environment* – for example, geography;
3. variations due to the *resources being used* – poorer results may be the result of poor quality or inappropriate mix of resources (such as an outdated configuration of capital stock);
4. variations due to *different accounting treatments* – there will always be some flexibility in the way that data conventions are interpreted;
5. variations due to *data errors* – the quality of data might vary substantially between systems;
6. variations due to *random fluctuation* – some health outcome measures are highly vulnerable to such fluctuation, outside the control of the system;
7. variations due to *different priorities* regarding objectives – some systems may choose to place a greater emphasis on (say) inequalities at the expense of total health outcome;
8. variations due to *differences in the effectiveness* of the system in achieving chosen objectives – the key issue of interest here.

The principal purpose of developing a composite indicator of performance is to cast light on the extent to which a system is efficient in the sense that it produces outcomes in some preferred mix (influence 7) delivered effectively (influence 8). Account should therefore be taken of the other six influences on a composite measure before any inference on performance is drawn. This issue is treated more extensively in the technical appendix.

A particularly difficult issue for the development of any measures of health system performance is the treatment of contextual considerations (influences 1 and 2). That is, to what extent should a performance measure seek to adjust for differences in environment that affect the difficulty of the task confronting the health systems under scrutiny? The response to this problem depends very much on the purpose of the analysis and the definition of the system. If the intention is to examine health system performance in the broadest sense, it might be argued that virtually all determinants of health are to some extent amenable to influence by the system. No adjustment for contextual issues such as lifestyle or diet is therefore necessary. If, at the other extreme, the interest is (say) in the performance of the health *care* system, then it may be essential to consider the context in which the system performs, and over which it has no control. Very careful adjustment for exogenous factors such as (say) prevalence of smoking may therefore be necessary.

Even if the boundaries of the health system of interest can be satisfactorily defined, there remains a technical problem as to how to treat exogenous influences on performance in any analysis. In the productivity literature there are a number of schools of thought (Fried *et al.*, 1999). One approach is to treat them as another (albeit uncontrollable) input to the production process (one-step modelling); another is to model the production process without reference to exogenous factors, and then examine the extent to which the scores obtained can be explained by putative exogenous influences (two-step modelling). The two-step procedure is likely to be more practical and transparent in most circumstances.

In some circumstances, adjustment for exogenous circumstances may be unnecessary. For example, the English health care funding formula is designed to offer health authorities the opportunity to deliver some standard level of services if they were to adopt standard policies and have a standard level of efficiency. That is, the funding formula is designed in principle to *enable* health systems to exhibit equal levels of performance, given their different environmental circumstances (Smith *et al.*, 2001).

Therefore if the funding formula is doing its job as intended, and if we were able to capture all relevant aspects of performance in the composite, there is no need to include costs or environment in any efficiency models. Through the funding formula, local health systems have in principle been given the means to provide equal quality services, and efficiency should therefore be judged only in the sense that observed outputs (or outcomes) vary between systems.

Of course the funding formula may be seriously flawed, and the "standard" level of service may refer to factors other than performance measures available for the composite, but these possibilities may be relatively secondary. If so, no costs or environmental factors need be included in the composite. Flaws in the funding formula and omitted output measures could then be explored by a second stage analysis that explores systematic environmental influences on efficiency as measured by the unadjusted composite.

3.6. Analytic approaches to inferring efficiency

Most of the discussion to date has focused on the problem of combining measures of system performance (or attainment) into a single composite measure. In order to develop estimates of system *efficiency*, it is necessary to examine the composite measure (and any environmental influences) in conjunction with a measure of the resources devoted to the health system. In some respects this may appear to be a trivial exercise. For example, the ratio of the composite measure to system expenditure might in some contexts be considered a reasonable indicator of efficiency.

However, any attempt to adjust for environmental influences on performance requires more thoughtful deployment of analytic techniques. To that end, econometricians and management scientists have developed two broad approaches to inferring the production possibility frontier from observed data: stochastic frontier analysis (SFA) and data envelopment analysis (DEA) (Coelli *et al.*, 1998). A technical treatment of these techniques is beyond the scope of this paper. The general principle is that in one way or another the performance of the health system should be modelled as a function of expenditure and any relevant environmental factors. The success with which a particular system exceeds (or falls short of) predicted performance indicates its relative efficiency.

There have been countless applications of SFA and DEA to health and health care. However, there are numerous technical judgements that must be made in any application, leading to enormous scope for debate and challenge regarding the results obtained. Furthermore, even narrowly constrained technical choices can dramatically affect judgements on efficiency (Jacobs, 2001). It is therefore

307

unsurprising that there are few if any examples of these approaches being used to inform operational policy towards improving efficiency in individual institutions (Hollingsworth, 1999).

4. Conclusion

A striking feature of all four examples outlined above is the high profile they secured in the popular media. Journalists therefore clearly believe that there is a mass audience for rankings of health systems based on composite indicators of performance. There is therefore strong *prima facie* evidence that the composites are fulfilling an important public role where the publication of individual performance indicators fails.

The arguments for developing composite indicators of performance (as distinct from separate consideration of the component indicators) are:

- They place system performance at the centre of the policy arena;
- They can offer a rounded assessment of system performance;
- They enable judgements to be made on system efficiency;
- They facilitate communication with ordinary citizens and promote accountability;
- They indicate which systems represent the beacons of best performance;
- They indicate which systems represent the priority for improvement efforts;
- They may stimulate the search for better data and better analytic efforts across all of health care;
- In contrast to piecemeal targets based on individual performance measures, they can offer local policy makers the freedom to set their own priorities, and to seek out improvements along dimensions of performance where gains are most readily secured.

Against this, the use of composite indicators (in preference to piecemeal scrutiny of individual performance measures) can lead to seriously dysfunctional outcomes:

- By aggregating individual measures of performance, composite indicators may disguise serious failings in some parts of some systems;
- As measures of performance become more aggregate, it becomes increasingly difficult to know to what to attribute poor performance, and therefore what remedial action to take;
- The individual elements used in the composite indicator are often contentious;
- A composite that seeks to be comprehensive in its coverage may have to rely on very feeble or opaque data in some dimensions of performance;
- A composite that ignores dimensions of performance that are difficult to measure may distort behaviour in undesirable ways;
- Current methodology on calculating weights is seriously inadequate;
- The weights used in composite indicators reflect a single set of preferences, yet all the evidence suggests that there exists great diversity in preferences amongst policy makers and ordinary citizens – in short, the principle of a composite indicator is centralist and does not respect alternative viewpoints.

In deciding whether to develop composite indicators the touchstone should of course be the extent to which the expected benefits outweigh the costs, including the potential dysfunctional responses noted above (Smith, 1995). In this respect, Williams (2001*a*) urges policy makers to consider the decisions that a putative composite indicator would inform.

However this paper has not sought to examine the political context within which composite indicators are applied. Rather, I have concentrated on the technical issues associated with composite indicators. The discussion has identified a number of important unresolved issues, of which three of the most important are the development of a set of weights, the treatment of exogenous influences on system performance, and the modelling of efficiency. I discuss these in turn.

Whatever method is used to derive weights, there is likely to be considerable variation in the preferences reported by different respondents. No consensus will exist regarding the weights to be used to form the composite. This should not preclude use of a composite, but does indicate the dangers of presenting any composite as "objective". At best, it indicates a set of priorities that has been informed by popular or expert judgement. For this reason, it may be more appropriate for composites to be developed by those with legitimate political authority (such as democratically elected national governments) rather than researchers, the media, or non-governmental organisations.

The treatment of exogenous influences on system performance is at a very rudimentary stage of development. There is widespread agreement that local circumstances have a profound influence on measured system performance. Some of these influences can be readily handled. For example, many performance measures are routinely adjusted for the age and sex profile of the relevant population. For individual conditions, risk adjustment methodology is progressing, albeit with variable levels of success (Iezzoni, 1997). However, experience with risk adjustment for more strategic measures of performance is more limited.

Methodology for estimating productive efficiency has achieved an advanced stage of technical development (Coelli *et al.*, 1998). However, the numerous technical judgements that must be made in any application of productivity techniques suggests the need for a careful audit trail and extensive sensitivity analysis and peer review before conclusions can be drawn. The methods are moreover often highly vulnerable to data errors and misspecification (Newhouse, 1994; Smith, 1997). And there are important issues of principle regarding the usefulness of the techniques still to be resolved (Stone, forthcoming).

In summary, there are strong arguments in principle for seeking to report composite indicators of health system performance. However, the practice of developing indicators is in its infancy, and many of the attempts to date have been seriously inadequate from a technical perspective. The danger is that premature publication will lead to seriously adverse responses from health systems. The hope is that the high profile that composite indicators enjoy in the popular press can be translated into heightened research endeavour and a more satisfactory methodology.

Appendix

TECHNICAL APPENDIX

I first consider the means whereby health systems secure their objectives. These means can be defined as *programmes*. Suppose there are just two objectives of system performance. Then – for a given level of expenditure – different programmes might in general secure different mixes of the two outcome measures, P_1 and P_2. For example, in Figure 1 implementation of programme A would favour outcome 1 relative to outcome 2, programme C emphasizes outcome 2, whilst programme B is intermediate. Note that (assuming programmes are divisible and exhibit constant returns to scale) anywhere along the straight line joining A and B can be achieved by implementing an appropriate mix of programmes A and B.[3]

The dotted line joining A and C is everywhere inferior to the lines AB and BC, so an efficient health system should choose segments AB and BC in preference to the line AC. If we progressively add more programmes to the diagram, we might eventually arrive at a curve FF, which economists refer to as the *production possibility frontier*. This indicates, for every feasible level of outcome 1, the maximum level of outcome 2 that can be achieved, given the technological choices available to the health system and a fixed level of expenditure. It can be thought of as the efficient frontier for the chosen level of expenditure, and is illustrated in Figure 2.[4]

The precise point on the curve FF at which a health system should seek to perform depends on relative valuations of the two outcomes. We assume that both outcomes are "goods", and that therefore more of each is better.[5] However, in general different observers will adopt different relative valuations of the two outcomes. This can be illustrated by the two indifference curves I_1I_1 and I_2I_2 in Figure 2, which reflect two competing views of the preferred level of system production. The slopes of these curves at the points of tangency with FF reflect the relative valuations of the two system outcomes. In this case, individual 1 places a higher relative valuation on outcome 1 than individual 2. There will in general be no agreement on what constitutes the preferred mix of outputs from a health system.

The use of a linear composite indicator of the sort set out above suggests that choice of system should be guided by maximizing a linear function of the two outcome measures. The parallel lines in Figure 3 indicate different values of the composite indicator, with scores increasing towards the top right hand corner. Choice of the point P^* on the possibility frontier would be optimal this example, giving a composite score indicated by the line C_1C_1. Given the weights used in the composite indicator, choice of any other point on the frontier would be considered inferior (reflecting the economist's concept of allocative inefficiency).

Figure 1. **Production possibilities with three programmes**

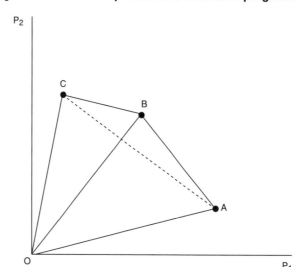

Figure 2. **The production possibility frontier: different preferences lead to different weights**

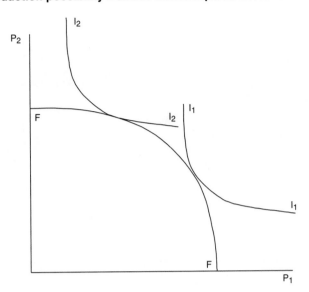

Moreover, few health systems will be precisely on the possibility frontier. Rather, each will exhibit some level of inefficiency, which leads to observed outcomes lying within the area indicated by the efficient frontier (technical inefficiency). In the context of the diagram, the point X indicates one realized level of performance in the health system. According to the composite indicator, this secures a level of system efficiency indicated by the line C_2C_2, reflecting the fact that a) the chosen mix of outputs diverges from the optimal and b) performance lies within the frontier. The measure of system efficiency can be represented by the ratio of the composite scores indicated by lines C_2C_2 and C_1C_1, the extent to which performance falls short of the maximum attainable and desired. It is the product of technical and allocative efficiency.

Of course in practice many commentators would argue that any realistic composite indicator of health system performance should comprise more than two components. However, the principles set out above remain valid for higher levels of dimensionality. See the end of the appendix for a more general treatment of the problem.

Figure 3. **Composite scores indicated by the lines C_1C_1 and C_2C_2**

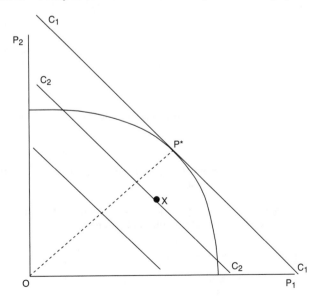

Figure 4. **Observed performance of five systems with identical expenditure and environment**

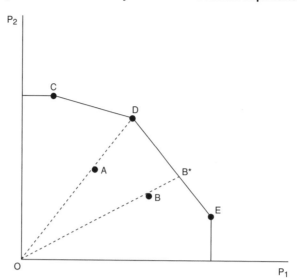

Notice that – although we cannot in general secure a consensus regarding the ranking of health systems – there may be circumstances in which all will agree that some systems perform better than others. Figure 4 illustrates with five systems with identical expenditure levels and environmental circumstances. Under most assumptions about preferences, system A is unambiguously inferior to system D in the sense of being technically inefficient. Furthermore, system B is inferior to a linear combination of systems D and E, represented by the point B*. However, the ranking of the systems C, D and E lying on the observed frontier depends on the relative weights we choose to apply to outcomes 1 and 2. We cannot rank these systems without introducing a composite indicator that reflects preferences for outcome 1 relative to outcome 2.

As the expenditure on the health system increases, so we would expect the production possibility frontier to expand outwards. However, given variable returns to scale in production, we would not necessarily expect the expansion to be entirely symmetric (at different levels of activity, improvement in some outputs may be easier than in others). Furthermore, we would not in general expect an individual's relative weights to remain constant as the production frontier expands. For example, at low levels of expenditure, very rudimentary outcomes, such as saving lives, might be weighted most heavily, whilst issues such as the quality of survival might become weighted more heavily as expenditure increases.

In the same way, some systems must operate in more adverse environments than others, in the sense that external circumstances make achievement of a given level of attainment more difficult. This means that – for a given level of expenditure – the production possibility frontiers of different systems will not in general be identical. The frontiers for systems operating in difficult environments will lie inside those of more favourably endowed systems.

A more general model

For a more general treatment, consider an additive composite indicator of the form:

$$C_i = \sum_j \alpha_j P_{ij}$$

where α_j is the weight attached to constituent performance indicator j, P_{ij} is the score of unit i (health system i) on indicator j, and C_i is the resultant composite score of unit i.

Suppose that each health care system i is seeking to maximize its composite score subject to a budget constraint X_i. Then if the n performance measures were independent, the first order conditions require that:

$$\alpha_j \frac{\partial P_{ij}}{\partial x} = \lambda_i \quad \text{for each performance measure j}$$

That is, unit i should invest in improving measure i up to the point where the marginal benefit is inversely proportional to the weight α_j attached to indicator j.

In practice, any initiative to improve health care performance is likely to have an influence on more than one performance indicator. That is, the performance indicators cannot be considered to be independent. Suppose then that there are K possible programmes designed to improve performance. Then optimization problem for health system i is to choose how much expenditure x_{ik} to assign to programme k, leading to the first order conditions:

$$\sum_j \alpha_j \frac{\partial P_{ij}}{\partial x_{ik}} = \lambda_i \quad \text{for each programme k.}$$

In the special case of constant returns to scale, the composite score is optimized by solving the following linear programme.

$$\text{maximize} \quad C_i = \sum_j \alpha_j P_{ij}$$

$$\text{subject to} \quad P_{ij} = \sum_k \beta_{kj} x_j \quad \text{for } j = ,..., N$$

$$\sum_k x_k = X$$

which can be rewritten as

$$\text{maximize} \quad C_i = \sum_j \sum_k \alpha_j \beta_{kj} x_j$$

$$\text{subject to} \quad \sum_k x_k = X$$

This is a linear programme with one constraint. It will therefore have an optimal solution with only one non-zero x_k: namely that which maximizes the value of

$$\sum_k \alpha_j \beta_{kj}$$

NOTES

1. Twenty-four indicators were reported, but only 22 used in construction of the composite.

2. The WHO measure of efficiency is rather confusingly referred to as system "performance". In this paper I reserve the use of the expression performance to refer to the attainment of goals.

3. In general, programmes are likely to exhibit variable returns to scale. This will not compromise the general argument set out in this section.

4. Note that this use of the expression "production possibility frontier" is not the same as the conventional use made in industrial economics. In particular, the two outputs are not direct substitutes, as any health system programme might contribute (in different proportions) to the production of *both* outputs. Rather, the frontier merely indicates the mix of outputs that is technically achievable, given current organisational technology.

5. In contrast to the conventional assumptions of the theory of economic goods, citizens might care about the *balance* between P_1 and P_2, if for example they represent the health enjoyed by different groups of the population. This concern with equity might lead to the need to adapt some of the forthcoming discussion, but at this stage I would prefer to treat equity as just another objective that can in principle be accommodated within the composite indicator.

REFERENCES

ALMEIDA, C., BRAVEMAN, P., GOLD, M. *et al.* (2001),
"Methodological concerns and recommendations on policy consequences of the World Health Report 2000", *Lancet*, Vol. 357, pp. 1692-1697.

APPLEBY, J. and MULLIGAN, J. (2000),
How Well is the NHS Performing? A composite performance indicator based on public consultation, King's Fund, London.

APPLEBY, J. and STREET, A. (forthcoming),
"Health system goals: life, death and ... football", *Journal of Health Services Research and Policy.*

CANADIAN INSTITUTE FOR HEALTH INFORMATION (2001*a*),
Health Care in Canada 2001: A Second Annual Report, Canadian Institute for Health Information, Ottawa.

CANADIAN INSTITUTE FOR HEALTH INFORMATION (2001*b*),
Health Indicators 2001, Canadian Institute for Health Information, Ottawa.

CHANNEL FOUR (2000),
The Sick List: the NHS from best to worst, www.channel4.com/plus/sick_list/:

COELLI, T., RAO, D. and BATTESE, G. (1998),
An Introduction to Efficiency and Productivity Analysis, Kluwer Academic Publishers, Boston.

CROMBIE, I. and DAVIES, H.T.O. (1998),
"Beyond health outcomes: the advantages of measuring process", *Journal of Evaluation and Clinical Practice*, Vol. 4, pp. 31-38.

DOLAN, P., GUDEX, C., KIND, P. and WILLIAMS, A. (1996),
"Valuing health states: a comparison of methods", *Journal of Health Economics*, Vol. 15, pp. 209-231.

FRIED, H., SCHMIDT, S. and YAISAWARNG, S. (1999),
"Incorporating the operating environment into a nonparametric measure of technical efficiency", *Journal of Productivity Analysis*, Vol. 12, pp. 249-267.

GAKIDOU, E., MURRAY, C. and FRENK, J. (2000),
Measuring preferences on health system performance assessment. GPE Discussion Paper 20, World Health Organization, Geneva.

HOLLINGSWORTH, B. (1999),
"Efficiency measurement of health care: a review of non-parametric methods and applications", *Health Care Management Science*, Vol. 2, pp. 161-172.

HOLMES, N. and PENNINGTON, B. (2001),
"Medicare: too little, too late", *Harpers*, Vol. 84, May.

IEZZONI, L. (1997),
Risk Adjustment for Measuring Healthcare Outcomes, Second Edition, Health Administration Press, Chicago.

JACOBS, R. (2001),
"Alternative methods to examine hospital efficiency: data envelopment analysis and stochastic frontier analysis", *Health Care Management Science*, Vol. 4, pp. 103-115.

JENCKS, S. F. *et al.* (2000),
"Quality of medical care delivered to Medicare beneficiaries", *Journal of the American Medical Association*, Vol. 284, pp. 1670-1676.

KAPLAN, R. and NORTON, D. (1992),
"The balanced scorecard – measures that drive performance", *Harvard Business Review*, pp. 71-79.

LI, T. and ROSENMAN, R. (2001),
"Cost inefficiency in Washington hospitals: a stochastic frontier approach using panel data", *Health Care Management Science*, Vol. 4, pp. 73-81.

MARSHALL, R. (1999),
"The Maclean's Health Report", *Macleans*, Vol. 112.

MARSHALL, R. (2001),
"Where we get the best health care", *Macleans*, Vol. 114, pp. 31-36.

MURRAY, C. and FRENK, J. (2001),
"World Health Report 2000: a step towards evidence-based health policy", *Lancet*, Vol. 357, pp. 1698-1700.

MURRAY, C., LAUER, J., TANDON, A. and FRENK, J. (2000),
Overall health system achievement for 191 countries. GPE Discussion Paper 28, World Health Organization, Geneva.

MURRAY, C., FRENK, J., EVANS, D., KAWABATA, K., LOPEZ, A. and ADAMS, O. (2001),
"Science or marketing at who? A response to Williams", *Health Economics*, Vol. 10, pp. 277-282.

NAVARRO, V. (2000),
"Assessment of the World Health Report 2000", *Lancet*, Vol. 356, pp. 1598-1601.

NAVARRO, V. (2001),
"World Health Report 2000: response to Murray and Frenk", *Lancet*, Vol. 357, p. 1701.

NEWHOUSE, J. (1994),
"Frontier estimation: how useful a tool for health economics", *Journal of Health Economics*, Vol. 13, pp. 317-322.

OECD (2000),
OECD *Health Data*, Paris.

RYAN, M. and FARRAR, S. (2000),
"Using conjoint analysis to elicit preferences for health care", *British Medical Journal*, Vol. 320, pp. 1530-1533.

SHAW, R., DOLAN, P., TSUCHIYA, A., WILLIAMS, A., SMITH, P. and BURROWS, R. (2001),
"Development of a questionnaire to elicit public preferences regarding health inequalities", Occasional Paper, Centre for Health Economics, University of York, York.

SMITH, P. (1995),
"On the unintended consequences of publishing performance data in the public sector", *International Journal of Public Administration*, Vol. 18, pp. 277-310.

SMITH, P. (1997),
"Model misspecification in data envelopment analysis", *Annals of Operations Research*, Vol. 73, pp. 233-252.

SMITH, P., RICE, N. and CARR-HILL, R. (2001),
"Capitation funding in the public sector", *Journal of the Royal Statistical Society*, Series A, Vol. 164, pp. 217-257.

STONE, M. (forthcoming),
"Questions of efficiency in public services: is the state of the art really state of the art'?", *Journal of the Royal Statistical Society*, Series A.

TOWNSEND, P. (1987),
"Deprivation", *Journal of Social Policy*, Vol. 16, pp. 125-146.

WILLIAMS, A. (2001*a*),
"Science or marketing at WHO? A commentary on World Health 2000", *Health Economics*, Vol. 10, pp. 93-100.

WILLIAMS, A. (2001*b*),
"Science or marketing at who? Rejoinder from Alan Williams", *Health Economics*, Vol. 10, pp. 283-285.

WORLD HEALTH ORGANIZATION (2000),
The World Health Report 2000. Health systems: improving performance, World Health Organization, Geneva.

Part V

APPLYING PERFORMANCE INDICATORS
TO HEALTH SYSTEM IMPROVEMENT

Chapter 15

APPLYING PERFORMANCE INDICATORS
TO HEALTH SYSTEM IMPROVEMENT

by

Sheila Leatherman[*]

> *"Knowing is not enough, we must apply*
> *Willing is not enough,we must do."*
> Goethe.

Abstract

The cycle of performance measurement and management begins with explicitly establishing goals which are reflected in the adoption of specific performance indicators, followed by analysis and actions aimed at producing change to improve performance in a variety of dimensions such as equity, access, effectiveness, efficiency and social responsiveness. The application of performance indicators may involve simply reporting data to actors for accountability purposes, or it may involve, in addition, taking action to stimulate change.

This paper will first summarize some evidence on the use and impacts of public release of health care performance data, based largely on the American experience (as described in "Dying to know: Public Release of Information about Quality of Health Care" by Marshall *et al.*, co-published by The Nuffield Trust and Rand, 2000). Some of the main conclusions from this review of evidence from the United States are that: first, currently available report cards are rarely read by individual consumers, and do not seem to have much influence on their decisions to choose health care providers; but second, and although physicians and provider organisations tend to be critical of performance reports, provider organisations seem to be the most responsive to publicly disclosed data.

The paper will then outline a further range of levers that might be used to try to improve performance, where available indicators suggest room for improvement. A careful diagnosis of the underlying causes of problems in the health care system is needed to select the appropriate intervention. Possible approaches, grouped within five categories, will be discussed: external oversight, provider knowledge enhancement, empowering consumers, incentives and regulation.

Significant challenges exist in using performance indicators to create intentional change in health care systems. First, the state of the art is embryonic, meaning that there is an insufficient evidence base for understanding what works, under what circumstances, and with what intended and unintended consequences. Secondly, the costs – both direct and indirect – are daunting. Thirdly, the complexity of the health care sector, and the multiplicity of audiences and actors, means that there are likely to be both intended and unintended consequences of any approach. Recognizing these caveats, and the inherent limitations of any one approach, implies the need to carefully employ a blend of approaches with complementary effects.

---

[*] Adjunct Professor, School of Public Health, University of North Carolina; Senior Advisor, The Nuffield Trust, London, England; Sr. Associate, Judge Institute of Management Studies, University of Cambridge, England.

319

---

1. Defining performance

Understanding the role performance indicators may play in improving the delivery and outcomes of health care requires an understanding of the scope and magnitude of performance issues in health systems. Additionally, the judicious use of performance indicators to predictably effect desired changes requires an understanding of the evidence on the effectiveness of, and the challenges in implementing, specific transformation strategies or levers for change.

Three countries – Australia, United Kingdom and the United States – will be used to illustrate the nature of these issues and challenges. These countries offer interesting comparisons as they range from the nationalized monolithic NHS, to the pluralistic private sector oriented system of the United States, with Australia having characteristics of both (McLoughlin *et al.*, 2001).

Though performance is described and evaluated in many ways, a consensus on the principal domains is emerging and evident in the work of international organisations like WHO and OECD, as well as the performance frameworks being implemented by individual countries. The domains of effectiveness, efficiency, responsiveness and equity are commonly included in describing key dimensions of health care performance. Discrete dimensions are sometimes subsumed in broad definitions of quality such as the one developed by the Institute of Medicine in the US, which defines quality as "the degree to which health services for individuals and populations increases the likelihood of desired health outcomes and are consistent with current professional knowledge" (Institute of Medicine, 1990). To fully actualize this definition of quality, principles of equity and efficiency are inherent to population health, effectiveness is requisite for achieving outcomes, and responsiveness is an essential property at the individual level. It is performance in this broad definition of quality that will provide the context for examining applications of performance indicators in this paper.

2. Improving health system performance: a clear priority

Performance assessments may vary dramatically according to the methods and definitions used. Though legitimate debate exists regarding measurement techniques, there is little disagreement regarding the need to improve performance in health systems globally.

Despite the evidence of significant gains in some health status indicators, the peer-reviewed literature describes dramatic quality-of-care deficiencies including inappropriate care, safety problems and unjustified regional variation in practice patterns. Numerous surveys at both an individual country level, as well as cross-country comparisons, portray the formidable scale and scope of performance issues. Whether through the eyes of physicians, patients or purchasers/payers, concerns regarding eroding performance are rife. In a recent physician survey conducted in Australia, New Zealand, Canada, the United Kingdom and the United States, physicians reported a significant decline in quality in all five countries (Blendon *et al.*, 2001). When asked how their ability to provide quality care had changed over the past five years, significant numbers of physicians reported that it was worse; Australia 38 per cent, Canada 59 per cent, New Zealand 53 per cent, the United Kingdom 46 per cent and in the United States 57 per cent. Only one-quarter or less of the physicians in any country reported that their ability to provide high quality care had improved over the past five years. In a survey (1998-99) looking at attitudes of nurses across five countries – Canada, Germany, Scotland, England, the United States – 17 to 44 per cent reported that quality had deteriorated in the past year (Aiken *et al.*, 2001).

Lest these findings be discounted as simply the complaints of demoralized clinicians, we can look at public perceptions on the performance of health systems. In a survey conducted in 1998 (Australia, United Kingdom, United States, Canada, and New Zealand), the public indicated overwhelmingly that the health systems in their country required fundamental change or a complete overhaul (Blendon *et al.*, 2001). And, even more telling regarding public attitudes was data from a 1998 American Consumer Satisfaction Index (Lieber *et al.*, 1998) which placed hospitals between the US Postal Office and the Internal Revenue Service. This sobering assessment clearly indicates a mistrust of the American public in health care institutions, and provides one more dramatic data point to illustrate the pressing need to address performance issues.

The case is clear for placing a high priority on improving systemic performance and fostering accountability through public reporting of performance data. The cycle of performance measurement and management begins with explicitly establishing goals, which are reflected in the adoption of specific performance indicators, followed by analysis and reporting of data to various audiences through public and confidential means (Hurst and Jee-Hughes, 2001). Then, systematic implementation of actions must be aimed at producing change in multiple dimensions such as equity, access, effectiveness, efficiency and social responsiveness. A careful diagnosis of the underlying causes of problems in the health care system is needed to select the appropriate intervention.

The possible methods and approaches for performance improvement are numerous but the evidence basis is often scant or equivocal for selection. Furthermore, the levers for change will vary among countries (or even within different health care systems in the same country) depending upon factors such as underlying values, financing and organisational arrangements, professional culture, and the self-perception of the citizenry as active or passive participants in health care interactions. The selection of the intervention will depend upon who and what is the intended target for behavioral change; for example, providers (individual or institutional), professional bodies, citizens, or managers. Though identifying a "best method" to effect change may not be realistic, this paper will identify the range of possible approaches, discuss their strengths and limitations, and describe relevant country experiences.

3. Public reporting of performance indicators

Despite a growing movement of quality measurement and intervention efforts in many countries, there is minimal evidence that predictable and widespread improvements in quality are occurring. This fact, coupled by a political trend towards greater transparency in government and public services, has resulted in a movement calling for accountability in health care. Public reporting of performance data is one of the principal instruments used to realize this accountability.

Three models of accountability in health care have been described and apply to OECD countries in various combinations (Table 1). All rely on performance indicators, either explicit or implicit, to some degree.

The three models are economic, public and professional (Emanuel and Emanuel, 1996). The model of professional accountability, dominant in most health systems historically, views the physician-patient dyad as the operative focus of accountability with certification, accreditation, licensure and litigation as instruments for enforcement. Increasingly the professional model of accountability is regarded as insufficient, perhaps even imprudent, and thus this model is accompanied by one of the other two. The economic model, for which the United States is the clearest example, is predicated on the notion that *choice* and *exit* can be mechanisms of enforcing accountability in a marketplace. And thirdly, the public model views the citizen as receiving a public good with the role of the government to compel accountability through the instruments of "voice" and policy. In all of these models, objective measures of performance are increasingly relied upon, accompanied by a trend towards public reporting despite minimal evidence of its effectiveness for driving constructive behavioral or system change.

Table 1. **Models and instruments of accountability**

	Conception	Domain of patients	Mechanisms/ Instruments of accountability
Professional	Recipient of professional services	Patient, physician, prof. association	Licensure, certification, malpractice suit
Economic	Consumer of health care commodity	Marketplace and regulation	Choice and "exit"
Political	Citizen receiving public good	Government reforms and actions	"Voice" and government pressure

Source: Adapted from Emanuel and Emanuel (1996).

The four principle reasons for public disclosure can be summarized as the following; regulation including public accountability, purchasing or commissioning decisions, facilitation of consumer selection and choice, and provider behavior change (Marshall *et al.*, 2000*a*). The United States is regarded as a country with some of the longest experience (over a decade) in public reporting of health system performance data, producing a body of evidence to evaluate the role public reporting may play to improve health care systems. A review article, published in JAMA (Marshall *et al.*, 2000*b*) provides useful information (summarized below) regarding the evidence of effectiveness of performance data for these purposes and for the critical audiences including the public, providers, purchasers or payers and policymakers. Whilst the market context in the US may differ in allowing for more consumer choice, OECD countries face similar challenges in regulation, purchasing/ commissioning decisions and clinical practice, as well as a growing attention to individual responsiveness and patient-centered care.

3.1. *The public*

In summary, evidence from the US indicates that patients/consumers have used performance data only minimally, continuing to largely rely on word-of-mouth for information to make health care decisions (Bates and Gawande, 2000; Coulter and Cleary, 2001). There are numerous reasons why this may be occurring. Most of the performance data that is publicly disclosed was intended for other purposes and audiences and so is neither easily comprehended nor readily applied for decision making. For example, it simply may not be realistic to expect that the average person is going to take an interest in performance data about health care subjects that they think are not going to occur in their lives, such as CABG (coronary artery bypass graft) mortality rates, one of the most highly publicized performance measures in the United States. As a result performance information goes unused and poor quality goes unpunished, or even unnoticed by a large part of the public (Dowd and Finch, 2001).

Furthermore, despite erosion of public confidence regarding the health system at large, individuals in the United States still believe their doctor is good and so have little motivation to sort through voluminous performance data to decipher the meaning. It is only fairly recently that consumers (at least in the United States) have begun to realize that there are significant quality problems that represent potential hazard to them. Designing performance data specifically with consumers in mind, that is understanding the salient data needs and formatting issues, may dramatically influence the uptake of data by consumers. The use of comprehensible performance indicators may be the most pragmatic format for delivering information.

3.2. *Providers*

A second key audience is providers, both institutional providers (hospitals, NHS trusts, health plans) and individual providers (physicians and other clinicians). Experience in the US has involved governmental initiatives, at both federal level (Medicare) and state level authorities, as well as voluntary initiatives through collaborative peer efforts at regional levels. Summaries of the literature indicate that institutions do, in fact, pay attention to, and use performance data in three ways; to improve appropriateness of care processes, to identify poor performers, and to alter processes or structures to be responsive to patient stated preferences or complaints (Marshall *et al.*, 2000*a* and 2000*b*; Legnini *et al.*, 2000). Whether the actual public release, as opposed to the use of data in confidential peer review, is the principal driving factor is debatable. Case studies have noted improvements in care in circumstances where public reporting occurred as well as when peer review was conducted in more confidential settings (addressed in Section 4).

Over the past twenty years, considerable experience with the use of data in peer review and public reporting has been published. One of the most successful, and highly studied initiatives was in New York State where the State Health Department published post-CABG (coronary artery bypass graft) mortality rates. The rate of decline in mortality in New York was twice the average national rate of decline in the first five years of the program (1987-92) and New York had the lowest risk-adjusted mortality of any state in the US by the fourth year of the program (O'Connor and Eagle, 1998). In the first three years alone the risk adjusted mortality rate fell 41 per cent (Chassin, 2001). These changes have been attributed to the actions taken by the hospitals and clinical staff, including changes in leadership, curtailment of operating privileges and intensive peer review. Market forces, including selection by consumers and payers, were not viewed as contributors to the significant change though it is important to acknowledge that in the early years media attention was fierce and drew attention to outliers (Chassin, 1997 and 2001). Impressive as these successes are, the program has not proved to be generalizable either by replication in New York with other clinical conditions, or emulated by other states.

There are other successful applications of performance indicators to changing health system performance in the US. For example, following the introduction of health plan reporting requirements for various process measures in selected conditions including post myocardial infarction, the rates of beta-blocker prescribing rose from 62 per cent in 1996 to 85 per cent in 1999 (Ayanian and Quinn, 2001). Evidence from the US does provide a basis for using performance indicators to drive provider and system change. To date, the evidence would best support using published performance data to effect institutional provider behavior, and to accompany data disclosure with additional levers for change.

3.3. Purchasers/Payers

A third audience for performance indicators is purchasers or payers. Since employers are the dominant buyers of health care in the US, they theoretically have both the motive and clout to buy health services or insurance coverage based on performance. To date, despite considerable attention to the competitive marketplace as a driver of discipline to improve performance, the reality lags beyond the rhetoric. There are notable initiatives of large employers and business coalitions who purportedly make value-based decisions in buying health care; that is, balancing cost with benefit. However, the common practice in purchasing or commissioning services is that price trumps all other performance data. Two large studies (Gabel *et al.*, 1998; Hibbard and Jewett, 1997) collectively looked at over 1500 employers across the US. The authors concluded that the use of performance data by employers was limited, explained in part because the data was not adequately packaged to be comprehensible and useful to these buyers. Reliance on purchasers and payers to improve performance through use of indicators as a basis for selection has not proven to be a reliable strategy.

3.4. Policy makers

Finally, a fourth key audience is policy makers at national and local levels who are responsible for regulation of the health services sector. Policy can be dramatically influenced by performance indicators as was demonstrated in the following examples from the United States and the United Kingdom as reported by Anderson and Hussey in *Health Affairs* (2001). The decision of Prime Minister Tony Blair to invest significant new resources into the NHS, was influenced by data showing Britain to be spending at a lower percentage of GDP than most northern European countries. Another example is the United States, which was influenced by international performance data to train more general practitioners when the data showed that the United Stated trains a higher proportion of specialists than most European countries (Anderson and Hussey, 2001).

New initiatives using explicit performance indicators are emerging in the form of national reports, issued by government, on the performance of health systems in several countries. The United Kingdom, in 1999 adopted a Performance Assessment Framework (NHS Executive, 1999), for publicly reporting NHS performance. The American Congress has mandated that a federal agency (Agency for Healthcare Research and Quality) develop a National Quality Report, comprised of multiple performance domains-including safety, responsiveness, and effectiveness (Institute of Medicine, 2001). The prototype of this report is to be released in 2003. And, in Australia, similar efforts have been underway since 1994 with the National Health Ministers' Benchmark Group, which produced three national reports in 1996, 1998 and 1999 (National Health Ministers' Benchmarking Working Group, 1996, 1998 and 1999).

323

4. Applications of performance indicators

In trying to identify reliable means for ameliorating performance, a natural reflex is to assume that more money and resources are the first solution to be considered. The case of the United States may be most dramatic to refute this assumption. The United States, where 1.1 trillion dollars is annually spent (13.1 per cent of GDP) (see National Health Expenditure Projections, 2001), ranked 37th on the WHO country assessments (World Health Organization, 2000), largely based on the low ratings in the equity domain. Even more striking, is the fact that despite the United States consistently having the highest health spending per capita and as a percentage of GDP (OECD, 2000), its relative performance on OECD indicators has not improved from 1960-1998 and has actually had the greatest relative decline in life expectancy at birth for females and infant mortality (Anderson and Hussey, 2001).

Though indisputable that the performance of health systems is linked to resourcing decisions at the macro and micro levels, this paper will focus on other applications of performance indicators for changing systems and human behaviors. Possible approaches can be grouped within five categories, as depicted in Table 2. This paper will briefly discuss each category and select applications, of emerging interest and reliance, to discuss in more depth.

Table 2. **A categorisation of interventions for changing system and provider behavior**

External oversight	**Knowledge/skill enhancement of providers**
– External review/Inspection	– Peer review and data feedback
– Accreditation, licensing and certification	– Use of guidelines and protocols
– Setting performance targets	
Patient engagement/empowering consumers	**Incentives**
– Providing performance information to consumers for choice	– Financial (pay for performance)
– Enacting patient charters/patient rights legislation	– Non-financial
Regulations	
– Government regulation	
– Professional/self regulation	

Source: Author.

4.1. *External oversights*

i) *External review and inspection*

External review, oversight and inspection are fundamental to performance monitoring and accountability. Accreditation, licensing and/or certification are the instruments used to assure, at least, minimum standards of compliance and competencies. All OECD countries have systems in place to accomplish these functions through a blend of government and professional mechanisms (Hurst and Jee-Hughes, 2001). Increasingly, countries are using explicit, rather than implicit, performance indicators and expanding the types of indicators from a traditional focus on structure, to incorporate process compliance and outcome indicators.

New investments for standard setting and oversight are evident in the UK and Australia. In each country, national bodies have been established to be responsible for an agenda of setting performance targets, monitoring performance through newly defined reporting procedures, and working to identify and implement effective change strategies. In the United Kingdom, three new bodies have been established. The first, the Commission for Health Improvement, is based on the model of the National Audit Commission, and is charged with regular review of all NHS agencies in a four year period, as well as being authorized by the Secretary of State for Health to have investigative powers in situations requiring an independent inquiry (McLoughlin *et al.*, 2001). Secondly, a new body, just established in 2001, called The National Clinical Assessment Authority will independently evaluate poorly performing doctors, when local efforts are inadequate. A third new national entity will have specific responsibilities for setting performance targets and monitoring performance in the areas of safety and error reduction (described later) (see Department of Health, 2001a). Likewise, Australia has also invested in new infrastructure for performance monitoring and oversight. The National Health Performance Committee (NHPC), established in 1999, has responsibility for developing and maintaining a national performance framework for the whole of the health system, as well as to support benchmarking and provide comparative performance data in population health outcomes, risk factors and health system measures (National Expert Advisory Group on Safety and Quality in Australian Health Care, 1999).

ii) Setting performance targets

Performance indicators can be used to make policy priorities explicit, thereby defining expectation, facilitating accountability, and focusing resources. This may be done at two levels; firstly, defining national priorities, and secondly, identifying specific performance targets within those priorities. Setting explicit performance targets has been in effect for nearly two decades in the NHS, largely focused on utilization and cost indicators (Hurst and Jee-Hughes, 2001). Both Australia and England have identified the need to focus on improving performance in specific priority disease areas and within specific population groups. Accordingly, Australia has had a system of identified national health priorities since 1996; namely asthma, depression, diabetes, cardiovascular and injury, with reports describing the best available data in most of the national priority areas (Commonwealth Department of Health and Family Services and Australian Institute of Health and Welfare, 1998a, 1998b, 1999a, 1999b, 1999c; Australian Institute of Health and Welfare and Dept. of Health and Family Services, 1997).

One case study for examining the effectiveness of setting priorities and specific performance targets will be the newly defined initiatives in the UK and Australia to improve safety and reduce the incidence of adverse events and medical errors. Reducing the risk of harm is not only the right thing to do for patient care as part of a professional ethos, it also has grave implications economically for health care systems. Recently, the National Audit Office in England reported that the outstanding claims for alleged clinical negligence in NHS hospitals totaled 3.9 billion pounds (US$5.6 billion) As part of the ambitious program set out in spring 2001, and described in the report titled *Building a Safer* NHS, the Department of Health in England identified four categories of serious harm with measurable targets; for example, reduction by 40 per cent of prescribing errors by 2005 (Department of Health, 2001b).

4.2. Knowledge/Skill enhancement

Performance deficiency among clinicians poses a challenge for diagnosing the problem with enough accuracy to select and implement an effective corrective action. Fundamentally, it is critical to understand whether the deficient behavior is a problem of will, skill, a knowledge gap or a systems problem. Of course, it is likely to be a combination of these factors. Performance indicators can play a role in education and providing feedback to providers.

Knowledge deficiencies may be best understood as simply deriving from an inability to master new knowledge at the rate and complexity it is being produced. Even well-intentioned and highly-motivated clinicians have to grapple with the volume of evidence that is constantly becoming available. In the mid 1960s about 100 articles from randomized clinical trials were published. By the 1990s, approximately 10,000 articles from randomized clinical trials were annually published. In the past five years alone, nearly half (49 per cent) of all the extant medical literature has been published (Chassin, 1998). This knowledge gap results in a knowledge lag meaning the time lapse between identification of more efficacious treatments and incorporation into routine practice. This time lag has been estimated to be in the range of 15-20 years, and even then the adoption of evidence into practice is very uneven (Balas and Boren, 2000). Furthermore this failure to translate research into practice is not only manifest in complicated clinical conditions or the use of emerging technologies and pharmaceuticals, but also in the most routinely treated medical problems like the common cold. For example, researchers in several different studies showed that physicians continue to prescribe antibiotics for the common cold in

40-60 per cent of office visits even though there is no evidence that antibiotics are effective for the cold virus (Mainous *et al.*, 1996; Gonzales *et al.*, 1997; Nyquist *et al.*, 1998).

The challenge for addressing this problem of knowledge deficiency, particularly when well understood as a continuous need for facilitating rapid uptake of published evidence into daily patient care, is complicated by a dearth of understanding as to powerful and predictable interventions. Clinical guideline use and peer reviews are two of the most common applications of performance indicators.

i) Clinical guidelines/protocols

Performance indicators, embedded in guidelines and protocols at a level understandable and actionable by clinicians, are widely used to improve clinical decision making. Performance measures may be more easily digested by physicians as they often are produced in a simple format defining critical process or outcome measures, thus facilitating the translation of evidence into practice.

There are significant challenges in the use of performance indicators to guide practice, and the acceptance of protocols and guidelines by physicians is likely to differ from country to country. In England, a recent British Medical Association survey of more than 100 doctors found that 70 per cent did not believe that the newly established national body (National Institute for Clinical Evidence) which is developing the evidence basis for guidelines and protocols is acting independently, Furthermore, 75 per cent said they disagreed with at least one of the newly developed decisions and 85 per cent said that they would ignore the Institute's guidance if they thought it was wrong (*Reuters Health Headline*, 18 May 2001).

The development of clinical guidelines and protocols is a necessary but not sufficient condition. Published research, to date, has not shown that the use of clinical guidelines and protocols alone have been effective in changing physician behavior (Greco and Eisenberg, 1993; Schuster *et al.*, 1998; Cabana *et al.*, 1999; Hayward, 1997; Lomas *et al.*, 1989). However, recent research is encouraging in the demonstration that practice guidelines incorporated into computer decision support systems shows potential. In two separate meta-analyses, totaling data from 39 studies, the use of computer generated prompts showed effectiveness in improving preventive services and drug prescribing (Balas *et al.*, 2000).

ii) Peer review and feedback of performance data

This section will focus on use of performance indicators by peers for individual or comparative appraisal in a confidential setting. The experience in the US of one large multi-state consortium of physicians in New England is instructive and has been used to argue that the public disclosure of performance data is not necessary as a lever for change. In this consortium, comparative data was not publicly reported, but instead shared among physicians as peers for quality improvement education. Over two years, the risk-adjusted mortality rate for CABG was reduced 24 per cent from what would have been expected based on previous experience (O'Connor and Eagle, 1998).

More broadly, literature documents few systematic and sustained improvements using data by hospital or medical groups and though there are some notable exceptions, most have had rather modest improvements (Chassin, 1997).What explains the relatively little activity by physicians to use data in a quest for performance improvement? A number of obstacles need to be addressed, most notably; lack of public demand for marked improvement, perverse payment incentives, inadequate education and training, and lack of effective information technology.

For physicians to be able to assume leadership positions for performance improvement, they will at minimum need data to be routinely available and credible. Better information regarding effective intervention strategies and improvement methods, and expert help in organisational change, will also be required (Becher and Chassin, 2001).

4.3. Patient engagement/Empowering consumers

During the past five years, improving the patient's experience of health care has become a more visible priority in many OECD countries. There are two applications of performance indicators at the level of the individual citizen; the first is in the role of potential consumer of services, and secondly, as a patient.

Firstly, there are increasing efforts by governments to define the health care system as a public service with the citizen as a consumer having rights and responsibilities. In England, this has taken the form of articulating the modernization programs for the "new NHS" using language of "a health service designed around the patient". Newly committed resources and initiatives to promote citizen and patient empowerment include making information more readily available by 1-800- nurse lines, an electronic medical library providing access for the consumer to medical information shared with the clinical professionals (Coulter, 2001), as well as publicly reporting high level performance indicators.

In the United States, patients rights legislation has been an area of high emotion and fiery rhetoric, but relatively little legislative success at the federal level. At the state level, various bills have been enacted to assure patients increased access to emergency care, clear appeals processes when turned down for treatment eligibility, protections of patients for continuity of care and protection of physicians from being "gagged" by health plans, meaning restricting physicians' ability to candidly discuss all treatment options with patients (even if insurers will not pay for the services). Legislative and regulatory inaction has fueled patient empowerment advocates to demand performance indicators allowing for more informed consumers who presumably will be able to decrease their risk exposure.

Patient empowerment is both theoretically and pragmatically sound. Programs to empower patients are not just politically correct, they can be effective at rationalizing resources. Evidence to support the importance of patient education is available. There is now a body of literature documenting the salutary effects of giving information to patients who have better outcomes, choose less risky procedures and avoid equivocal treatments (Coulter, 2001). This should increase our confidence that patients can not only make constructive use of performance data but also be reliable informants for performance assessment, such as in the NHS where systematic collection of data on patient perceptions will be part of the comprehensive performance framework (NHS Executive, 1999).

4.4. Incentives

i)   Financial

Pay for performance is a concept of increasing interest in both publicly financed and private pay health care systems. Payment policies can strongly influence how both institutional providers (hospitals, health systems) and individual providers (physicians and other health care professionals) deliver health services (Hillman, 1991). The task is essentially one of designing and implementing funding mechanisms to reduce suboptimization in payment. There is some evidence to indicate that certain payment mechanisms are associated with particular practices. Capitation has been associated with providing fewer services and fee-for-service in encouraging the provision of more services, however the use of payment for objectively measured performance has relatively little research (Kindig, 1998).

Paying for results, or rewarding high quality of care, is not a new concept. For example, it has been applied in various countries to promote preventive services such as immunization where there is universal agreement on the evidence basis. Though mortality from vaccine-preventable diseases is very low in most developed countries, WHO estimated that 20 000 avoidable deaths occurred in 1994 and rates of immunization in the United States remain so low that it is unlikely that the country will reach the target immunization rates set out in *Healthy People* 2010. For years, the NHS has been successful in paying general practitioners additionally for reaching target rates of immunizations. In Australia, incentives have included cash to parents and doctors and fast food vouchers to children. And in the US, managed care has experimented with various payment mechanisms to reward reduction of unnecessary procedures while reinforcing primary prevention (Anderson and Hussey, 2001).

The second major task for applying performance indicators to designing incentives is removing financial barriers to improving care. For example, if a performance target is identified for the reduction of unnecessary procedures, then payment methods must, at minimum, eliminate the financial barrier. To illustrate, in the case of reduction of unnecessary hysterectomies and C-sections, a loss of income for those hospitals most successful at achieving the target might occur. A fee-for-service payment method would reward the payer, as opposed to the hospital, which loses revenues.

The judicious use of financial incentives requires careful design in two ways; reinforcing positive performance through additional payments and removing payment mechanisms that perversely effect desired performance.

ii)   Non-financial incentives

Though the word incentives is usually equated with money, there are other forms of incentives such as recognition, reductions in oversight, reputation enhancement, and increased professional satisfaction or institutional esteem.

A new incentive system being implemented in the UK is called "earned autonomy". It will reward high performing institutions with greater autonomy and direct access to financial resources, while the lower performers will be required to demonstrate intent to change and be subjected to more external vigilance. Explicit performance indicators and patient survey data will be used to judge performance (Secretary of State for Health, 2000).

4.5. Regulation

Countries worldwide are facing the same challenge of balancing the strengths and weaknesses of professional self-regulation with governmental regulation. Whilst recognizing that professionalism is possibly the best quality assurance that patients can have, there is an acknowledgement that the degree of reliance heretofore exhibited is no longer regarded as sufficient or prudent. Both government and the professions have a shared responsibility to the public, and many countries are experimenting with the design of complementary roles and responsibilities.

Health systems are restructuring in ways that fundamentally change the nature and scope of professionalism. In the United States, the predisposition of the public to be wary of government interference is changing to an environment where the public looks to the government for protecting basic rights and enforcing accountability. This is being done through a concatenation of federal and state legislative and regulatory actions. Many of these actions are based on performance indicators including reporting requirements, accreditation and licensure. Even in the United Kingdom, where the NHS has long been a centralized system with regulation inherent to the management structure, significant regulation is being introduced for monitoring and inspection, as well as new systems and requirements for annual appraisal and revalidation (every five years) of physicians (based on explicit performance indicators).

One illustrative area (previously mentioned) where government regulation is being increased in England is in patient safety and reduction of adverse events. *Building a Safer* NHS, a Department of Health paper recently published, estimates that 850 000 adverse events that effect one in ten hospitalized patients occur per year in the NHS and reported that there has been no real understanding or systematic approach to the identification and reduction of adverse events in England or in other countries worldwide (Department of Health, 2001*b*). The United Kingdom, Australia and the United States are becoming exceptions to this observation as each country is addressing the concern at a national policy level as well as investing in new infrastructure and capacity to reduce the risk of error and occurrences of adverse events. These national initiatives require reporting of performance against explicit indicators. In England, a National Patient Safety Agency was announced in April of 2001 to facilitate learning from a new national reporting system which will collect and analyze data on medical error and adverse events.

5.   The way forward

The use of performance indicators is a growing trend, and is supported by conventional management theory, a growing body of research, as well as policy imperatives. Table 3 shows the key

Table 3. **Key strategies for improving performance of providers, professional groups, policymakers, the public and purchasers/commissioners**

Targets for performance change	Key strategies for change					
	Performance reporting	Accreditation and inspection	Incentives	Patient empowerment	Regulation	Knowledge/Skill enhancement
Providers	X	X	X		X	X
Professional bodies	X				X	X
Public	X		X	X		X
Payers and contractor purchasers	X	X			X	
Policy makers	X					

Source: Author.

strategies for change and their target audiences, being implemented in Australia, the United Kingdom and the United States. In every country multiple interventions are being used. Careful selection of strategies is called for given the costs inherent in implementation, and continuing uncertainly regarding conditions for most effective application. Recognizing these caveats, and the inherent limitations of any one approach, implies the need to carefully employ a blend of approaches with complementary effects.

Significant challenges exist in using performance indicators to create intentional change in health care systems. First, the state of the art is embryonic, meaning that there is an insufficient evidence base for understanding what works, under what circumstances, and with what consequences. Secondly, the costs, both direct and indirect, are daunting, particularly in developing the necessary information infrastructure which is deficient in many countries. Thirdly, the complexity of the health care sector, and the multiplicity of audiences and actors, means that there are likely to be both intended and unintended consequences of any approach. For example, the public reporting of performance data may have positive effects in terms of reducing the asymmetry of information between consumers and physicians and in compelling improved performance by institutions. However, it is also likely to require additional resources to implement and may result in tunnel vision, erosion of consumer trust and the reluctance of providers (both individual and institutional) to provide health services to higher risk patient populations if outcome data may look worse (Leatherman and McCarthy, 1999).

The state of the art of performance measurement and reporting has made dramatic advances in the past decade but is still deficient to support widespread diffusion, predictable systematic application, and routinely fair and accurate assessments.

The investment of new resources into building capacity will be required, The potential of performance indicators to guide and compel improvement will not be fully realized until the state of the art is dramatically changed to make performance data more useful to target audiences. This will not only require better research and development but also investment in the areas of informatics and information infrastructure. Even in the US, where, arguably, relatively more has been spent on information capabilities, the health care industry lags behind other industries in IT investment. According to a US Department of Commerce report (1999) the health care industry ranked 38th out of 53 industries surveyed in informatics and information technology (US Department of Commerce, 1999).

The design of a comprehensive strategy for intentional improvements in performance requires prudent choices of what levers for change should be implemented. Identification of the various key stakeholders and target audiences is necessary. Selection of intervention strategies should be guided by policy imperatives and research on effectiveness. Table 4 suggests a broad set of interventions, all based on some usage of performance indicators, which constitute a reasonable set of activities for any country to consider implementing. A multiple intervention strategy is necessary given the diverse set of actors and purposes, as well as the caveats requiring evidence of effectiveness for any single lever.

329

Table 4. **A set of levers for change using performance indicators in an intentional multiple intervention strategy**

Intervention	Target audience	Purpose/Intent
Performance reporting	Public	– Accountability – Providers and treatment choices
	Providers	– Behavior and systems change
	Policymakers	– Inform regulations
Knowledge enhancement – Guidelines – Protocol – Electronic learning/prompts	Providers Public	– Increase evidence-based practice – Shared decision-making – Informed selection/choices
Oversight/regulation	Public	– Safety, quality and access
	Providers	– Compliance and competency
	Managers	– Financial and quality stewardship
	Policymakers	– Facilitate accountability/transparency
Incentives – Financial – Non-financial	Providers Managers	– Improve quality/effectiveness – Efficiency and responsiveness

Source: Author.

Actualizing the contribution of performance measurement and management to systematically improving health systems is both a matter of will and skill. There must be the will of countries to develop a coordinated and sustained strategy to achieve consensus on performance priorities and to implement improvement strategies. There must also be the skill to undertake capacity building in requisite competencies and infrastructure.

REFERENCES

AIKEN, L.H., CLARKE, S.P., SLOANE, D.M., SOCHALSKI, J.A., BUSSE, R., CLARKE, H., GIOVANNETTI, P., HUNT, J., RAFFERTY, A.M. and SHAMIAN, J. (2001),
"Nurses' reports on hospital care in five countries", *Health Affairs*, Vol. 20, No. 3, pp. 43-53, May-June.

ANDERSON, G. and HUSSEY, P.S. (2001),
"Comparing health system performance in OECD countries", *Health Affairs*, Vol. 20, No. 3, pp. 219-232, May-June.

AUSTRALIAN INSTITUTE OF HEALTH AND WELFARE AND DEPT. OF HEALTH AND SERVICES (1997),
First Report on the National Health Priority Areas, AIHW No PHE1, Canberra.

AYANIAN, J.Z. and QUINN, T.J. (2001),
"Quality of care for coronary heart disease in two countries", *Health Affairs*, Vol. 20, No. 3, pp. 55-67, May-June.

BALAS, E.A. and BOREN, S.A. (2000),
"Managing Clinical Knowledge for Health Care Improvement", *Yearbook of Medical Informatics*, National Library of Medicine, Bethesda, MD, pp. 65-70.

BALAS, E.A., WEINGARTEN, S., GARB, C.T., BLUMENTHAL, D., BOREN, S.A. and BROWN, G.D. (2000),
"Improving preventive care by prompting physicians", *Archives of Internal Medicine*, Vol. 160, No. 3, pp. 301-308, Feb. 14.

BATES, D.W. and GAWANDE, A.A. (2000),
"Error in medicine: what have we learned?", *Annals of Internal Medicine*, Vol. 132, No. 9, pp. 763-767, May 2.

BECHER, E.C. and CHASSIN, M.R. (2001),
"Improving quality, minimizing error: making it happen", *Health Affairs*, Vol. 20, No. 3, pp. 68-81, May-June.

BLENDON, R.J., SCHOEN, C., DONELAN, K., OSBORN, R., DESROCHES, C.M., SCOLES, K., DAVIS, K., BINNS, K. and ZAPERT, K. (2001),
"Physicians' view on quality of care: A five country comparison", *Health Affairs*, Vol. 20, No. 3, pp. 233-243, May-June.

CABANA, M.D., RAND, C.S., POWE, N.R., WU, A.W., WILSON, M.H., ABBOUD, P.A. and RUBIN, H.R. (1999),
"Why don't physicians follow clinical practice guidelines? A framework for improvement", *Journal American Medical Association*, Vol. 282, No. 15, pp. 1458-1465, Oct. 20.

CHASSIN, M.R. (1997),
"Assessing strategies for quality improvement", *Health Affairs*, Vol. 16, No. 3, pp. 151-161, May-June.

CHASSIN, M.R. (1998),
"Is health care ready for Six Sigma quality?", *Milbank Quarterly*, Vol. 76, No. 4.

CHASSIN, M.R. (2001),
"Measuring and improving quality: exhortation to achievement", Invited paper for the US/UK collaboration meeting The Commonwealth Fund and the Nuffield Trust, London, pp. 510, 565-591.

COMMONWEALTH DEPARTMENT OF HEALTH AND FAMILY SERVICES AND AUSTRALIAN INSTITUTE OF HEALTH AND WELFARE (1998*a*),
National Health Priority Areas Report on Cancer Control 1997, AIHW Cat. No. PHE 4, DHFS and AIHW, Canberra.

COMMONWEALTH DEPARTMENT OF HEALTH AND FAMILY SERVICES AND AUSTRALIAN INSTITUTE OF HEALTH AND WELFARE (1998*b*),
National Health Priority Areas Report: Injury and Prevention and Control 1997, AIHW Cat. No. PHE 3, DHFS and AIHW, Canberra.

COMMONWEALTH DEPARTMENT OF HEALTH AND FAMILY SERVICES AND AUSTRALIAN INSTITUTE OF HEALTH AND WELFARE (1999*a*),
National Health Priority Areas Report: Diabetes Mellitus 1998, AIHW Cat. No. PHE 10, DHFS and AIHW, Canberra.

COMMONWEALTH DEPARTMENT OF HEALTH AND FAMILY SERVICES AND AUSTRALIAN INSTITUTE OF HEALTH AND WELFARE (1999*b*),
National Health Priority Areas Report: Mental Health 1998, AIHW Cat. No. PHE 13, DHFS and AIHW, Canberra.

COMMONWEALTH DEPARTMENT OF HEALTH AND FAMILY SERVICES AND AUSTRALIAN INSTITUTE OF HEALTH AND WELFARE (1999c),
National Health Priority Areas Report: Cardiovascular Health 1998, AIHW Cat. No. PHE 9, DHFS and AIHW, Canberra.

COULTER, A. (2001),
"Patient engagement. Invited paper for the US/UK collaboration meeting", The Commonwealth Fund and the Nuffield Trust, London.

COULTER, A. and CLEARY, P.D. (2001),
"Patients' experience with hospital care in five countries", *Health Affairs*, Vol. 20, No. 3, pp. 244-252, May-June.

DEPARTMENT OF HEALTH (2001a),
Organization with a Memory, HMSO, London.

DEPARTMENT OF HEALTH (2001b),
Building a Safer NHS, HMSO, London.

DOWD, B. and FINCH, M. (2001),
"Employers as catalysts for health care quality: theory and practice", unpublished paper prepared for the Agency for Healthcare Research and Quality Conference, March.

EMANUEL, E.J. and EMANUEL, L.L. (1996),
"What is accountability in health care?", *Annals of Internal Medicine*, Vol. 124, No. 2, pp. 229-239, Jan. 15.

GABEL, J.R., HUNT, K.A. and HURST, K. (1998),
"KPMG Peat Marwick. When employers choose health plans: Do NCQA accreditation and HEIDIS data count?", The Commonwealth Fund, New York.

GONZALES, R., STEINER, J.F. and SANDE, M.A. (1997),
"Antibiotic prescribing for adults with colds, upper respiratory tract infections and bronchitis by ambulatory care physicians", *Journal of American Medical Association*, Vol. 278, pp. 901-904.

GRECO, P.J. and EISENBERG, J.M. (1993),
"Changing physicians' practices", *New England Journal of Medicine*, Vol. 329, No. 17, pp. 1271-1273, Oct. 21.

HAYWARD, R.S. (1997),
"Clinical practice guidelines on trial", *Canadian Medical Association Journal*, Vol. 156, No. 12, pp. 1725-1727, June 15.

HIBBARD, J.H. and JEWETT, J.J. (1997),
"Will quality report cards help consumers?", *Health Affairs*, Vol. 16, pp. 218-228.

HILLMAN, A.L. (1991),
"Managing the physician: rules versus incentives", *Health Affairs*, Vol. 10, No. 4, pp. 138-146, Winter.

HURST, J. and JEE-HUGHES, M. (2001),
"Performance Measurement and Performance Management in OECD Health Systems", Labor Market and Social Policy Occasional Papers, No. 47, OECD, Paris.

INSTITUTE OF MEDICINE (1990),
Medicare: A Strategy for Quality Assurance, in K.N. Lohr (ed.), National Academy Press, Washington, DC, p. 21.

INSTITUTE OF MEDICINE (2001),
Envisioning the National Health Care Quality Report, in Hurtado, M.P., Swift, E.K. and Corrigan, J.M. (eds.), National Academy Press, Washington, DC.

KINDIG, D.A. (1998),
"Purchasing population health: aligning financial incentives to improve health outcomes", *Health Services Research*, Vol. 33(2 Pt 1), pp. 223-242, June.

LEATHERMAN, S. AND MCCARTHY, D. (1999),
"Public disclosure of health care performance reports: experience, evidence and issues for policy", *International Journal for Quality in Health Care*, Vol. 11, No. 2, pp. 93-105.

LEGNINI, M.W., ROSENBERG, L.E., PERRY, M.J. and ROBERTSON, N.J. (2000),
"Where does performance measurement go from here?", *Health Affairs*, Vol. 19, No. 3, pp. 173-177, May-June.

LIEBER, R.B., GRANT; L. and MARTIN, J. (1998),
"Now are you satisfied? The 1998 American Customer Satisfaction Index", *Fortune*, Vol. 137, No. 3, pp. 161-168, Feb. 16.

LOMAS, J., ANDERSON, G.M., DOMNICK-PIERRE, K., VAYDA, E., ENKIN, M.W. and HANNAH, W.J. (1989),
"Do practice guidelines guide practice? The effect of a consensus statement on the practice of physicians", *New England Journal of Medicine*, Vol. 321, No. 19, pp. 1306-1311, Nov. 9.

MAINOUS, A.G., HUESTON, W.J. and CLARK, J.R. (1996),
"Antibiotics and upper respiratory Infection: do some folks think there is a cure for the common cold?", *Journal of Family Practice*, Vol. 42, pp. 357-366.

MARSHALL, M., SHEKELLE, P., BROOK, R. and LEATHERMAN, S. (2000),
"Dying to Know; Public Release of Information about Quality of Health Care", Co-Published by The Nuffield Trust (London) and RAND (Santa Monica, CA), Nuffield Trust Series No. 12, July.

MARSHALL, M., SHEKELLE, P., LEATHERMAN, S. and BROOK, R. (2000),
"What do we expect to gain from the public release of performance data? A review of the evidence", *Journal American Medical Association* 2000, Vol. 283, No. 14, pp. 1866-1874.

McLOUGHLIN, V., LEATHERMAN, S., FLETCHER, M. and WYN OWEN, J. (2001),
"Improving Performance Using Indicators; Recent Experiences in the United States, the United Kingdom and Australia", *International Journal for Quality in Health Care*, invited article, pending publication, Fall.

NATIONAL EXPERT ADVISORY GROUP ON SAFETY AND QUALITY IN AUSTRALIAN HEALTH CARE (1999),
Implementing Safety and Quality Enhancement in Health Care; national actions to support quality and safety improvement in Australian health care, Department of Health and Aged Care, Australia.

NATIONAL HEALTH EXPENDITURE PROJECTIONS 2000-2010, March 2001,
www.hcfa.gov/stats/nhe-proj/proj2000/proj2000.pdf.

NATIONAL HEALTH MINISTERS' BENCHMARKING WORKING GROUP (1996),
First National Report on Health Sector Performance Indicators; public hospitals – the state of play, Commonwealth Department of Health and Aged Care, Australia.

NATIONAL HEALTH MINISTERS' BENCHMARKING WORKING GROUP (1998),
Second National Report on Health Sector Performance Indicators, Commonwealth Department of Health and Aged Care, Australia.

NATIONAL HEALTH MINISTERS' BENCHMARKING WORKING GROUP (1999),
Third National Report on Health Sector Performance Indicators, Commonwealth Department of Health and Aged Care, Australia.

NHS EXECUTIVE (1999),
"Quality and performance in the NHS. High level performance indicators", Whitehall, London, June.

NYQUIST, A., GONZALES, R., STEINER, J.F. and SANDE, M.A. (1998),
"Antibiotic prescribing for children with colds, upper respiratory tract infections, and bronchitis", *Journal of American Medical Association*, Vol. 279, pp. 875-877.

O'CONNOR G.T. and EAGLE, K.A. (1998),
"How do we know how well we are doing?", *Journal of the American College of Cardiology*, Vol. 32, No. 4, pp. 1000-1001.

OECD (2000),
OECD *Health Data*, Paris.

SECRETARY OF STATE FOR HEALTH (2000),
The Department of Health, HMSO, London.

SCHUSTER, M.A., MCGLYNN, E.A. and BROOK, R.H. (1998),
"How good is the quality of health care in the United States?", *Milbank Quarterly*, Vol. 76, No. 4, pp. 509, 517-563.

US DEPARTMENT OF COMMERCE (1999),
"The Emerging Digital Economy II", Economic Statistics Administration, Office of Policy Development, Washington, DC. Online at *http://ecommerce.gov/eds/report.html*.

WORLD HEALTH ORGANIZATION (2000),
"Health systems improving performance", *World Health Report*, Geneva.

Part VI
SUMMARY AND CONCLUSIONS

Chapter 16

MEASURING UP: LESSONS AND POTENTIAL

by

Jean-François Girard[*] and Étienne Minvielle[**]

A mere summary of the proceedings would not adequately convey the importance of the conference organised by the OECD in Ottawa. What was said there reflected so much breadth of experience, and was presented in so much depth, that such a synthesis is impossible. This chapter will seek to report on the conference differently and in three ways.

The first is to place the research and the practices that were presented in their historical perspective – that of the history of performance measurement and improvement over the past decade. By doing so, we can grasp the magnitude of what has been accomplished in ten years – accomplishments that have enhanced the legitimacy of *undertakings* to measure and improve performance (Section 1).

Whilst acquiring legitimacy, this process simultaneously revealed its full complexity. The dimensions of performance to be assessed are many – efficiency, effectiveness and equity, to name only the main considerations – and they involve linkages that are still not clearly established. Lessons learned from experiences show that there are many outstanding challenges, including: defining a coherent analytical framework; co-ordinating measurement efforts and actions taken in response; and ensuring the validity of the measurement instruments used. The second way to convey the importance of the conference is to report on the state of the art in thinking about the challenges involved in instituting systems of performance measurement and improvement (Section 2).

The third key observation relates to the central role of the political arena. This role is justified by the issue at hand – the health of our populations. It is also justified by the fact that health system performance is relevant to everybody. In other words, the effort to measure and improve performance is also an affirmation of democracy in the realm of health, which it is government's role to uphold and preserve. This chapter also seeks to describe these new forms of democracy and public management that underpin the development of the process (Section 3).

In making this overview, we have used on judgement in selecting for comment those topics which we felt to be critical. We trust that speakers who do not find all the subtleties of their remarks reproduced herein will forgive us.

1. A legitimate undertaking

All of the remarks made at the conference underscore a clear change in the very concept of performance and performance measurement in the field of health over the past decade. This change

[*] Rapporteur-Général, Conseiller d'Etat et Président, Institut de recherche pour le développement, France.

[**] Assistant Rapporteur-Général, Center for Health Economics and Administration Research, INSERM/CNRS, France.

Acknowledgements: This report could not have been written without the help of the rapporteurs of the parallel sessions, and that of Gaétan Lafortune and Kristell Le Cerf from the OECD Secretariat and François Sauvé from Health Canada. We would like to thank them sincerely.

can be summed up as follows: the abandonment of a fatalistic vision that saw health system performance as non measurable.

This vision was firmly entrenched only a few short years ago. In 1990, for example, it was stressed in the introduction to the OECD report entitled *Health Care Systems in Transition: The Search for Efficiency* (p. 9) that "Systems' performance cannot be easily evaluated because of our inability to measure health outcomes" (see Introduction by George J. Schieber and Jean-Pierre Poullier).

1.1. A *watershed decade*

Ten years later, whilst there are still no simple answers to the definition of the concept of performance, or how it should be made operational, the steps taken have cast it in an entirely new light.

- First, concerning *the very concept of performance*. All of the dimensions now considered testify to an enlargement of the concept. From that of an output (a term that often connotes an accounting approach centred on volume of activity), the concept of performance is becoming more multidimensional. This shift is evident in the incorporation, along with efficiency, of dimensions of quality (in the sense of safety, effectiveness of care, quality of services rendered and quality as perceived by patients and the people around them) and equity as cornerstones of performance. What is most notable is not so much the inclusion of these dimensions as the determination to measure them and to consider them within the same framework of performance analysis. This last point can be seen, for example, in the design of the numerator of the efficiency ratios proposed by the OECD (see Part I, Chapter 2), which in turn is largely inspired by the WHO (Part III, Chapter 9). The volume of production or activity is no longer seen as the benchmark criterion; it has been replaced by quality, construed as improvements in health outcomes or the system's responsiveness to patients' expectations.

- Second, concerning *the non-measurable nature of certain key aspects of health system performance*. Clearly, changes are often incremental and many difficulties remain, but there have undeniably been major strides in the capacity to measure the various dimensions of performance: the expanding scope of "outcome research", the generalisation of costing and technical and allocative efficiency measures; the expansion of work on patient-perceived quality and the responsiveness of services; the safety and quality of processes in general; and lastly, work in the area of equity measurement. These strides are also reflected in the development of comparative approaches at all levels, both internationally – through the complementary work of the OECD and the WHO in particular – and at national and sub-national levels. While such measurements existed prior to 1990, the last decade has seen a sharp acceleration in the capacity to measure dimensions that had seemed ill-suited to such analysis, and to comprehend the linkages involved (Part II, Chapter 7).

- This change in both the concept and the ability to measure has been accompanied by a third change: an enlargement of *the scope of performance analysis*. This enlargement can be seen at a number of levels, through the incorporation of: an integrated vision of the health care system in which hospital performance is viewed in a broader context of human services (while its immediate role is still acknowledged); long-term care alongside acute care (Part IV, Chapter 13); lastly, and obviously, social, environmental and economic considerations alongside the health care system.

The acknowledgement of this shift, in respect both of the concept and scope of analysis and of the capacity to measure, shows the magnitude of the progress made in recent years. The result is a multidimensional vision of performance that makes it a fully-fledged public health issue.

1.2. The *underpinnings of legitimacy*

This shift obviously testifies to the profound changes in health systems and how the performance of these systems is perceived. How else, for example, could one explain the increasing weight that is given to socio-economic determinants in explaining health outcomes? Or the priority that is given to long-term care? At the same time, this shift constitutes a response to expectations. Two expectations would appear to justify the development of indicators of health system performance: the need to support improvements in health systems and the need for greater public accountability. It is the high level of these expectations that gives the undertaking its legitimacy.

i) Supporting the improvement of health systems

Better measurement can contribute to better health systems at many levels, as noted several times during the conference. At a general level, such measurements of performance can serve as a sort of "compass" for governments. Allan Rock, the Canadian Minister of Health, stressed the potential contribution of such an approach by noting that "we know what goes in, but we know too little about what happens with the huge amount of resources spent on health care". Clive Smee, in his presentation of the British experience (Part II, Chapter 3), also reminded us that policy decisions were often based on a narrow view of performance measurement and could therefore have unwanted side effects. A balanced set of performance measures can thus help achieve better resource allocation in a context of rising demand due to an ageing population, the reduction of health care inequalities, the harnessing of technological innovation and continued health reforms. In all these areas, better measurement can prompt changes in the practices of actors within health systems, the inertia of whom was pointed out by André-Pierre Contandriopoulos.

Within health services, measurement can help improve performance, as was shown by the experiences of the Netherlands (Part II, Chapter 6) and Sweden (Part II, Chapter 4), especially in conjunction with quality improvement campaigns (CQI/TQM, evaluation of professional practices). Lastly, it can help improve performance through a population analysis that identifies the social and economic determinants of risk-generating behaviour and can be used to devise preventive action.

Adding to these various potential contributions are at least two others that are less direct: attempts to define more clearly territorial jurisdictions – a sensitive issue *par excellence* – and attempts to improve the evidence base for future reforms, in particular those related to the overall design of the health system, as pointed out by Roy Romanow, head of the Commission on the Future of Health Care in Canada.

ii) Accountability

The past decade has also been marked by demands from the public to make the various components of health systems more transparent. These demands voiced by users/consumers/patients, or more precisely by citizens, as pointed out by Bernard Kouchner, the French Minister of Health, have pushed their way into what was already a crowded debate among government, public and private insurance funds, administrators (both purchasers and suppliers of health care), health care professionals, the media and the courts.

In this groundswell of opinion, two facts warrant mention:

- In response to public interest, the media have in many cases latched onto the subject by proposing rankings, with the attendant danger that their drive to report striking information will supplant the objective of transparency. Nevertheless, at least their actions have prompted governments, scientific and professional communities and other players in the system to develop their own measurement tools.

- This demand for transparency is generally accompanied by a desire that civil society be involved in health care choices. That involvement is indispensable to the debate, but more problematic when it comes to decision-making, and how far it should be taken is a sensitive issue. In any event, the demands are a clear sign that measuring health system performance is more than a question of public dissemination of information and has come foursquare into the public domain.

From this brief overview, it emerges that the development of ways to measure health system performance derives its legitimacy from the responses it brings to demands to improve these systems and make them more transparent. The conference organisers knew what they were doing when they brought together the three themes of measurement, improvement, and democratic debate about health system performance.

This legitimacy explains the magnitude of the initiatives that can be seen in OECD countries. Undertaken by governments, international organisations, professional associations and independent bodies, these initiatives have reached varying stages of advancement, quite unrelated to the performance of the individual countries' health systems. These activities lend a character of universality to the process of measuring and improving performance. Whilst this implies that all countries, including developing countries, should be involved, it raises the issue of designing a single approach that could be applicable to all. We shall see that experience in fact suggests a need to tailor the approach to the particularities of each health system, although as pointed out by John Hutton, Minister of State for Health in the United Kingdom, there is also a need to recognize the importance of developing a core set of common indicators to be able to draw lessons from international comparisons.

In any case, it would appear that everything is conspiring to bring us into an era of intensive efforts to measure and improve performance, creating new challenges and new objectives. Just as its legitimacy is becoming more evident, the observation of practices and relevant research is showing the full complexity of the task at hand.

2.   A difficult undertaking

By presenting a range of initiatives now underway, the Ottawa conference also made it possible to take stock of what is known on the subject. This assessment showed both the pitfalls to be avoided and the prerequisites for coherent development. These can be summed up in three major challenges, each of which, in its own way, shows the difficulty involved.

2.1. *What is the proper framework for performance analysis?*

From the outset, it is necessary to establish a framework for performance analysis, since to measure performance implies an ability to circumscribe the scope of analysis and to know where to situate each of its components. But there are no obvious answers here.

This statement may seem surprising, given the recent plethora of definitions and publications on the subject of performance. This work has shed a great deal of light: *inter alia*, the recognition of efficiency, effectiveness and equity as the cornerstones of performance; the positioning of notions of effectiveness and responsiveness as the cornerstones of quality (Part I, Chapter 2); the breakdown of various forms of equity considerations, and especially access to the system (Part III, Chapter 11); and expansion of the notion of responsiveness to embrace a compilation of facts regarding actual patient experiences in addition to mere patient satisfaction surveys (Part III, Chapter 10). Closer scrutiny, however, shows that the concept of performance can still mean many different things and that the boundaries are difficult to draw. For example, the notions of efficiency and equity, as they relate to those of effectiveness and responsiveness, suggest different approaches in the analytical frameworks of the WHO, the OECD and the Canadian Institute for Health Information. Likewise, while the conventional distinction between a health care system and a health system is well established, matters become more delicate when one tries to sort out the principles by which to justify choices between competing claims on public expenditure.

These examples testify to the many choices that are made during the often imperceptible phase of circumscribing and "carving up" the scope of performance. It is difficult to perceive what the right outcome of these choices might be. Any attempts to impose a unique analytical framework would certainly be detrimental, given the current state of our knowledge. But to develop no framework at all would be just as detrimental. There is a middle ground where we could cultivate the twin virtues of any measurement tool: to assist decision-making, but also to provide educational value, by shedding light on the very concept of what would be the "right" framework for analysing health system performance. In this regard, as was noted by Julio Frenk, Minister of Health in Mexico, the framework developed by the WHO set in motion this learning process, which might otherwise never have taken place.

If such care must be taken in tracing these boundaries, it is because more is involved than a mere question of semantics: it is a definition of the conditions of action. The choices that are made determine

– often implicitly – the nature of the actions taken by governments and providers. Therefore, the process for making these choices is a first difficulty that must be overcome to avoid confusions of what one seeks to promote through the measurement of health system performance.

2.2. What should be the development strategy?

As shown by the accounts of each country's experience, undertakings to measure and improve performance entail formulating a strategy for subsequent development. This strategy can be formulated at various levels – health care professionals, hospitals and other care-dispensing institutions, government agencies and other organisations, or population groups. But taken as a whole, the strategy concerns the health system and must therefore be considered at a national level. At that level, a first issue is whether it is possible to secure the coherent development of performance measurement and improvement given the multiple initiatives that exist at a local level. In other words, what connection can there be between undertakings at national level and approaches that are more microscopic? What architecture can be envisaged that consolidates undertakings at different levels and from different perspectives?

i) Constructing an architecture

Many difficulties can impede the construction of that architecture. For example, David Naylor (Part I, Chapter 1) evokes the risk that a macroscopic perspective will develop, seeking to pull "big policy levers" (generally financial levers), whereas the real changes often take place at far more microscopic levels. Similarly, much has been said about the scant involvement of care providers and managers in performance measurement undertakings. They often remain sceptical of the reliability of performance indicators, feel the process is of little relevance to them and fear that the fallout will be unfair.

At the same time, different analysis point to the same need for co-ordination amongst a plurality of approaches to performance measurement and improvement. In this co-ordination exercise, it is probably illusory to consider one element of information alone. The Swedish experience illustrates this aspect through the distinction that is made between information conveyed to professionals, policy-makers and the citizenry. On the other hand, it would seem relevant to consider a balance between national undertakings and local ones. Experience in different countries converges to underscore this point through descriptions of top-down and bottom-up approaches and the degree of decentralisation of strategies that have been implemented. Following the observations of Edward Sondik on behalf of the Secretary of Health and Human Services in the United States, it seems to us that there even emerges from the deliberations a certain consensus that measurement should serve two purposes. First, a national perspective on measurement is taking shape, with strong local anchoring, striving to develop an official framework based on a "hard core" of indicators, which would support international comparisons. This perspective is based on the territorial division of powers within a country and is therefore not incompatible with a decentralised approach. Second, there is a clear drive to take action at the level of health care organisations and professionals directly involved, based on peer group comparisons and feedback on performance information (Part II, Chapter 6).

ii) Providing a scientific basis

In this overall architecture, whatever level is selected, it will involve a series of steps, from formulation of the unit of measurement to its utilisation with an aim of improving performance. Depicted as a cycle (Part I, Chapter 2), and even perhaps as a virtuous circle between the measurement stage and that of improvement, this series of steps entails overcoming a variety of methodological obstacles, as follows.

341

• Setting the objectives for measurement

This first step follows from what was stated above. At this stage, the unit of measurement must be formulated with a view to the explicit objectives (Part I, Chapter 1 and Part II, Chapter 3) and the intended audience (Part V, Chapter 15), which requires frequent ranking of priorities (Part II, Chapters 3 and 4). At the same time, another critical parameter is the length of time, set in advance, over which the measurement will be taken: sufficiently long to detect significant trends; sufficiently short to keep conservative attitudes or stalling tactics from developing.

• Constructing indicators

This step is replete with methodological considerations that will ultimately determine the validity of the measurement. First and foremost, this validity is heavily dependent on the integration capacity of information systems and standardisation of data collection methods – a vital prerequisite to comparison (Part II, Chapter 7), on the international level in particular (Part III, Chapter 8). It also hinges on the technical qualities, in the strict sense, of the measurement. This involves the well-known criteria of reproducibility, validity, specificity and sensitivity, and the required methods of adjustment. These aspects determine the reliability of the measurement instruments developed, as illustrated by the example of the RAI presented by Naoki Ikegami and collegues (Part IV, Chapter 13). When such measurements are aggregated into composite indicators, the weighting method that is used represents another aspect, the pitfalls of which were shown by Peter Smith (Part IV, Chapter 14). Lastly, another key technical issue is the sensitive problem of how to interpret any observed variations. Interpretation can prompt efforts to break down results so as to estimate the relative share of each variable in explaining overall differences (Part III, Chapter 9). It also poses the question of cause and effect between measurements of processes and practices and measurements of outcomes. Controlling for the process variables need not always feed through to outcomes, making the study of linkages between the two types of measurement frequently risky.

• Routine measurement

This step, which is often neglected, involves the shift from an experimental undertaking to routine measurement. Between the two phases, many aspects need to be managed, including: conditions for acceptance by the parties involved, means of conveying the information gathered (the importance of how and in what format data are reported), the resultant rating methods (in the NHS experience, a system of stars was deemed more neutral than using traffic light colours – red, orange or green – to rate establishments on their performance), manageability of measurement, and the necessary human and financial resources (in this regard, the time required to develop measurement systems was cited frequently).

• Using performance measures

With this final step we come full circle. Here the interface between the measurement and the proposed improvement initiative takes shape – another process that is fraught with pitfalls. For example, David Naylor (Part I, Chapter 1) stressed the risks arising from the time lag between corrective actions and their reflection in the measurements. Likewise, the British experience shows how focusing exclusively on one unit of measurement and one performance objective – in this case, waiting times – can lead to undesired behaviour instead of corrective action, with surgeons making choices not according to medical urgency but on a first come, first served basis (Part I, Chapter 2). Gérard de Pouvourville (Part IV, Chapter 12) also showed the paradox that can link measurement and action in the example of the tracking of post-heart bypass mortality that was developed in New York State: measurements of mortality rates by establishment appear difficult to interpret in terms of quality of care, despite sophisticated adjustment techniques.

These various pitfalls show that it is not easy to achieve the virtuous circle of measurement and improvement. Some indicators seem to lend themselves to the task better than others. From a technical standpoint, units of measurement involving responsiveness to patients' expectations, and those involving processes (such as waiting times) and the monitoring of practices seem easier to develop than those involving health outcomes (the problem of reliability, linked in particular to adjustment issues). At the same time, indicators such as those on the mortality and survival rates associated with a given disease are the ones that usually raise the greatest expectations.

But in general, regardless of the type of indicator that is used, there is no clear-cut formula for developing a system of performance measurement and improvement. The strategies adopted are shaped by the choice of incentives. Many speakers stressed the overriding importance of these incentives. By type, they can be considered at the institutional level or at the level of health care professionals (peer group analysis). They can be financial or of some other type (Part V, Chapter 15). Above all, their successful application would seem heavily dependent on their suitability to the context, and more specifically the extent to which they ensure that the often divergent interests of the parties involved are aligned.

2.3. How does performance become public?

Implicit in this question is an acknowledgement of citizen participation in this undertaking to measure and improve performance. But once it is acknowledged that performance should be in the public domain, two new challenges arise: disseminating in a targeted way information to the general public, and constituting a democratic debate on performance.

i) From expertise to public dissemination of information

It would appear for now that the information that is conveyed on performance has little impact on the public at large. The reasons that have been cited for this are that citizens discover the importance of the information only gradually, that they are often overwhelmed by the density of it, that they prefer the opinions of people they know, and that their preferences are not well known. There is also a certain conflict between the goals of expert assessment and democratic debate. On the one hand, the relevance of the information produced is based on expert scientific assessment, which tends to make it complex and detailed. On the other hand, public dissemination of the information assumes that it will be understood by large numbers of people, which can lead to the reverse pressure for aggregation and simplification – a process that can be of dubious validity (Part I, Chapter 1). All of these reasons suggest a need for improved ways to communicate the information to the general public.

Initiatives undertaken in this area were presented by a number of speakers. They involved educating and motivating citizens, improving the availability and access to communication supports, and incentives to use them (Part II, Chapter 5). They also involved the identification of intermediaries and mediators who can help citizens in making choices and in educating them (Part I, Chapter 1; Part IV, Chapter 12). All of these actions are designed to support a debate that is still in its infancy, judging by how little this information is being used at present. There is a need finally to assess the effectiveness of each of these actions in moving towards this democratic objective and in building citizens' perceptions thereof.

ii) The constitution of a democratic debate and its consequences

The assumption that information about performance measurement could be readily accessible to the general public is a condition *sine qua non* for the constitution of a democratic debate on the subject. At the same time, as we have already mentioned, the emergence of this debate is not just an issue of disseminating information. It also reflects a groundswell of popular opinion and, more broadly, of new relationships between the parties to health systems. Alongside citizens, health care professionals, policy-makers and managers (purchasers and providers alike) are also interested in this debate. Each is being prompted to forge new relationships and to play new roles. In this new-style pattern of social interaction, a degree of perplexity can sometimes be detected behind the optimistic messages.

Citizens are therefore asserting their role as fully-fledged participants in the system, if not as co-decision-makers (Part V, Chapter 15). As consumers, citizens select health care professionals and services. As citizens, they are also entitled to access all data, even the most "sensitive" data, which allow them to formulate clearer opinions on system components. While these changes are obviously eminently warranted, some speakers highlighted the difficulties involved in reconciling them with efforts to improve performance. For example, health care professionals or managers may hesitate to expend their energy identifying sources of potential improvement if they know that the general public will see them merely as highlighting current malfunctions. These same professionals may also feel a loss of autonomy associated with their involvement in improvement efforts, prompting some to emphasise their essential role as self-regulators of the system. But then how must we interpret the message of Janne Graham (former Chairperson of the Consumers' Health Forum in Australia) when she says us that self-regulation usually leads to a lack of regulation?

It is clear, then, that the construction of this democratic debate inevitably gives rise to certain tensions. Without calling the principle of the debate into question, drawing attention to these tensions serves to underscore that the means employed to achieve this objective merit careful consideration, especially in the case of systems that are having problems recruiting enough people to health care professions.

From these three major challenges – defining a coherent analytical framework, formulating a development strategy and organising a democratic debate – it is clear that the path leading to the use of performance measurement to make improvements and achieve transparency is a demanding one. If we avoid tackling any of the challenges discussed above, there is a major risk that measurements will be irrelevant, inoperative or invalid, that inappropriate actions will be taken, or that all this will have little impact on the citizenry. To embark upon the undertaking is to acknowledge its importance; it also entails taking certain precautions.

2.4. *Precautions to be taken*

The first of these precautions involves the use of rigour. While no concession should be made regarding methodological rigour, it must not slide towards excessive perfectionism either. As David Naylor pointed out, it is better to measure approximately than not to measure at all. Methodological rigour must always be combined with the virtues of pragmatism.

As a corollary, a second precaution involves the humility that anyone embarking upon such an undertaking should assume. This humility should apply at every step along the way, but it is probably most essential in setting the objective of measurement. Without succumbing to the seductive reductionism (Part I, Chapter 1) that could lead to the creation of a single composite indicator, there should be a real concern not to develop too many indicators.

There is a need to allow time – in most cases years – to set the system in place. But on the other hand, there is a need to yield tangible results in a not-too-distant future. Between the Charybdis of impetuousness and the Scylla of immobility, a quest for gradual maturation constitutes a third precaution that must be taken.

A fourth precaution is to maintain a high level of confidence between the various parties to the system. The word "trust", which was used often during the conference, underscores the need for fairness in using the information. We have shown how the dissemination of performance measurements causes roles to be redefined. This entails the construction of a new pattern of social interaction, in which the degree of trust amongst the players will clearly be a key success factor.

Lastly, a final precaution – but by no means the least important – is to take the particular circumstances of each country, and more specifically of each health care system, into account. Here, the first consideration is how a system is funded. Each is based on its own particular preferences and requires a different approach to the integration of performance results in terms of quality. For example, competition on quality between health care providers would be conceivable in a free-market model like that of the United States. It would not, however, be appropriate for universal health insurance models with a single payer in a dominant position, such as the one that has been developed in France, where the objective is theoretically to ensure identical quality, regardless of which health care provider a patient chooses.

Systems also differ in the way they are organised. In the United States, for example, the existence of managed care networks implies different performance measurement techniques to those found in systems that focus on hospitals alone. Similarly, the extent to which these networks are decentralised, and the degree of autonomy that is left for professionals, determine how the system evolves. Such distinctions, which are tied in with historical contexts and socio-cultural values, suggest that caution is needed when comparing the performance measurement systems that have been developed in each country. None would seem justified in the absolute: their profiles are shaped by prevailing conditions and the nature of the change in question. In other words, to bring about change in conjunction with performance measurement entails customised management, the effectiveness of which can be judged only in relation to the specific context.

3. A political undertaking

Instituting performance measurement is a political undertaking in more than one sense. It is public. It concerns a community asset underpinned by values. And lastly, it involves a large number of players, whose interests are not necessarily convergent. All these factors conspire to make the process preponderantly a political one. Public policy-makers must ensure the democratic expression of the process – health care democracy – to be construed not as a special form of democracy, but as the application of the principle of democracy to the realm of health.

At the same time, this political role serves to nurture the process. In this regard, the Ottawa conference, culminating with a Ministerial roundtable, unleashed a vision that can serve as a basis for planning such a public undertaking. This vision will require investments that everyone agrees are vital to the consolidation of the process of performance measurement and improvement. A number of countries in the vanguard in this area have moved beyond a vision, implementing practices that can serve as benchmarks for other countries. It is these visions and practices that we shall report on here.

3.1. Consolidating international comparative approaches

Measurement implies comparison. First and foremost is the international level, which enables each country to situate its performance in relation to others. Judging from existing work, there would seem to be two approaches to international comparisons: an integrative approach and a specific one, by disease. The first is reflected in work by the OECD and the WHO. The second is centred on comparison of practices and results specific to particular diseases, which can offer an interesting alternative, in particular by showing up, at least in part, differences that would otherwise go unobserved (Part III, Chapter 8). In any event, development would appear to hinge on the methodological issues addressed in Section 2 above, especially concerning the availability of information. But here, lessons are surely to be learned from the work done in the realm of quality, a vast range of work that should not be hindered by semantic debates over the terms performance, quality and effectiveness.

3.2. Developing an "infostructure"

This investment in information and its infrastructure emerged as an indispensable prerequisite to the development of performance measurement initiatives. It involves: improving data collection and standardisation methods; developing information systems and the ability to link them together (e.g. linkages between the accounting systems of hospitals and private doctors; the tracking of health care episodes); and the quality of information supports, based on the computerisation of systems and the use of Internet networks. The Canadian experience, which made the quality of its infostructure an overriding objective through the central role of Statistics Canada and the Canadian Institute for Health Information, shows the importance of this investment. It constitutes a benchmark that could be an inspiration to many other countries.

345

3.3. Developing multi-disciplinary research

Methodological difficulties, which were discussed at length during the conference, call for a great deal of expertise. Without such expertise, the rigour that is required for performance measurement and improvement initiatives will always prove inadequate.

Expertise needs to be developed in such diverse fields as measurement methodology, approaches to instituting measurement, ways of presenting and reporting results, linkages between measurements and actions and the effectiveness of various ways to disseminate information to patients. It is justified by the consideration of three major issues: analysis of the links between health care outcomes and the actions or practices put in place; the acknowledgement of the variables that explain differences in performance results; and the disclosure of patients' preferences in their use of health services.

These findings show the importance of making the necessary investment in research. In an OECD context, investment primarily involves economic analysis, at the heart of many research topics (e.g. reducing the asymmetry of information to promote more enlightened choices on the part of consumers, and knowledge of the redistributive effects of economic policies on the health and well-being of the population). In addition, this investment involves other social sciences, including management sciences (e.g. for the understanding of ways to institute the measurement and improvement initiatives) and sociology (to help put comparisons in context, formulate ways to report results or ascertain characteristics of certain practices or high-risk behaviours). The list of fields could be extended, even beyond the social sciences (life sciences, epidemiology). It shows the need to harness multi-disciplinary efforts for health service performance measurement and improvement. In fact, while the efforts are focused to a large extent on economics, they fall within the broader context of health service research.

3.4. Educating citizens to a culture of measurement

The above discussion emphasises that an undertaking to measure and to improve health system performance could be likened to the creation of a new field of knowledge – one that is multi-disciplinary. Adding to this knowledge is a new form of power: the power derived from mastery of knowledge, dear to the French philosopher Michel Foucault (in *La Volonté de Savoir*, 1977). "Measuring up", in this case, means ensuring that this knowledge – and thus the power it confers – is shared democratically.

This democratic sharing of knowledge entails developing new ways to educate citizens. It would be out of place to reiterate all of the points relevant to this educational effort that were raised, and that we have tried to incorporate, insofar as they underlay so much of what was said at the conference, but let us cite two overriding principles. First, this education entails the existence of mediators, so that it can be organised according to citizens' requirements. The role of new partners such as associations of health care consumers (i.e., non-specific to any particular disease) is certainly essential, in particular for providing the means necessary for dissemination, but also for developing this educational effort based on the citizen's point of view. The next step is of course to train these representatives in measurement issues. Here, let us note the large scale of their participation in the work of organisations specialised in this field, as was the case in Ottawa. Let us also note that people will become educated about measurement more effectively if it affects them close to their daily lives.

3.5. Designing institutional arrangements

Apart from the benefits of being able to use international comparisons, there is also a political responsibility to develop a comparative monitoring system on a national level, and in some cases to provide a wake-up call.

This responsibility entails an institutional mechanism to reconcile centralised undertakings and incentives for the development of approaches that are more decentralised, as discussed above. Regardless of how a health system is organised, it would appear in fact that some themes lend themselves more readily to centralised management: the definition of a "hard core" of indicators to provide the basis for comparisons at the national level; legal aspects, associated with the dissemination of information; and iatrogenic risks and medical errors falling within the realm of health-related safety.

More generally, an initial outline of what could be meant by an "ideal" performance measurement and improvement mechanism emerges from what has been said above:

- There would be independent bodies (or bodies drawing upon the resources of bodies already existing in the area, such as licensing organisations), based on substantial representation of professionals and citizens, and they would take on multi-disciplinary expertise. These bodies would either be centralised or established at a more decentralised level, depending on how the health system was set up.

- Their primary missions would be to:

  - Formulate recommendations on data collection and standardisation; statistical processing; and the linkage between performance measurements and quality enhancement efforts;

  - Define indicators for use in comparisons on a national level;

  - Provide incentives, *e.g.* via calls for tenders, for the development of comparative analysis of establishments or professionals, in co-operation with professional associations and unions representing health care establishments;

  - Develop a system of accreditation centred on the measurement of quality;

  - Develop programmes to disseminate information to the general public, while putting emphasis on the evaluation of their effectiveness;

  - Develop quality enhancement incentive systems.

- These bodies would be provided with a substantial infostructure that would enable them, *inter alia*, to gather the information needed for international comparative analysis.

- Lastly, they would be given the funding needed to embark upon multi-year programmes.

In constructing this scenario, we have probably strayed a little too far in projecting the future. But let us note simply that whilst this projection in no way incorporates all of the options cited over the course of the conference, it symbolises the recognition that health system performance evaluation is a pillar of government action. In this regard, it requires substantial financial and human investment, commensurate with the political responsibility involved.

4. Conclusion

In the light of all of these deliberations, one might well doubt that there is any single best path to the measurement and improvement of health system performance. Such an undertaking needs to overcome obstacles of all sorts (scientific, institutional and political), in some cases taking unexpected turns. But the goals are very important ones: to show that health system performance is no longer beyond the reach of measurement, and to affirm that improving that performance is a democratic imperative.

In this context, the presentations and discussions that we have tried to summarise seem especially timely in affirming the legitimacy of the undertaking, seeking to make sense of the complexity inherent in its development, and beginning to anticipate the challenges associated with its use. They invite all health care professionals to take up new challenges and commit themselves to following a new path. Let us wager that history will show that the November 2001 Ottawa conference made a decisive contribution in pointing the way.

MINISTERIAL ROUNDTABLE:
LEADERSHIP, SUCCESSES AND CHALLENGES

Chapter 17

MEASURING HEALTH SYSTEM PERFORMANCE AND THE IMPACT ON POLITICAL DECISION-MAKING: THE VIEWS OF OECD MINISTERS

by

Julio Frenk, *Minister of Health, Mexico,* John Hutton, *Minister of State for Health, United Kingdom,* Bernard Kouchner, *Minister of Health, France,* Allan Rock, *Minister of Health, Canada,** Edward Sondik, *Director, National Center for Health Statistics, United States* (on behalf of Tommy Thompson, *Secretary of Health and Human Services, United States*)

Introduction

The Ottawa conference concluded with a Ministerial Roundtable to discuss successes and challenges in measuring health system performance and its impact on political decision-making. The Secretary-General of the OECD, Donald Johnston, invited Ministers to share their thoughts on three questions:

- to what extent can performance reporting become a key instrument in health policy and management?
- what are the potential benefits and risks of releasing public performance reports?
- can countries improve performance by sharing information and, if so, how best to go about it?

The opening remarks of each Minister were followed by a lively period of "questions and answers" with conference participants.

1. Opening remarks by Allan Rock, Minister of Health, Canada

The federal and provincial governments in Canada are actively working to strengthen publicly-funded health services in order to provide quality health care to all Canadians. In 2000, Health Ministers developed a short list of needed actions which was then adopted as a shared plan by First Ministers. This action plan included significant increases to federal cash transfers to provinces to help fund health care. It also included plans to increase the number of doctors and nurses, broadened home and community care, better management of pharmaceutical costs, and changes in the way that front-line services are organized and delivered.

There are two features of this recent First Ministers' agreement that are of particular relevance to this conference. First, there is a specific commitment by all governments to measure and report on the performance of our health care system. All governments acknowledge that we know far too little about what happens to the Can$100 billion a year that Canadians spend on health care. We spend over Can$3 000 annually for health care per capita. This is about 10 per cent of Canada's GDP. So Canadians have a vested interest in seeing that their investment is being managed properly.

Canada's First Ministers committed to provide comprehensive and regular public reporting on health system performance and on progress toward stated priorities, and also to develop and use

---

* Minister of Health, Canada, until January 2002.

comparable indicators to measure health outcomes and quality of services, with third-party verification. First Ministers specifically committed to reporting on waiting times for key services, patient satisfaction, hospital re-admissions, access to 24-hour and 7-day front-line services, home and community care services, the adequacy of public health surveillance, and protection and promotion activities. The first public report will be released in September 2002.

We believe that this commitment to measurement and reporting will allow Canadians to know whether governments are making progress in their efforts to improve the Canadian public health system. It will also permit system managers to make more informed choices, making it easier to identify best practices so they can be shared more rapidly. It will also make all governments more accountable, not to each other but to the public.

Governments need to respond to the dual challenge of improving the performance of health care systems and reporting openly on that performance, as a means of preserving public confidence in those systems. Of course, we could offer the public an enormous amount of data on system performance to show that our health care system is working well, but if people do not see that information as credible, they will not believe us and our efforts will be worthless. As Janne Graham (former Chairperson of the Australian Consumers' Health Forum) said during this conference, if our efforts in performance measurement become simply an academic exercise, we will not have achieved our goals. We must make our work relevant to patients and to the general public. To help us achieve that goal, we have reached another important political commitment in Canada. The federal and provincial governments have committed to the creation of a citizen's council on the quality of health care. This citizen's council will be composed of regular citizens from across the country. Each will bring their lay perspective, and their important role will be to assure that the information provided in public performance reports is objective, relevant and readable, so that these reports truly respond to the quality preoccupations of Canadians.

A second important feature of the recent First Ministers' agreement in Canada is a commitment to strengthen our national health infostructure, including a specific commitment to develop electronic patient records. First Ministers agreed to develop common data standards to ensure compatibility of health information networks, while stringently protecting privacy and the confidentiality of health information. In support of its commitment, the Government of Canada has already made a very substantial financial contribution toward the design and development of electronic patient records. We know that this process will be lengthy and costly, but we also have in our sights the enormous benefits of this technology – benefits for patients and providers alike as all relevant health information is consolidated into a single accessible electronic file. By making this information more easily accessible to all caregivers, these electronic records should help avoid costly duplication of services and mistakes, and improve responsiveness and quality.

At the same time, electronic patient records will provide some definite benefits to health researchers, by providing them with integrated information about clinical outcomes, prescription practices and disease patterns. The electronic patient record is intended to complement our very significant increased investment in health research in recent years. Two years ago, Canada replaced the old model of medical research with a new model of health research. We created the Canadian Institutes of Health Research which are virtual institutes without bricks and mortar. The essence of the innovation is that these virtual institutes combine in a coherent way the four pillars of health research – bio-medical inquiry, clinical investigation, health services research and health determinants research. The Government of Canada is making investments in research and data collection because we believe that balanced investment in health research, fueled by good data, will yield the knowledge and insights we need to undertake a programme of continuous improvements. Data is to research what fuel is to an engine. By making investments in both research and data collection, while protecting the privacy of health information, we believe we will more quickly produce the knowledge and the insights we need to both improve health care and the health of Canadians.

2. Opening remarks by Julio Frenk, Minister of Health, Mexico

I would like to start by thanking the Canadian government and especially my esteemed colleague, Minister Allan Rock, for inviting me to this conference. By hosting this conference, Canada once again shows the leadership it has exerted for decades in innovating in the organisation and financing of health systems. I would also like to thank the OECD and especially Secretary-General, Donald Johnston, for his leadership in organising this important meeting. It is one more example of the extremely valuable contribution that the OECD has made down the years to develop a very sound basis of knowledge and evidence for health policy.

In these remarks, I would like to briefly share the way in which the new Mexican government has been using performance assessment as a very key element in formulating and implementing health policy. But before describing our new national health policy, let me begin by sharing with you where I come from in terms of looking at performance assessment.

Prior to becoming Minister of Health, I was responsible at the World Health Organisation for developing the conceptual framework for health system performance assessment. As David Naylor and others during this conference have pointed out, the 2000 *World Health Report* has sparked a great deal of interest and debate. There is no doubt that the measurement side of this exercise can be improved and is in fact in the process of being improved. But I think the exercise has made some important contributions already in terms of the conceptual framework, which we have adopted now at the national level in Mexico. First of all, this framework has a very clear outcome orientation. The key question is: what are health systems for? We are all investing huge and growing amounts of resources into our health systems, and we need to know what we are getting out of this investment. A clear orientation around the intrinsic goals of health systems, the goals that are valued by societies, is a first important contribution of this exercise.

Second, it put forward the notion of performance as a "relative" concept, in which we think of performance as the attainment of those goals but relative to the resources that are invested and the level of development of a country. This approach, I think, empowers policy-makers. Until now, most international comparisons were based only on the absolute attainment of different health status measures. For instance, one would compare countries on the basis of infant mortality or life expectancy at birth, and obviously one would find that poorer countries did not attain the results observed in richer countries. In a sense, there was a certain unfairness in comparing, say, Swaziland to Switzerland and finding that indeed, given the level of development and the amount of resources invested in health, the attainment of goals was very different between these two countries. But when you actually take goal attainment, for example in terms of health gains, and make it relative to the amount of resources invested and the level of socio-economic development, you still find enormous variations across countries. These variations hold true even for countries that are spending the same amount of resources in health systems and are at the same level of development. These findings are an empowering message to policy-makers because they suggest that there is a lot that we can learn from each other. The message is no longer "wait until you become like an advanced industrialised country and then your attainment of goals will improve". Rather, the message is "taking into account your limited resources and your current level of development, there are still huge variations in terms of health outcomes compared with other countries". This has the potential to engage countries in a process of shared learning.

How do we take this concept from an international perspective and make it relevant to national decision-making? Let me briefly describe what we have done in Mexico. Mexico is a large, middle-income country, which underwent a major political transition in July 2000. It then became a normal democratic country, with the longest ruling party in the world at that time losing the election. We have had a very peaceful, but fundamental political transition since then.

In that context, the question of democratization becomes a key question, not just at the time of the election but also in every field of public policy. And indeed, the title of our national health programme is "The Democratization of Health Care in Mexico." Democratization not only offers a set of values that we stand for, such as freedom of justice, of representation and participation, but it also offers practical guidelines for governing. One of them is the basic principle of accountability. The democratization process has raised the question of: how to move from the full exercise of political and civil rights to the full exercise of social rights, including health care rights? and how to account for the resources that are invested to achieve that social citizenship?

That is why the point of departure in formulating our six-year programme has been an orientation on the attainment of goals relative to resources, by adapting the WHO framework to what we want the health system to achieve for the citizens of Mexico. In other words, we begin with the end in mind. In this way, performance assessment not only becomes a tool for retrospective evaluation of what happened but can also become a tool for prospective target-setting and therefore for telling citizens what the government, in conjunction with the whole society, intends to achieve in quantifiable terms.

That is what we have done in a very thorough exercise. We have identified three fundamental challenges: equity, quality and financial protection. Equity because a characteristic of large, middle-income countries like Mexico is the persistence of enormous disparities. Quality both in its technical dimension, which translates in the attainment of better levels of health, and also in its interpersonal dimension, which means enhancing the responsiveness of the health system to the legitimate expectations of the population. And finally, fair financing, meaning that people are protected from catastrophic expenditures. The national health programme sets out a target of reducing what are now extremely high levels of catastrophic expenditure because half of the population in Mexico is not covered by social insurance.

Let me finish with a very quick reflection on the use of performance assessment. While a part of the WHO framework is dealing with goals, the other part deals with the functions of the health system. One of these key functions is stewardship. As countries like Mexico have rapidly devolved the function of providing care to lower level territorial units – in our case, the states – the federal level retains as a central mission the stewardship of the system. I believe that a key component of effective stewardship is performance assessment. I would even suggest that, in the public sector, each level of government should become a source of performance assessment of lower levels, all the way to the facility level, in order to allow improvement of performance through peer comparison and to use that information to guide some resource allocation decisions. This does not mean a "top down" approach. We certainly need a "bottom up" generation of good and transparent information to make this assessment possible. But I do think that a comprehensive system of performance assessment, going from the macro systemic level all the way to the facility level, in which you build a system of "checks and balances" and peer comparison, can be a very powerful tool for the function of stewardship. We are now moving towards achieving this objective in Mexico. We have established a new area in the Ministry of Health whose work focuses specifically on performance assessment. And we are starting now to assess the performance of health systems at the state level.

In conclusion, let me say that I believe that performance assessment has a clear and practical value in helping to achieve the goals of health systems. It can also play a key part in achieving greater accountability, and therefore be a key component of democratic governance through a culture (an ethos) of service to people. Comparison is essential to shared learning, as this conference is showing. And I also believe that this process of shared learning will bring us closer to the joint pursuit of one of the few remaining truly universal aspirations which is the improvement of health for everyone.

3. Opening remarks by John Hutton, Minister of State for Health, United Kingdom

I am delighted to have this opportunity to discuss these important issues which are common to all our countries as we focus on improving the health care services available to our people. In the United Kingdom, we have been actively developing a range of new performance measurement indicators since 1997. And it is true to say, as I am sure this has also been the experience of other countries, that we are still working on how we can improve the quality, reliability, and relevance of the data that we are assembling.

Our experience in the United Kingdom thus far suggests that assessment measures have three very important potential benefits. First, if we get the assembly of data right and if we can get our performance management information working effectively, we have the opportunity to make better decisions. We now have more and better evidence on the effect of policies that we are introducing, so there is an opportunity for policy-making itself to be made more effective. This is certainly a fundamental objective.

Second, performance assessment is very important not just for policy-makers but for service deliverers as well, by offering them an opportunity to speed up the learning curve. If performance measurement is done in a timely and effective manner, we can get more rapid feedback on what different providers are doing and how well our national health service in the United Kingdom is coping with expected changes. Unsuccessful policies and practices can be identified more quickly, while we can spread successful policies and practices more rapidly across our service.

Third, and this is perhaps the most difficult area of all for politicians, the decision-making process itself actually comes under better public scrutiny. With more data in the public domain, Ministers become subject to more external challenge. This is a necessary discipline. Given all the challenges and the expectations that now are heaped upon us in the field of health care, we are indeed interested in making sure that demanding consumers can become responsible partners, as we look to improve the efficiency of health care delivery.

Overall, better performance measurement can therefore lead to better informed decisions. It should help lead to better value for money for the taxpayer and consumer alike. And in our context in the United Kingdom, it can also hopefully lead to stronger support for public health care provision, which we consider to be of fundamental importance to make sure that the values of equity and fairness are kept to the forefront. It is very important that we continue to strive to ensure that we have a balanced overall assessment that can truly inform consumers, not mislead them, and that can help improve performance and encourage innovation and change rather than inhibit them. The UK government is committed to promote such a "balanced score card" approach to performance assessment, and this conference is making a significant contribution to our endeavours in this field.

Looking to the future, we have learned a lot already from our experiences, but I think there is much more that we need to do. I would suggest that there are three areas where in the future we will need to work together more effectively. First, we need to continue the process of sharing and learning from our respective efforts in the development and implementation of national performance assessment frameworks. This learning process is very important. Second, we will need to consider together the development of a better framework of common performance indicators that would enable better international comparisons of our health care systems. This is obviously a complicated task, but it is one that deserves our attention. Third, we need to do further research on the effectiveness of performance management tools themselves.

My final message is that politicians in all countries are struggling at the moment with what might be described as a rising tide of public cynicism about our declarations, including any statements that health care services are improving. In the current public environment, it is going to be very important that we make sure that the quality of our data is as reliable and independently verifiable as possible. In the United Kingdom, we are looking at ways to ensure that this process remains "immune" to public scepticism about the reliability of that information. Politicians will always obviously tell you that their health care systems are getting better! It is very important that these statements be credible. One of the most important benefits of better performance indicators will therefore be to provide reliable information to the public, and also to keep Ministers on their toes regarding the choices and the priorities attached to the complex range of issues associated with improving modern health care systems.

4. Opening remarks by Bernard Kouchner, Minister of Health, France

I should like to begin by noting a fact: nothing in our countries is more political than health. It has become – and will be tomorrow – the most highly political area of government policy-making. Health and the practice of medicine used to be areas that people liked to think of as neutral territory, but illness is not neutral. It is our citizens' number one concern. All of the ministers present here today know that they are amongst the most called-upon members of their governments. In front of my Ministry, demonstrations take place every day. Some days, it is representatives of private clinics that demonstrate in France, while on other days it is public hospitals. Let me therefore make a first observation: let us stop talking about medical neutrality. There is nothing neutral about health. It is infinitely political, in the noblest sense of the word.

I share with the OECD and all of the participants in this conference a comprehensive and multidimensional approach to performance. Obviously, we cannot judge our systems' performance in terms of life expectancies alone. There are many factors to be taken into account. Moreover, it must not be forgotten – even if this is not the main focus of the conference – that we live in a world that is divided into at least two vast halves: rich countries – those that can talk about the performance of the health care economy and how best to organise that economy; and then the other half of the world, which needs our help rather than our talk. We must stand with them and not be selfish.

With regard to the performance of health systems in the developed countries, one must consider first the financial contributions to our systems, since it would be difficult to discuss their strengths and weaknesses without taking their levels of funding into account. If one sacrifices one, two, three, four or five more percentage points of GDP to health care expenditures, one is obviously in a better position to meet people's expectations. It is therefore necessary, in assessing performance, to factor in the percentage of gross domestic product that is devoted to health care spending, although clearly that is not enough.

It is also important to report publicly on performance indicators that are both diversified and related to key system goals and issues. France does not know how to do this well. France does not have a poor health care system, but it certainly has an inadequate evaluation system, because this has not been part of the French tradition. That tradition, built upon impenetrable medical power and a lack of medical competition, led people to believe that to go to a given hospital for a given operation was the same thing anywhere across the country. This is not true.

In recent years, we in France have created instruments to improve how performance is measured and monitored, in particular by establishing a national agency for health care accreditation and evaluation (*Agence nationale d'accréditation et d'évaluation en santé*). But there is room for further improvement. Formulating evaluation tools is a very lengthy process, first of all because doctors do not like to be compared to each other. It is lengthy also because patients do not like their doctors to be compared to each other either. Patients do not tend to judge a system in its entirety, but focus only on their own anxieties and their own personal health outcomes. The most frequent ways for people to assess a system's performance are not very objective. Patients are very adamant and very quick to attack the government about a health care system but never their own doctors, because to attack one's own doctor is to attack oneself and one's own anxiety.

Obviously, we must try to make performance indicators as visible and transparent as possible. For the moment, in France, comparisons between hospitals are more likely to be published in the press than by government authorities. What is new and encouraging, however, is that the performance ratings by journalists are based on figures provided by the Ministry. This shows clear progress in data collection.

The only way to make further strides in this direction is to share our difficulties and our performance with the public, and with patient associations in particular, in a fully transparent manner. In the French health insurance system trade unions play a very important role, but patients, for their part, are not very well represented. We must increase the representation of patients in discussions on the health care system and health insurance, because it is with patients' money and that of their families that we can bring the system forward. We must try not to take any decision without consulting patients' associations and associations of health care professionals; some day, I hope, maybe these associations might even have decision-making power.

A far-reaching debate on performance must also incorporate the very important issue of inequality in the realm of health. Clearly, this encompasses access to the system, and especially the way in which patients in any given area can get access to health care services. Because I view public health as a package which goes from information to prevention to care, it is especially sad to see a persistence of major inequalities *vis-à-vis* diseases in the various regions of France. French research into inequalities shows that non-medical factors, such as socio-economic circumstances, regional conditions, nutrition and alcoholism, play a very important role. Differences in socio-economic circumstances in France may not result in unequal access to care, yet therapeutic outcomes (*e.g.*, in terms of life expectancy following treatment) are influenced by a patient's living conditions. It is therefore important to be extremely careful in our reasoning about the impact of socio-economic inequalities on health.

A system of care (or, more broadly, a health system) may be efficient economically, but that is not enough if access to the system is fraught with inequalities. This is why the French government passed an anti-exclusion law that increases the chances that sick people afflicted by economic or sociological difficulties can access the health care system. We have also paid special attention to disease prevention amongst the young, for instance by launching regional programmes for access to prevention and care (PRAPS). These young people had no information, or any possibility of obtaining information, on elementary aspects of public health. It is distressing to note that this situation persists, even if new mechanisms are helping to improve prevention.

Furthermore, despite the fact that France had very broad sickness coverage, until very recently between two and four million people had limited access to the system. We therefore instituted universal sickness coverage, which was adopted two years ago. It means that the number of people having direct access to health care at all levels, with the government paying 100 per cent of the bills, has increased from three million to five and a half million today (for people who are less disadvantaged, about 75 per cent of these expenditures are reimbursed in France).

Another important point concerning performance improvement is the absolute need for a transparent and democratic debate. Improving the health system will always cost more money. Our only allies, if we do not wish to overspend our means, are the citizens and patients. It is with them that the spending must be determined. A health care democracy is built with citizen participation. This health care democracy is of course intertwined with just plain democracy, but it is something very special. It is not true, for example, that being in a democratic country is enough to ensure access to health care. However, a health care democracy takes a very long time to construct. We recently passed a patients' rights act. Amongst other things, this law ensures that patients have direct access to their medical records; people may therefore find out what they are suffering from, if they choose to do so. The law also affords new possibilities for patients to discuss therapeutic options and to make decisions for themselves.

I do not have the time to delve deeply into the issue of hospital safety. I shall mention only the need to reform medical studies if we want to make the system more transparent, because unless doctors are a part of that transparency it will be very difficult to change the old habit of concealing information and decisions. I also believe in reparations for medical accidents. In France, these reparations will be financed with the aid of a government fund and accident insurance, and they will cover therapeutic accidents, whether anyone is at fault or not.

Health care democracy cannot therefore be instituted unless performance is measured better than it is today, and unless that information is shared with patients. I also believe that we cannot go on working in the rich countries only. We can no longer tolerate, nor will patients themselves tolerate, that the bulk of the sick people are in the south whilst the treatments are in the north. After inventing "Doctors Without Borders" we must now invent "Patients Without Borders".

5. Opening remarks by Edward Sondik, Director, National Center for Health Statistics, United States (on behalf of Tommy Thompson, Secretary of Health and Human Services, United States)

Secretary Tommy Thompson sends his apologies for being unable to participate in this Ministerial Roundtable, and asked if I would present his thoughts on performance measurement and the importance of collaborative international efforts.

The Secretary wants me to emphasise first that the events of September 11th brought home what we frequently take for granted, that is, the importance of personal and professional relationships. He is grateful for the overwhelming expressions of support from his colleagues at this Roundtable and around the world. That support is noted and appreciated by staff at the Department of Health and Human Services and the people of the United States.

The discussions we have had on health system performance during this conference represent another advantage of the close relationships among the nations represented here in Ottawa. Discussion and collaboration on an international scale has helped and will continue to help all of us exchange methods, best practices and research findings that will improve our health system performance.

Why focus on health system performance? Simply because we want to improve health and because we want to make the best use of our resources, the human resources involved and, in the United States, the over US$1 trillion spent on health each year. We want to provide information to health care providers so that they can improve their practices. We want to know how to reward clinicians and institutions providing the highest quality care. We also have a very important duty to provide the data and analyses that can help the public make the best possible decisions. We also want to identify our health gaps and get the information we need to help us close those gaps. And we most certainly hope the information affects political decisions by directing resources to those issues that need the most attention.

The United States is committed to ensuring that Americans have access to the highest quality health care. The public has a right to know if its health system is not performing up to the highest standards. To measure and improve health care quality, the Congress has mandated an annual national quality report. Gregg Meyer mentioned this initiative earlier in this conference. The report will be the product of government working with the private sector. It will cover four dimensions: our health system's safety, its effectiveness, its timeliness and its patient-centeredness (*i.e.*, the extent to which health care providers are actually focussed on patients' needs). That report, which is due in 2003, will include a broad set of performance measures to be used to monitor the nation's progress toward improved health care quality.

We are also committed to reducing disparities in health. These disparities are all too evident with, for example, the life expectancy of white Americans at 77 years but that of black Americans at only 71 years. To help improve these unfortunately longstanding problems, we are developing a series of national disparities reports to more fully understand the causes and monitor our progress in improving health for all Americans. This is another set of measures that will be integrated with the quality measures. Both the quality and disparities reports are crucial in helping us to identify and understand our system's performance gaps.

Let me raise another dimension of performance: disease prevention and health promotion. Our healthy people programme is now entering its third decade of setting a comprehensive programme of quantitative goals, now with 28 focus areas and over 400 goals linked to morbidity and mortality reduction. Every goal is linked to a data source, so that we can measure progress. Frequent public progress reports are the hallmark of the programme. This healthy people programme is totally consistent with the cycle of performance measurement and management that Jeremy Hurst from the OECD Secretariat presented at the beginning of this conference.

We have also identified a list of some 20 health measures that we call "leading health indicators". These indicators – related to obesity, tobacco, alcohol, responsible sexual behaviour, drug use, environmental quality, etc. – represent major factors influencing health. They will give us an efficient capsule view of progress in overcoming major health problems.

In the United States, our approach to measuring our health system performance is as diverse as the system itself. WHO has proposed using a single comprehensive indicator to measure the health system performance of an entire country. We don't have a single measure of efficiency per se. And we have not settled on a single measure in part because we feel the need for the richness of multiple measures that are "actionable", meaning that they can lead to policy-setting or to informing clinical decision-making. These measures need to be sufficiently sensitive so that we can measure progress. We also need to be able to disaggregate our measures to monitor progress for our diverse population groups. And finally, we need to be sure that these measures are as transparent as possible, so that health professionals, the public and Congress can understand their importance. We see this set of measures as a "basket" of performance indicators.

To improve health care quality, we must also clearly ensure the dissemination of evidence-based clinical information and realistic measures of provider performance and patient outcomes. International comparisons such as those encouraged at this conference provide even more opportunities to compare these measures and to develop new ones. This is a clear benefit to all of us.

To conclude, despite differences in health care financing and delivery systems across OECD countries, we are all pursuing the answers to the same question: how do we improve the quality of health care and keep our patients safe? Secretary Thompson encourages us to collaborate to advance international discussions on this vital issue. These discussions help each of us view our systems through different prisms. There is no end to the insights we can gain.

6. Open discussion: Ministers' responses to questions from conference participants

Question 1: **Do you consider providers generally (not just physicians) as barriers to the kind of performance measurement and improvement efforts that you are looking for, or do you consider them as partners?**

Bernard Kouchner, Minister of Health, France: Health care providers should of course be part of the team. It is impossible to consider any strategy for change and improvement without them being part of it. But one of the practical difficulties is that providers are not united. The different views between, for example, unions representing general practitioners and those representing different groups of specialists are difficult to overcome. In addition, one should be careful about only listening to health care providers, or else one would end up doubling the health care budget!

Allan Rock, Minister of Health, Canada: And what's wrong with that! More seriously, the only time I ever heard a physician express concern about public reporting of performance measures was when that person felt that we were going to look at their performance simply by publishing unadjusted data. This would of course be very unfair. Important variables affecting clinical outcomes, such as the severity of cases, should be taken into account. As long as we properly adjust performance indicators to reflect such important differences in risk, I don't think there is much concern with public reporting. In the United States and in England, there is a great deal more performance reporting at the hospital or even at the surgeon level than is the case now in Canada. We can learn from these experiences. We also need collaboration with the professions. In general, I find enthusiastic endorsement by health care providers in Canada about the process of performance measurement and reporting.

Julio Frenk, Minister of Health, Mexico: The issue of how to involve providers in efforts to account for the responsiveness and outcomes of health care is indeed a very critical one. If we think about what health care is about, in the end, the core event is an encounter between a provider and a patient (or a population, if we are including also non-personal health services). Obviously, finding out the quality and outcome of that encounter is very complicated, not least because that encounter occurs with enormous asymmetries of information. If we think only of personal health care, most patients do not have the necessary information to judge the potential for high quality care. This is where performance assessment can help to redress such imbalances. I would also add that comparative performance assessment is entirely within the ethos of medical professions. The main issue, I would suggest, is not performance assessment itself, but rather what happens with that information – for instance, whether it is used to guide decisions by the population or used to reward good performance.

Many health systems suffer from the fact that the final allocation of resources now is insensitive to performance. It is driven by bureaucratic or other forces, but not by performance measures. To the extent that we can make performance information also part of the way resources are allocated, then I think we can use performance assessment to align the necessary incentives to improve health care for patients. Again, this is not an element foreign to the best traditions and ethos of the medical and nursing professions.

359|

John Hutton, Minister of State for Health, United Kingdom: As other Ministers have said, the medical professions should clearly be partners in efforts to measure and improve performance. It would be impossible to achieve these objectives through a process that would be antagonistic. We are certainly trying to avoid this in the United Kingdom. There are at least two ways to avoid potential conflicts. First, the issue of data quality and reliability is fundamental. We have to work with the medical professions to make sure we release accurate data. Second, we also need to see these performance measurement efforts in a wider context. This wider context should include the support and incentives for on-going performance improvement. We need not only to develop proper appraisal systems and re-certification exercises, but also to support these efforts with the necessary investment in training and continuous professional development. The whole purpose of the performance assessment exercise is to improve quality, not just from the patient's perspective, although this is obviously crucial, but also from the perspective of health care professionals. The process of collecting performance data should lead to a better situation for health care professionals too. We need to look at performance assessment as an exercise that is going to add value, rather than simply make life more complicated.

Edward Sondik, Director, National Centre for Health Statistics, United States: Let me just point out an important information gap that we have in the United States. Peer review is a very important part of the continuous improvement process, and this works quite well in hospitals and other institutions. However, an enormous part of medical care in the United States takes place in individual doctor's offices. And this is an area where it is very difficult to really understand and monitor outcomes, even with current surveys. This has to be a priority target for us to better understand that process.

Question 2: **Can you share some further thoughts on the political processes needed to sustain health care improvement? In particular, is there a need to better structure the participation of consumers in health care quality debates, following perhaps the experience of the Australian Consumers' Health Forum?**

Bernard Kouchner, Minister of Health, France: First, an initial comment on the notion of "consumers". This is a concept that I do not like very much, because it is somewhat difficult to work with. Who are the consumers? Patients? Patients' families? Everyone? At the very least, it is a notion that needs clarification. Having said that, in the French system, the "consumer" has the choice of obtaining care in private or public establishments. Both systems – private and public – co-exist, and people may choose one or the other. At the end of the day, however, it is the same social security contributions that pay the bills. In a sense, it's paradise ... but a paradise that is not easy to manage!

I have already mentioned the very great importance that I attach to increasing the participation of patients and patients' associations in discussions about health care quality. A note of caution, however: "consumers", just like professionals, cannot be the only ones to decide. Trade-offs and policy decisions will still be necessary. These policy decisions must of course be guided with input from professionals, consumers and patients' associations. At some point, however, choices have to be made, and you can't get a litre out of a pint pot. The government's only money is the money that comes from the population. It is therefore necessary to calculate and to choose.

Julio Frenk, Minister of Health, Mexico: I agree with Bernard Kouchner that the concept of "consumers" with respect to health care is a little bit problematic. In a sense this is probably the only area of economic activity where people as users of services really perform three roles. First, they are the raw material upon which "producers" (physicians and nurses) work. Second, they are "consumers" in the sense that they are actually going out there and purchasing some services and expecting "value for money". And third, they are also "co-producers" through very concrete actions such as compliance. There is no other "production function" where there is such a multiplicity of roles. Therefore, I think we need to move away from a confrontational framework of providers versus consumers, and think rather in terms of "joint production" decisions.

One normally does not want to impose therapeutic decisions on populations. We value the autonomy of people to participate in the decision-making process. I do agree therefore with the point that we need explicit structures to manage the complexity of this very unique interaction between patients and providers. The first requirement is to share information because that interaction is now based on profound information asymmetries. Second, there is also a need to have incentives that are well-aligned with objectives, and this is where performance assessment can play a fundamental role at all levels. And third, there is a need for explicit institutions to redress conflicts between patients and providers, in ways that are not as onerous as judicial litigation, but rather through other mechanisms of conciliation and mediation.

John Hutton, Minister of State for Health, United Kingdom: It is important to keep in mind that we represent different health care systems with different political processes. In the end, how different actors are actually involved in discussions on health care quality is a matter of choices for individual countries and societies to make. However, regardless of the specific choices that are being made, any effective system of performance assessment will inform not only the political decision-making process, but will also promote greater accountability between different orders of governments and between governments and their electorates. In the United Kingdom, we have a universal health care system which operates within a very clear framework of accountability and political responsibility. The development of performance assessment measures will better hold Ministers accountable for their decisions. And as we all know, the ultimate method for citizens to hold Ministers accountable is actually to vote them out of office! Furthermore, we are also going to legislate soon in the United Kingdom to create stronger structures, including legal structures, by which the voice of patients and the public can be heard within the decision-making process of our national health service. One should not forget that the public "owns" the national health service; it is their health care system. So they should have a much stronger voice within the system. That is what we are committed to do, building on other measures that we have taken to improve the responsiveness of the health care system.

Allan Rock, Minister of Health, Canada: In Canada, the political process of involving citizens in discussions on health care quality has recently been initiated. As I mentioned briefly in my opening remarks, there is a federal and provincial commitment now in Canada to create a citizen's council on health care quality. This council will be composed of people without a personal stake in the health care system apart from their status as consumers and patients. The role of the council will be to make sure that the information being gathered in public performance reports is objective, readable and of real value to the average citizen. It will also be to make sure that those performance reports are discussed in the context of quality from the consumers' perspective. We are now working with the provinces towards the final design of that council in order to achieve these goals.

Question 3: **How do we continue to encourage medical innovation as we are improving our systems of measurement?**

Bernard Kouchner, Minister of Health, France: Of course it is necessary to improve the system of measurement, but above all it is necessary to improve the system itself. Measurement has educational value; it seeks to demonstrate, compare and prove. But it is very possible for systems to get better without any improved measurements. The entire health system has been transformed within 20 or 30 years. Cancer care, for example, is no longer the same. The diagnosis and treatment of breast cancer in particular have made extraordinary progress in the past few years. Just a short time ago, day surgery did not exist. These are improvements we can no longer neglect, and that must be offered to people. But all this is more expensive.

John Hutton, Minister of State for Health, United Kingdom: The issue of encouraging change and innovation is a very important issue as we develop modern systems of performance assessment. Medicine is continuously changing and innovating. This reality must be a fundamental feature of how we develop and try to improve our health care systems. We want services to change and to improve. We want to be able to incorporate the latest technologies, drug treatments, surgical procedures as quickly as possible into our health care system, because that obviously is in the best interests of patients. Therefore, we need to make sure that performance assessment measures do not act as a brake on innovation and change. They should neither act as a way of consolidating or locking what one could loosely describe as conservative traditions in medicine. In the United Kingdom, our objective in

361

developing performance assessment systems is clearly to encourage innovation and the rapid diffusion of new procedures and techniques, as opposed to inadvertently inhibit beneficial change. I don't think any of us yet has the magic solution about how to avoid potential pitfalls. This is an area where international collaborative research will be very important.

7. Final observations by Allan Rock, Minister of Health, Canada

Listening to my colleagues, it is quite clear that our agendas are almost identical. The performance of health care systems has become one of the main policy issues in all our countries. In this context, it is particularly important to develop and share widely reliable measures of key aspects of the performance of our health systems, if we want these policy discussions to be based on facts.

This leads me to a final point about international work. We have talked about national health information systems to measure performance. But I would also like to emphasise the importance of an international system. The OECD and WHO are presently working on comparing different aspects of health system performance across countries. It would be really helpful if we could have common international standards and common indicators, so that we spoke one single language in comparing performances across countries. How much easier it would be for all of us to look for best practices if comparisons were based on a set of common and reliable indicators. Perhaps that can be a goal we strive for as a follow up to this meeting.

This conference has been of singular value to Canada as the host country, and we have been very grateful for this opportunity to learn and share experiences with you all.